Biomedical Applications of Microfluidic Devices

Biomedical Applications of Microfluidic Devices

Edited by

Michael R. Hamblin
Distinguished Visiting Professor, Laser Research Centre, University of Johannesburg, South Africa

Mahdi Karimi
Cellular and Molecular Research Center, Iran University of Medical Sciences, Tehran, Iran
Department of Medical Nanotechnology, Faculty of Advanced Technologies in Medicine, Iran University of Medical Sciences, Tehran, Iran
Oncopathology Research Center, Iran University of Medical Sciences, Tehran, Iran
Research Center for Science and Technology in Medicine, Tehran University of Medical Sciences, Tehran, Iran

ELSEVIER

ACADEMIC PRESS
An imprint of Elsevier

Academic Press
125 London Wall, London EC2Y 5AS, United Kingdom
525 B Street, Suite 1650, San Diego, CA 92101, United States
50 Hampshire Street, 5th Floor, Cambridge, MA 02139, United States
The Boulevard, Langford Lane, Kidlington, Oxford OX5 1GB, United Kingdom

Notices
Knowledge and best practice in this field are constantly changing. As new research and experience broaden our understanding, changes in research methods, professional practices, or medical treatment may become necessary.

Practitioners and researchers must always rely on their own experience and knowledge in evaluating and using any information, methods, compounds, or experiments described herein. In using such information or methods they should be mindful of their own safety and the safety of others, including parties for whom they have a professional responsibility.

To the fullest extent of the law, neither the Publisher nor the authors, contributors, or editors, assume any liability for any injury and/or damage to persons or property as a matter of products liability, negligence or otherwise, or from any use or operation of any methods, products, instructions, or ideas contained in the material herein.

Library of Congress Cataloging-in-Publication Data
A catalog record for this book is available from the Library of Congress

British Library Cataloguing-in-Publication Data
A catalogue record for this book is available from the British Library

ISBN: 978-0-12-818791-3

For information on all Academic Press publications
visit our website at https://www.elsevier.com/books-and-journals

Publisher: Mara Conner
Acquisitions Editor: Fiona Geraghty
Editorial Project Manager: Joshua Mearns
Production Project Manager: Prem Kumar Kaliamoorthi
Cover Designer: Mark Rogers

Typeset by SPi Global, India

To the love of my life, my beautiful wife Angela without whom this book would not have been possible.
Michael R. Hamblin

Contents

Contributors xv
Preface xvii

CHAPTER 1 An overview of microfluidic devices **1**
Saeid Maghsoudi, Navid Rabiee, Sepideh Ahmadi, Mohammad Rabiee, Mojtaba Bagherzadeh, and Mahdi Karimi

1.1 Introduction 1
1.2 Chemical synthesis 8
1.3 Drug delivery 10
1.4 Cell biology 12
1.5 Biosensors 13
References 14

CHAPTER 2 Microfluidic devices: Synthetic approaches **23**
Shahin Aghamiri, Navid Rabiee, Sepideh Ahmadi, Mohammad Rabiee, Mojtaba Bagherzadeh, and Mahdi Karimi

2 Cleanroom 24
2.1 Classification 24
2.2 Cleanroom concepts 24
2.3 Cleanroom equipment 25
2.4 Materials 25
2.5 Deposition methods 27
2.6 Lithography 28
2.7 Etching techniques 29
2.8 Types of molding 30
2.9 3D printing 31
2.10 Stereolithography 33
2.11 Fused deposition molding 33
References 34

CHAPTER 3 Microchannels for microfluidic systems **37**
Behzad Nasseri, Samet Akar, and Erdinc Naseri

3.1 Introduction 37
3.2 Cross-section geometry in microchannels in microfluidic systems 38

3.3 Channel design for different flow regimes (turbulent and laminar flow).......50
3.4 Phase study in microfluidic devices and microchannel patterns.......51
3.5 Hydrodynamic behavior of the flow in microfluidic systems.......54
3.6 The velocity development in the microchannels.......55
3.7 Hydrophilicity and hydrophobicity effects in microfluidic systems.......59
3.8 Physical specifications of channels in microfluidic systems.......60
3.8.1 Effect of friction coefficient of the microchannels in microfluidic devices.......60
3.8.2 Roughness effects in channels of microfluidic devices.......62
3.9 Biomedical applications of transport phenomena in microfluidic systems.......62
3.10 Pathogen detection by microchannel devices using nanotechnology.......64
3.11 Soft microchannels in biomedical applications.......66
3.12 Reusable microchannels in biomedical applications.......66
3.13 Conclusions.......69
References.......70

CHAPTER 4 Microarray technologies.......77
Mohammad Rabiee, Azin Rostami, Navid Rabiee, and Mojtaba Bagherzadeh

4.1 Introduction.......77
4.2 What are microarrays?.......78
4.2.1 DNA microarrays.......81
4.2.2 Protein microarrays.......85
4.2.3 Cell microarrays.......88
4.3 Microfluidic arrays.......89
4.3.1 Advantages of microfluidic array technology.......89
4.3.2 Disadvantages of microfluidic array technology.......90
4.3.3 Fabrication of microfluidic arrays.......91
4.3.4 Automated microfluidic arrays (lab-on-a-chip systems).......93
4.3.5 Examples of microfluidic arrays.......95

4.4 Conclusion 95
References 96

CHAPTER 5 Microfluidics: Organ-on-a-chip 99
Shahin Aghamiri, Navid Rabiee, Sepideh Ahmadi, Mohammad Rabiee, Mojtaba Bagherzadeh, and Mahdi Karimi

5.1 Traditional systems drawbacks 100
5.2 Microfabrication principles 101
5.3 Significant organ-on-a-chip platforms 102
5.3.1 Lung-on-a-chip 102
5.3.2 Intestine-on-a-chip 102
5.3.3 Blood vessel-on-a-chip 103
5.3.4 Heart-on-a-chip 103
5.3.5 Liver-on-a-chip 104
5.3.6 Tumor-on-a-chip 106
5.3.7 Bone marrow-tumor-on-a-chip 107
5.3.8 Brain-tumor-on-a-chip 108
5.4 Conclusion and future perspectives 110
References 111

CHAPTER 6 Microfluidic devices for pathogen detection 117
Sepideh Ahmadi, Navid Rabiee, Mojtaba Bagherzadeh, and Mahdi Karimi

6.1 Introduction 117
6.2 Sample preparation for microfluidics devices 120
6.3 Microfluidic devices integrated with different technologies for the detection of pathogens 121
6.3.1 Biosensor-based microfluidics 121
6.3.2 Optical-based microfluidics 124
6.3.3 Fluorescence-based microfluidics 125
6.3.4 Chemiluminescence-based microfluidics 125
6.3.5 Plasmonic-based microfluidics 127
6.3.6 Colorimetric-based microfluidics 130
6.3.7 Electrochemical-based microfluidics 132
6.3.8 PCR-based microfluidic systems 134
6.3.9 Mass spectrometry-based microfluidics 138
6.4 Conclusions 139
References 142

CHAPTER 7 Microfluidic devices and drug delivery systems **153**
Mohammad Rabiee, Negar Namaei Ghasemnia, Navid Rabiee, and Mojtaba Bagherzadeh

7.1 Introduction to microfluidics 153
7.2 Fabrication of the microfluidic device 155
7.2.1 Geometry 155
7.2.2 Materials 155
7.3 Applications of microfluidic devices 156
7.4 Microfluidic devices in drug delivery systems 157
7.5 Microfluidics in the fabrication of drug delivery carriers 158
7.5.1 Self-assembled drug carriers 159
7.5.2 Droplet-based carriers 161
7.5.3 Nonspherical carriers and particles 163
7.6 Effective parameters for the production of carriers 165
7.7 Carrier materials 165
7.8 Examples of immobilization of drugs using microfluidic technology for drug delivery 167
7.9 Benefits of using microfluidics in drug delivery systems 168
7.10 Direct drug delivery via microfluidic systems 169
7.10.1 Localized drug delivery 169
7.10.2 Skin anatomy and transdermal drug delivery 171
7.11 Microfluidics for drug delivery: Cellular and organ level 175
7.11.1 On-site analysis 175
7.11.2 Protein crystallization 176
7.12 Organ-on-a-chip 177
7.13 The role of microfluidic technology for cancer cell studies 178
7.14 Autonomous and smart integrated drug delivery microfluidic platforms 178
7.15 Conclusions and future directions 179
References 180

CHAPTER 8 Microfluidic devices for gene delivery systems **187**
Sepideh Ahmadi, Navid Rabiee, Mojtaba Bagherzadeh, and Mahdi Karimi

8.1 Introduction 187
8.2 Microfluidic devices for production of nonviral vectors (micro/NPs) 189

8.3 Continuous flow systems 192
8.4 Droplet-based microfluidic devices 193
8.5 Microfluidic devices based on physical methods for genes transfection 196
8.5.1 Electroporation 198
8.6 Microinjection 199
8.7 Hydrodynamics-based transfection 200
8.8 Conclusions 201
References 203

CHAPTER 9 Microfluidic devices in tissue engineering **209**
Sajad Bahrami, Nafiseh Baheiraei, Mohammed Najafi-Ashtiani, Shirin Nour, and Mehdi Razavi
9.1 Introduction 209
9.2 Fabrication techniques in microfluidic devices 210
9.2.1 Etching 210
9.2.2 Thermoforming 211
9.2.3 Micromachining 211
9.2.4 Polymer casting 211
9.3 Materials used in microfluidic devices 212
9.3.1 Polymers 213
9.3.2 Hydrogels 213
9.3.3 Inorganic materials 213
9.4 Research progress in microfluidics-based tissue engineering 213
9.4.1 Scaffold fabrication using microfluidics 213
9.4.2 Stem cell-based microfluidics systems 215
9.5 Organomimetic prospects in microfluidics 217
9.5.1 Liver-on-a-chip 217
9.5.2 Gut-on-a-chip 219
9.5.3 Brain-on-a-chip 220
9.5.4 Kidney-on-a-chip 221
9.5.5 Heart-on-a-chip 222
9.6 Microfluidic models of cancer tissue 223
9.6.1 Cancer cells 2D and 3D culture and co-culture 224
9.6.2 In vitro models of tumor spheroids and tumor tissue 224
9.6.3 In vitro models of tumor including multiorgans 225
9.7 Conclusions and challenges 227
References 227

CHAPTER 10 Microfluidics in organic chemistry **235**
Beheshteh Khodadadi Chegeni
10.1 Introduction 235
10.2 Microfluidic devices used in organic chemistry 236
10.3 Effect of microfluidics on reducing by-products in organic synthesis 242
10.4 Effect of microfluidics on mass transfer in organic synthesis 244
10.5 Microreactors for the high-temperature synthesis 245
10.6 Effect of microfluidics on control of conversion and selectivity in organic synthesis 246
10.7 Multiphase microfluidic strategies for the synthesis of microparticles 247
10.8 Summary 249
References 249

CHAPTER 11 Microfluidic paper-based devices **257**
Akbar Hasanzadeh and Iman Hashemzadeh
11.1 Introduction 257
11.2 Fabrication techniques 257
11.2.1 Physical techniques 258
11.2.2 Chemical techniques 261
11.2.3 Fabrication techniques for 3D μPADs 264
11.3 Applications of microfluidic paper-based analytical devices 265
11.3.1 Biochemical detection 265
11.3.2 Immunological detection 267
11.3.3 Molecular detection 269
11.3.4 Other detection approaches 270
References 270

CHAPTER 12 Smartphone-based microfluidic devices **275**
Akbar Hasanzadeh
12.1 Introduction 275
12.2 Utilization of MS^2 for biomedical diagnosis 276
12.3 Detection of pathogens using MS^2 276
12.4 Analysis of genes 278
12.5 Analysis of food safety and environmental contamination using MS^2 279
12.5.1 Identification of heavy metal pollution 279
12.5.2 Identification of bacterial contaminants 281
12.5.3 Tests for pH, nitrate and nitrite 282

12.6 Applications of MS^2 for routine clinical testing 283
References 285

CHAPTER 13 Targeted delivery of nucleic acids using microfluidic systems **289**
Masoumehossadat Hosseini, Navid Rabiee, and Mojtaba Bagherzadeh

13.1 Introduction 289
13.2 Structure of nucleic acids 290
13.2.1 Primary structure 290
13.2.2 Secondary structure 290
13.2.3 The tertiary structure of nucleic acids 291
13.2.4 The quaternary structure of nucleic acids 291
13.3 Structures of natural and artificial nucleic acids 292
13.3.1 DNA chemical structure 292
13.3.2 RNA chemical structure 293
13.3.3 Aptamer chemical structures 293
13.3.4 Peptide nucleic acids 294
13.3.5 Locked nucleic acids (LNA) 295
13.4 Therapeutic potential of nucleic acids 295
13.4.1 DNA-based approaches 296
13.4.2 RNA-based approaches 297
13.5 Mechanisms in microfluidic systems 305
13.6 Applications of microfluidic systems to nucleic acid transfection 305
13.7 Future prospects for microfluidic systems related to nucleic acids 309
13.8 Conclusions 309
References 309

CHAPTER 14 Microfluidics: Future perspectives **319**
Arefeh Ebadati

14.1 Introduction 319
14.2 Future prospective in biology and health 319
14.3 Future prospectives in chemistry 321
14.4 Future industrial applications and commercialization 321
14.5 Closing words 322
References 322

Index 325

Contributors

Shahin Aghamiri
Student Research Committee, Department of Medical Biotechnology, School of Advanced Technologies in Medicine; Cellular and Molecular Biology Research Center, Shahid Beheshti University of Medical Sciences, Tehran, Iran

Sepideh Ahmadi
Student Research Committee, Department of Medical Biotechnology, School of Advanced Technologies in Medicine; Cellular and Molecular Biology Research Center, Shahid Beheshti University of Medical Sciences, Tehran, Iran

Samet Akar
Department of Mechanical Engineering, Çankaya University, Ankara, Turkey

Mojtaba Bagherzadeh
Department of Chemistry, Sharif University of Technology, Tehran, Iran

Nafiseh Baheiraei
Tissue Engineering and Applied Cell Sciences Division, Department of Hematology, Faculty of Medical Sciences, Tarbiat Modares University, Tehran, Iran

Sajad Bahrami
Department of Medical Nanotechnology, Faculty of Advanced Technologies in Medicine, Iran University of Medical Sciences, Tehran, Iran

Beheshteh Khodadadi Chegeni
Oncopathology Research Center, Iran University of Medical Sciences, Tehran, Iran

Arefeh Ebadati
Department of Medical Nanotechnology, Faculty of Advanced Technologies in Medicine; Oncopathology Research Center, Iran University of Medical Sciences, Tehran, Iran

Akbar Hasanzadeh
Department of Medical Nanotechnology, Faculty of Advanced Technologies in Medicine; Advances Nanobiotechnology and Nanomedicine Research Group (ANNRG), Iran University of Medical Sciences, Tehran, Iran

Iman Hashemzadeh
Department of Medical Nanotechnology, Faculty of Advanced Technologies in Medicine; Advances Nanobiotechnology and Nanomedicine Research Group (ANNRG), Iran University of Medical Sciences, Tehran, Iran

Masoumehossadat Hosseini
Faculty of Chemistry and Petroleum Sciences, Department of Chemistry, Shahid Beheshti University; Soroush Mana Pharmed, Golrang Pharmaceutical Investment Co (GPI), Golrang Industrial Group (GIG), Tehran, Iran

Mahdi Karimi
Cellular and Molecular Research Center; Department of Medical Nanotechnology, Faculty of Advanced Technologies in Medicine; Oncopathology Research Center, Iran University of Medical Sciences; Research Center for Science and Technology in Medicine, Tehran University of Medical Sciences, Tehran, Iran

Saeid Maghsoudi
Department of Medicinal Chemistry, Shiraz University of Technology, Shiraz, Iran

Mohammed Najafi-Ashtiani
Department of Physical Therapy, Faculty of Medical Sciences, Tarbiat Modares University, Tehran, Iran

Negar Namaei Ghasemnia
Biomaterials Group, Department of Biomedical Engineering, Amirkabir University of Technology, Tehran, Iran

Erdinc Naseri
Department of Cardiovascular Surgery, Park Hayat Hospital, Afyon, Turkey

Behzad Nasseri
Drug Applied Research Center, Department of Medical Biotechnology, Faculty of Advanced Medical Sciences, Tabriz University of Medical Sciences, Tabriz, Iran

Shirin Nour
Tissue Engineering Group, Biomedical Engineering Department, Amirkabir University of Technology (Tehran Polytechnic), Tehran, Iran

Mohammad Rabiee
Biomaterials Group, Department of Biomedical Engineering, Amirkabir University of Technology, Tehran, Iran

Navid Rabiee
Department of Chemistry, Sharif University of Technology, Tehran, Iran

Mehdi Razavi
Biionix™ (Bionic Materials, Implants & Interfaces) Cluster, Department of Internal Medicine, College of Medicine, University of Central Florida, Orlando, FL, United States

Azin Rostami
Biomaterials Group, Department of Biomedical Engineering, Amirkabir University of Technology, Tehran, Iran

Preface

Not so many years ago, the term "microfluidics" was largely unknown amongst laboratory scientists, and completely unknown amongst the general public. However, an unstoppable trend for miniaturization has revolutionized technology in all aspects of society and industry. Famously driven by Moore's law stating that "the number of transistors in an integrated circuit (computer chip) doubles every 2 years," the computer industry has become accustomed to producing ever more powerful devices in ever-smaller formats. The same trend is now being applied to devices that require a flow of liquids rather than a flow of electrons. So now we have a field called microfluidics, which can be regarded as an analogous development to microelectronics but producing chip-based devices intended for different purposes. This remarkable increase in broad interest in this subject has motivated us to compile this edited book to assemble both basic knowledge and research advances in one place.

The principal property that characterizes microfluidics devices, is the use of microchannels. One chapter covers the basic principles of design and synthesis of the actual microchannels, and another covers the synthetic approaches to prepare the materials themselves. It discusses how the devices are coupled to signal read-outs and calibrated. Some broad areas of application in the basic science areas of analytical chemistry and synthetic organic chemistry are covered. The major emphasis, however, is on biomedical engineering and biomedical science applications. These areas include tissue engineering, organ-on-a-chip devices, pathogen identification, and drug/gene delivery. Special chapters cover microarrays and paper-based microfluidic devices. To keep the coverage up-to-date one chapter addresses smartphone-based microfluidics devices, which have clear applications in less-developed countries for disease diagnosis and screening. Moreover, the rapidly expanding fields of genetic engineering and nucleic acid-based therapeutics are ideally suited for the use of microfluidics approaches, due to the highly-specific recognition system being able to occur in very small volumes of liquid.

The reader will notice that many of the authors of the chapters are based in Iran. This is an example of the remarkable rise in high-technology science that has taken place in Iran. Iran was ranked 4th in the world, behind China, United States, and India in terms of the number of nanotechnology publications. Microfluidics has always been closely associated with nanotechnology, although they are not necessarily the same thing.

The arrival of the COVID-19 pandemic in 2020 has made microfluidics even more relevant than it otherwise might have been. The requirement for inexpensive, rapid, and accurate tests for the presence of SARS-CoV-2 in biological samples is ideally suited for a microfluidics-based solution. Although the timing of this book did not allow us to have a chapter specifically dedicated to COVID-19 testing, there will undoubtedly be reports of microfluidics-based systems designed to solve this challenge to the whole world.

The commercial introduction of microfluidics devices, that are now manufactured by several major multinational companies as detailed in the book, augurs well for the wider dissemination of this approach in the years to come. Readers are encouraged to stay up-to-date as the very nature of the subject implies that advances in both basic science and biomedical applications of microfluidics will continue to be made, and may even increase exponentially in the years to come.

Michael R. Hamblin, Editor
Mahdi Karimi, Editor

CHAPTER

An overview of microfluidic devices

1

Saeid Maghsoudi[a], Navid Rabiee[b,*], Sepideh Ahmadi[c,d], Mohammad Rabiee[e], Mojtaba Bagherzadeh[b], and Mahdi Karimi[f,g,h,i]

[a]*Department of Medicinal Chemistry, Shiraz University of Technology, Shiraz, Iran*
[b]*Department of Chemistry, Sharif University of Technology, Tehran, Iran*
[c]*Student Research Committee, Department of Medical Biotechnology, School of Advanced Technologies in Medicine, Shahid Beheshti University of Medical Sciences, Tehran, Iran*
[d]*Cellular and Molecular Biology Research Center, Shahid Beheshti University of Medical Sciences, Tehran, Iran*
[e]*Biomaterials Group, Department of Biomedical Engineering, Amirkabir University of Technology, Tehran, Iran*
[f]*Cellular and Molecular Research Center, Iran University of Medical Sciences, Tehran, Iran*
[g]*Department of Medical Nanotechnology, Faculty of Advanced Technologies in Medicine, Iran University of Medical Sciences, Tehran, Iran*
[h]*Oncopathology Research Center, Iran University of Medical Sciences, Tehran, Iran*
[i]*Research Center for Science and Technology in Medicine, Tehran University of Medical Sciences, Tehran, Iran*
**Corresponding author. E-mail: nrabiee94@gmail.com*

1.1 Introduction

In the 21st century, the development of a new approach for the analysis and detection of many different biomolecules could address some insurmountable dilemmas. One judicious choice could be an innovative technology that can overcome these important issues in the life sciences. But which technology could break these barriers?

The complete dispersal and dissolution of samples in a liquid is a requirement for significant improvement in analytical detection approaches. The optimal solution may be to manufacture systems based on very small quantities (microliter or nanoliter) of fluids (liquid or gas), along with reducing the reaction time to mere seconds, together with miniaturized analytical technology for biomedical and chemical applications [1–3]. In the early 1950s, to get to grips with the issue of liquid sampling, microfluidics became an interdisciplinary field using micrometer-scale channels. According to George Whitesides [4], acknowledged to be the father of microfluidics, microfluidics is "the science and technology of systems that process or manipulate small (10^{-9} to 10^{-18} liters) amounts of fluids, has taken advantage of channels with

Biomedical Applications of Microfluidic Devices. https://doi.org/10.1016/B978-0-12-818791-3.00005-X

dimensions of tens to hundreds of micrometers." The development of microfluidics has revolutionized the science of chemistry [5], biology [6], analytical biochemistry [7], biotechnology [8], tissue engineering [9], and medicine [10] by allowing the flow and manipulation of minute quantities of liquids in a network of channels [11, 12]. Microfluidic devices have high reproducibility and robustness [13], use high surface-to-volume ratio (m^2/m^3) microchannels [14], with identical fabrication, good handling of droplets [15], improvement of mass and heat transfer, and minimal reagent consumption during optimization [16], as well as rapid analysis, high sensitivity, and good portability [8].

The history of microfluidics dates back to the mid-20th century when two scientists Golay and Van Deemter worked on gas chromatography and liquid chromatography, respectively. They figured out that for maintaining a high level of performance, the diameter of the open column and the packed column particle size should be reduced; hence columns began to be fabricated in the micrometer range. As a consequence, capillary electrophoresis became popular for the separation of diverse biomolecules [17]. Following these innovative studies, many groups of scientists put large amounts of time and energy into developing microfluidic devices for fluid transport, fluid metering, fluid mixing, for the concentration and separation of molecules within minuscule volumes of fluids [18]. These techniques were first performed in planar substrates surrounding channels with lengths, widths, and depths of approximately 10 mm, 100 μm, and 10 μm, respectively. In comparison to traditional devices that only focused to a limited extent on the physical properties, in microfluidic technologies, the focus is on viscosity, surface tension, and diffusion which becomes a matter of the utmost importance [19]. Surface tension in microfluidics is involved with: (i) passive pumping of fluids into the devices; (ii) user-defined patterned surfaces; and (iii) filtering of undesirable products. It is worth mentioning that gravitational forces are considered to be insignificant in microfluidic devices, due to the small overall dimensions of the devices [20].

This blooming field has been making great progress based on development reports. Its market value was approximately \$2.5 billion in 2017 and is projected to increase dramatically to \$5.8 billion by 2022 [21]. Microfluidic science has triggered a renaissance in the fields of drug discovery, drug delivery, biomedical engineering, and other lab-on-chip (LoC) applications, to which many studies have been devoted during recent decades. Due to the intrinsic ability of microfluidics to be beneficially coupled with a wide variety of devices onto a single chip in a straightforward, flexible, and ideally monolithically manner, they are becoming highly versatile for biomedical research, with many more opportunities compared to traditional laboratory techniques [18, 22]. For instance, the integration between microfluidics and electrophoresis in several publications has been reported. In this regard, Li et al. published many important papers that incorporated multiple fluidic, electronic, and mechanical devices or chemical processes onto a single chip-sized substrate [23]. Importantly, microfluidic devices open doors for the generation of micro- and nanoparticles with excellent size control, composition, morphology, and size distribution. Furthermore, in microfluidic devices, the low reaction volumes needed to be combined with the high heat and mass transfer rates, together make a variety of chemical reactions possible. These chemical reactions can be performed with higher yields, and under more harsh conditions than can typically be performed with conventional batch reactors [24]. For instance, in order to improve the chemical synthesis yield, one approach is to carry out the experiment at high pressure leading to a broader range of chemistries and processes. As a result, most solvents, precursors, and ligands will remain either liquid or become a supercritical fluid (at a temperature and pressure above its critical point) at temperatures needed for nanomaterial synthesis [25].

In order that a simple functional microfluidic device could be prepared, some tools are required including a syringe pump or a pressure source along with tubing attached to a microfluidic device typically installed on top of a microscope slide. Moreover, other components can be connected to the device making it either simpler or more complicated, such as a single cell-cultured inside a straight channel, or different cell-types cultured in networks of interconnected channels, respectively [26]. Using microfluidic devices, manual processing and bulky bench-top apparatus can be replaced with automated and multiplexed procedures. Nevertheless, many experts are reluctant to utilize commercial microfluidic devices owing to difficulties in working with them such as the need for external pumps and pneumatic fluid handling systems, requiring comprehensive training. This reluctance may lead them to use conventional instruments [27]. However, some marketed brands of analytical laboratory equipment have already used microfluidic components including Agilent, Caliper, Illumina, GE Healthcare, Shimadzu, and PerkinElmer.

Owing to the fact that microfluidic flow displays fewer eddies and vortices, producing laminar flow instead of turbulent flow, precise fluidic control can be more achievable. Laminar flow in microfluidics is characterized by the flow velocity, channel dimensions, and the properties of the fluidic channels [28]. Laminar flow allows convective mixing even though the ion exchange at the liquid-liquid interface is not restrained [29]. Moreover, this laminar flow leads to a narrow residence-time distribution, in addition to an increase in heat and mass transfer, which allow substantial control over the flow [30]. More practically, microfluidics with controllable flow and integration play an important role in obtaining rapid and more accurate, high throughput, and sensitive detection [31].

Since the 1990s, the practical applications of microfluidics has attracted more research in diverse scientific fields, including magnetism [32], high-throughput screening [33], drug screening [34], biosensors [35], cancer diagnosis [36], proteomics [37], and environmental monitoring [38]. At the same time, due to the rapid adoption of this critical technology, more challenges are emerging, specifically in those fields which deal with nanotechnology research. Microfluidics has been applied to many studies in which biological organisms have been included, such as pathogens [39], yeasts [40], plant cells [41] as well as mammalian cells [42]. As an example, the comprehensive applicationof microfluidicsinthe bioprospecting of microalgaeas an important source for biofuel production, and other components of microalgae (like pigments) were reported by Juang et al. [8].

Microfluidic devices have been fabricated on various substrates. In order to choose the best substrates, some principles should be taken into account such as machinability, surface charge, molecular adsorption, electroosmotic flow mobility, and optical properties [43]. Previously, silicon and glass materials were mainly employed to fabricate microfluidic devices, due to their high thermal conductivity and ability to withstand temperature gradients, respectively [44]. However, due to their unsuitability for fabricating devices in water, lack of compatibility with living mammalian cells [4], and complicated and high-priced components, they have been replaced with polymers. Master molds can be produced using inexpensive and transparent elastomers, in particular, polydimethylsiloxane (PDMS) that has attracted much attention for their efficient applications [45, 46]. It is worth noting that the introduction of PDMS has helped the development of more useful microfluidic devices for technological and biomedical studies. This new microfluidic technology has brought remarkable benefits including, safe molding processes [47], optically transparency, gas and water-permeability [48], rapid curing at relatively low temperatures [49], biocompatibility, ease of molding into (sub) micrometer dimensions, and the ability to interact with itself and with glass [50]. These properties have led to them being used in immunoassays and for the separation of proteins and DNA [51]. These devices are usually produced by soft lithography, which is an effective process used in separation and analytical sciences, creating a device by replica molding [31]. Nevertheless, this process has some drawbacks such as small molecule absorption (can affect critical cell signaling dynamics), high sensitivity to organic solvents, and problems with vapor permeability [52, 53].

Recently, microfluidic paper-based analytical devices have been described, not only because of their simplicity, biocompatibility, availability, high ability to be stacked, stored and transported, easy modification [54], but also due to their mechanical properties, comprising flexibility, lightness, and low thickness. Paper-based devices are simple, cheap, and user-friendly [55]. Microfluidic paper-based analytical devices (μPADs) contain hydrophilic/hydrophobic microchannel networks, resulting in the ability for fluid handling and quantitative analysis with excellent performance in applications in medicine, healthcare, and environmental monitoring [56]. These devices are highly disposable and biodegradable, cheap and ubiquitous, lightweight and readily transportable, and capable of wicking fluids by capillary action in the absence of any external power source [57]. More recently, applications of perfluorinated polymers, usually known as Teflon, have been reported for coating the microchannel surface to fabricating whole-Teflon chips and Teflon-hybrid chips [52]. Nonetheless, despite the rapid development of materials in microfluidics, the progress of novel miniaturized total analysis systems (μTASs) in biomedical research has not attracted much attention [58]. Hence, based on the advancement of LoC devices and innovations in manufacturing, automation, and control, the future perspective of μTASs requires deeper consideration and more experimental work. Indeed, LoC systems including the relevant microsystem families such as microfluidics, MEMS/NEMS, and μTASs should concentrate more on the challenges of integration, standardization, the economy of commercialization as well as the application of the intended systems, rather than the extra elaboration of advanced functionality [59].

Microfluidic continuous flow, microarrays, and droplet-based systems with superior fluid control, along with lower consumption of expensive reagents have been increasingly utilized in the miniaturization of large-scale chemical assays and analytical techniques [60]. These devices, which were initially introduced by the semiconductor industry, and were then extended to microelectromechanical systems (MEMS), generally known as μTASs or LoC technologies [58]. LoC systems based on μTASs usually combine several components to form a unified system including processes such as sample injection, mixing, storage, optical analysis, incubation, sample treatment as well as extraction for cell culture and perfusion, cell lysis, polymerase chain reaction (PCR), and screening assays [61].

More importantly, as nanoparticles have gained popularity throughout the scientific world, the invention of new approaches to produce better and more reproducible synthesis techniques has become important. Thus, batch synthesis techniques should be transitioned into continuous flow reactors, due to irreproducibility, poor size distribution, and low quality of nanomaterials varying from batch to batch [24]. Therefore, the advantages of microfluidics, including low reagent consumption, large surface-to-volume ratio, online single and/or multiphase flows, as well as increased reliability, have led to significant progress being achieved [16]. However, continuous flow microfluidic devices still suffer from problems such as Taylor dispersion, solute-surface interactions, cross-contamination, and the need for larger volumes of reagents and fairly long channel lengths. Accordingly, segmented flow platforms in which the reagents are contained in picoliter to nanoliter sized droplets, within a continuous and immiscible fluid can form droplets produced by combining two immiscible phases [62, 63]. Two major types of microfluidic devices, including microchannels and microcapillaries have been proposed for generating these particles. While the first type is produced by various microfabrication processes such as micromilling, micromachining, lithography as well as mold replication, the second type, microcapillary systems are created by more time-saving and cost-efficient processes, but require more harsh chemical conditions compared to microchannel-based devices, which need expensive and time-consuming procedures [64]. In parallel with the rapid development of microfluidics, various procedures have been implemented to organize the flow in microfluidic systems, including capillary driven test strips, pressure-driven systems, centrifugal microfluidic devices, electrokinetic platforms, droplet-based microfluidic systems, and noncontact dispensing systems [65]. Importantly, in order to transfer fluids in microfluidics systems, different driving forces are required such as electrostatic [66], centrifugal [67], optical [68], body force (such as gravity force) [69], magnetic [70], and surface tension [71]. Among these, droplet-based microfluidics, forming a colloidal and interfacial system, has been described in scientific studies for tackling the limitations of slow mixing and sample zone dispersion. These problems are evident in laminar flow microfluidic platforms involving both continuous-flow emulsion-based droplet microfluidics, and electrowetting-based droplet microfluidics [3, 72]. Droplet-based microfluidics can produce samples with a high throughput with a controllable size in which the droplets can be used as an extracellular matrix, simulating a 3D microenvironment

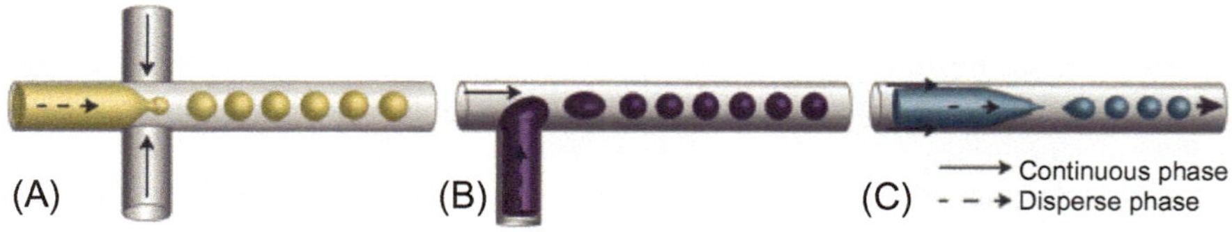

FIG. 1.1

Common types of microfluidics design. (A) Flow focusing, (B) T-junction, and (C) concentric capillaries.

Reprinted with permission from Zhang Y, Chan HF, Leong KW. Advanced materials and processing for drug delivery: the past and the future. Adv Drug Deliv Rev. 2013;65(1):104–20, Elsevier.

[73]. Furthermore, droplet-based microfluidic devices can have a variety of geometries, namely X- and Y-junctions, co-flow and comb geometry as well as droplet splitting/merging units for diverse applications [74]. Among these, T-junctions, for flow-focusing and concentric capillaries are the most popular and more common than others, see Fig. 1.1 [75].

In the droplet generation unit, the properties of immiscible fluids are utilized at the microscale to generate and manipulate droplets; in consequence. In order to generate droplets, microfluidic chips requiring accurate manipulation of fluidic elements on a small scale are needed [76]. The size of the droplet is managed through forming a balance between the flow rate and ratio of the two phases, although the viscosity of the dispersed phase, the channel and orifice diameter, and flow regimes can also influence the droplet size [77].

Digital microfluidic (DMF) describes a droplet-based microfluidic technique with a planar geometry [65], which can be established in either open or closed (sandwiched) configurations [78]. DMF works by the manipulation of discrete droplets on a substrate or nano- to micromolar fluid droplets on an open array of insulated electrodes. DMF is a microscale fluid handling process that allows the organized motion of fluids and can be an alternative to the conventional paradigm of mixing, reacting, and transferring fluids [79, 80]. Interestingly, in comparison with other single-cell analysis techniques, these systems do not require mechanical tubes, pumps, and valves and liquid motion can be obtained through the controlled application of voltages to an array of electrodes, via electrowetting on dielectric (EWOD or EWD) or dielectrophoresis (DEP) [81]. DMF has been extensively exploited as a disruptive methodology owing to the significant reduction in the volumes of analytes [82], the capability to be integrated with measurement techniques [83], intrinsic flexibility for laboratory applications [84], and the potential to integrate automated systems and external detectors for offline biological analysis [85]. Several publications have reported the integration between DMF and a variety of other systems, and most of them have provided an excellent alternative to the analytical toolbox, especially for analytes that are only available at very dilute concentrations in complex sample matrices [86, 87].

In order to address problems in traditional medical diagnostic procedures, microfluidic-based diagnostic devices have demonstrated better simplicity and sensitivity for rapid analysis compared to traditional diagnostic approaches [88]. Droplet microfluidics can provide high performance in clinical laboratory tests using minute volumes of reagents in a short time, mainly used in proteomic and nucleic acid-based diagnosis [3]. Among them, point-of-care (POC) diagnostic devices have been devised for helping medical scientists diagnose patients in less developed countries without access to standard laboratories. These devices also outperform previous diagnostic devices with remarkable advantages like portability, convenience, robustness, and low-cost as well as producing rapid results [74, 89]. Applications of polymer and paper-based microfluidic devices for the manufacture of POC devices have increased recently because they can pave the way for testing patients in their own locality without the need for travel to clinical centers. Also, POC devices can be used in the diagnosis of pregnancy, infectious disease, cardiac disease, human immunodeficiency virus (HIV-1) infection, diabetes, and also in screening for drug abuse in individuals and athletes [90, 91]. Specifically, this achievement is of critical importance for people living in resource-limited countries as they cannot easily travel to dedicated diagnostic facilities, whereas on-site diagnosis could yield more efficient medical treatments [92]. For example, up to half of the people in developing countries, including, mothers, newborns, and children suffer from a variety of infectious diseases; therefore, helping them is a priority issue. Hopefully, microfluidic-based POC devices can provide: (1) better access to faster and more accurate diagnostic instruments than were previously provided; (2) better epidemiological data that can be utilized for disease modeling; (3) introduction of better vaccines to improve the economics of healthcare systems; and (4) ability to employ minimally trained healthcare workers [93]. Microfluidic-based POC devices are considered an utmost priority for healthcare, molecular biology, cell culture applications, and analysis, because of their low instrument size, high sensitivity and efficiency, inexpensive processes, high throughput, rapid and easy method of use, easy fabrication, better sensing ability, and finally, continual monitoring of appropriate analytes [89, 94, 95]. Up to now, many companies have proposed microfluidic-based POC devices as cutting-edge solutions for improving LoC processes necessary for building an integrated POC diagnostic device [96, 97].

Methods for the fabrication of microfluidic devices can be classified into three categories: subtractive, additive, and molding (also known as formative) [98]. For instance, in additive microfabrication, materials are usually selectively added to a substrate using physical vapor deposition (PVD), while in subtractive microfabrication, the structure of interest is transformed by chemical or physical removal of some of the material, for instance by micromilling [99]. Not long ago, 3D microfluidics underwent an unprecedented expansion in fields such as MEMS and LoC technologies, where the fabrication of 3D microstructures used diverse methods and components. Among them, 3D printing microfluidics, also known as additive manufacturing (AM) or rapid prototyping (RP) have progressed dramatically [100–102]. These remarkable technological systems come with a reasonable price and environmentally friendly features [103], the ability to easily design unique bespoke one-off systems [104], fast iterative changes, and easy fabrication [105]. Fundamentally, 3D printed microfluidics are now able to overcome the problems of PDMS devices. For example, they can be implemented in a single step, and complicated structures can be made with just a few steps [106]. In this technique, a simple layer-by-layer fabrication procedure is employed because the main structure can be divided into several 2D cross-sections [107]. Additionally, easy fabrication procedures can bridge the gap between 3D computer designs and physical models [108]. One example is inkjet printing (IJP) where each droplet of ink is generated and deposited under digital control through manipulating the liquid flow [109]. Besides, these techniques are capable of cheap installation, rapid prototyping, with 3D digital design [110]. The most powerful technologies used for the manufacturing of 3D printed microfluidic devices are fused deposition modeling (FDM), stereolithography apparatus (SLA), and digital light processing (DLP) due to their low cost, high accuracy, and straightforward operation [102]. The increase in published articles concerning 3D printing has demonstrated a substantial contribution from researchers, which is expected to gather even more attention. For example, in one study, Boutelle et al. described a 3D printed microfluidic device combined with the Food and Drug Administration-approved clinical microdialysis probes and integrated with needle-type biosensors that showed great potential for monitoring real-time subcutaneous glucose and lactate levels in cyclists who were participating in a training regimen. Not only did this experiment indicate the promising benefit of 3D printing microfluidic devices that could be easily coupled with other systems, but it offered a rational design for future therapeutic applications [111]. However, the main reason why 3D printers have not been as widely used as expected, may be: (i) the roughness property leading to poor optical transparency [112]; and (ii) a shortfall in their spatial resolution to make systems that are literally microfluidic ($< 100 \times 100\,\mu m = 10{,}000\,\mu m^2$) [105].

As mentioned above, microfluidics are now applied to many scientific applications. In the next section we will summarize some of the important properties of microfluidic devices, as well as the advantages over some of the important competing devices.

1.2 Chemical synthesis

With regard to many advantages of microfluidics, namely the ability to offer controlled environmental conditions, continuous and laminar flow systems at the small scale, a diversity of applications in synthetic chemistry have been developed over the last few years, resulting in the possibility of them being routinely used in chemical laboratories [113].

Chemical synthesis has witnessed rapid growth over traditional batch-wise techniques. However, the limitations of conventional batch synthesis have exerted a heavy toll on the economics of chemical synthesis, particularly, in biomedical reactors. These problems range from unwanted and possibly toxic waste materials, poor reproducibility, costly procedures, and time-consuming to labor-intensive processes. Microfluidic devices, functioning as microreactors offer good mass and heat transfer performance have emerged in this field to produce high purity materials as well as providing safer and more efficient chemical reactions.

Several publications have reported different applications of microfluidics for chemical synthesis in both academic laboratories and in industrial development facilities [63, 114]. Microfluidics has brought about significant benefits for synthetic reactions including (i) much lower reagent volumes; (ii) high selectivity; (iii) greener credentials; (iv) rapid reaction kinetics; (v) small footprint and safe environment. Two dimensionless physical constants, the Reynolds number (*Re*) and the thermal Péclet number (Pe_L), should be considered for chemical synthesis in a microfluidic reactor. The Re is the ratio of inertial force to viscous force within a fluid, while the Pe_L is a dimensionless parameter that characterizes the microfluidic regime. If chemical reactions are completed in microfluidic reactors, a low *Re* shows that there is no turbulence and therefore, no back-mixing within the reactor. Moreover, Pe_L expresses the rate of heat transport by the moving fluid, Scheme 1.1 [115].

(inertial forces)/(viscous forces) = $\rho dv/\mu$

- Reynolds number

(advective)/(diffusive) = $dv\rho C_p/k$

- Thermal Péclet number

SCHEME 1.1

Equations of *Re* and PeL. ρ: density, d: characteristic dimension, v: fluid velocity, μ: dynamic viscosity, Cp: heat capacity, k: thermal conduct vity.

Microfluidics can allow synthetic chemistry to be closely coupled with many cutting-edge modern technologies, such as 3D printing, big data, and artificial intelligence [116]. In a chemistry laboratory, microfluidic devices can be coupled with different spectroscopic techniques such as X-ray, Uv–Vis, fluorescence, Fourier transform infrared (FT-IR), and absorption. Due to the lower sensitivity of chemical synthesis to changes in reaction conditions, a capillary tubing-based set up in a continuous flow platform is preferable, because it can be used in the scale-up optimization of the reaction [117]. More importantly, multiphase flows using microchannel networks enable chemical reactions by improving effective mass transfer between two immiscible fluids, resulting in being able to evaluate reaction mechanisms within short timescales and for synthesizing monodisperse nanoparticles. This is very useful for exothermic gas–liquid or gas–liquid–solid reactions that can take place under well-defined and isothermal conditions [118]. For example, Lee et al. synthesized an [^{18}F] fluoride-radiolabeled molecular imaging probe, 2-deoxy-2-[^{18}F] fluoro-D-glucose ([^{18}F] FDG), using an integrated microfluidic system. Multistep and sequential reactions allowed the synthesis of both [^{18}F] FDG and [^{19}F] FDG in a nanoliter-scale reaction vessel. These steps were: (1) dilute fluoride ion that was concentrated within miniaturized anion exchange; (2) exchange of solvent from water to dry acetonitrile (MeCN); (3) fluorination of the D-mannose triflate precursor; (4) exchange of the solvent back to water; and finally (5) acidic hydrolysis. This study reported a high radiochemical yield and purity along with a time-efficient synthesis procedure compared to conventional automated synthesis [119]. Furthermore, the use of harsh conditions such as performing reactions at high temperatures and pressures, as well as preventing leakage of hazardous and explosive materials, microfluidics could provide unprecedented advances for the controllable synthesis of micro-/nanostructured materials [120]. In this sense, miniaturized spiral-shaped microchannels with one or two inlets have been designed for the controllable flow synthesis of numerous reaction products [121–123].

In order to expand microfluidics systems in the biomedical industry, some crucial factors are required, in which the ability for scale-up is the top priority. Whether small flow reactors or continuous-flow reactors can be effectively used in a scaled-up chemical reaction is a matter of opinion, due to the scarcity of experimental examples, although a capillary tubing-based setup has often been recommended. Another question is the rate of the reaction, which should be faster than batch reactions in terms of heat and mass transfer. Most importantly, standardization of microfluidic systems must be optimized before they can replace traditional systems, and the optimization and simulation of microfluidics design, selectivity, assembly, and control of operational conditions should be taken into account. To address these issues, more experimental investigations must be carried out [115, 117, 124]. Another factor that limits the use of microfluidics is their low production capacity, which is difficult to successfully transition from laboratory studies to commercial manufacturing [125].

1.3 Drug delivery

Even though nanoparticle-based drug delivery has already made a big impact on biomedical technologies, some challenges that remain in traditional smart drug delivery system (SDDS) need improvements in areas such as mass production, chemical characterization, feasibility, and possible toxicity. Most of these questions need to be answered before any clinical trial phases can begin. The emergence of microfluidic platforms could advance the field of drug delivery, as well as that of nanoparticle synthesis, and allow these studies to be carried out in a versatile, large-scale, and controllable manner [126]. Several studies have been devoted to the applications of microfluidics for targeted and controlled drug delivery [127, 128].

The combination of microfluidics and controlled-release technology can produce biological agents that can be delivered in a sustained manner which could be indispensable in tissue engineering [129]. The advantages of microfluidic devices in drug delivery could include: (a) a tunable structure, diameter, and surface; (b) controlled release profile; (c) desired robustness; and (d) good adaptability [77]. More importantly, microfluidics enable SDDS to improve the drug encapsulation efficiency, allowing additionally loaded drug molecules in the same carrier for dual function responsiveness [130].

Droplet microfluidics with a narrow dispersion (less than 1% size variation) and no cross-contamination are promising tools for fabricating complex particles or particle-based materials that can be used as SDDS. Moreover, unprecedented advances in droplet microfluidics have allowed scientists to produce complex drug systems with uniform sizes, monodisperse size distribution, and beneficial properties. Drug delivery systems based on microfabricated devices can be in the form of emulsions, microparticles, microcapsules, or microgels [131]. In droplet microfluidics, diffusion and convection are controlled by the diffusion coefficient and device-dependent factors respectively and play a pivotal role in the mass-transfer rate [132]. Applications of PDMS-based microfluidic systems for the production of hydrogel microparticles, for cellular encapsulation and water-soluble drug delivery, have been increasing [132, 133]. Janus particles possess two different well-defined hemispheres each with diverse physical and chemical properties, and have been utilized at the inlet of the microfluidic channel for potential drug delivery applications [134]. Janus microencapsulated particles have the potential for targeted drug delivery; hence, many publications have been dedicated to the applications of Janus particles and microcapsule in microfluidics devices. Janus particles have two distinct regions of different surface structures, while microcapsules have a typical core–shell configuration [135]. Moffitt et al. developed a multiscale structure with a drug delivery capability using paclitaxel (PAX)-loaded polycaprolactone-*block*-poly(ethylene oxide) (PCL-b-PEO) polymeric nanoparticles (PNPs) using synthesis with flow-directed shear processing in a two-phase gas-liquid microfluidic reactor. They demonstrated that the flow-variable shear processing with an intermediate flow rate enabled tunable PNP sizes/morphologies and expanded the sustained release time to longer than 2 weeks, along with the best antiproliferative effects against cultured MCF-7 breast cancer cells. On the other hand, slow and fast flow rates led to lower levels of cytotoxicity due to the inappropriate particle sizes produced, Fig. 1.2 [136].

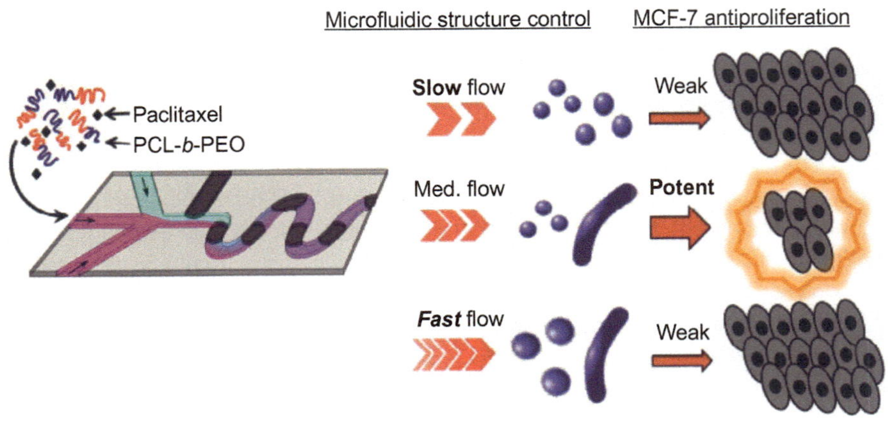

FIG. 1.2

Controlled release of PAX through two-phase gas-liquid microfluidic reactor [136].

Reprinted (adapted) with permission from Bains A, Cao Y, Kly S, Wulff JE, Moffitt MG. Controlling structure and function of polymeric drug delivery nanoparticles using microfluidics. Mol Pharm. 2017;14(8):2595–606.

1.4 Cell biology

Over the last decades, there has been an explosion in the numbers of papers investigating the use of microfluidics in cell biology, because of the suitable dimensions of the microfluidic channels to accommodate biological cells, and the ability to mimic the cellular microenvironment on the precise length and time scales [137]. Microfluidic techniques have offered great advantages for cellular research, such as cell culture, cell separation, and cell lysis. However, studies on PCR, immunoassays, organ-on-chip, stem cell research, analysis, and identification of circulating tumor cells (CTCs) have been more often reported [138]. These benefits can be attributed to complex 3D spaces that contain both physical and biochemical cues closely mimicking the in vivo microenvironment. Moreover, microfluidic devices can reproduce the concept of cellular confinement, which typically restrains cell movement within the interstitial spaces of tissue, and which is not fully reproduced in 2D culture assays [139]. Additionally, in the field of tissue engineering, microfluidic techniques have shown exceptional benefits including (i) simultaneous accomplishment of multiple assays; (ii) cellular control of the spatiotemporal distribution of physicochemical signals; (iii) analysis of cellular differentiation and functions [140]. In order to efficiently replicate the in vivo environment and address limitations of typical cell/stem cell culture approaches and tissue engineering procedures, various microfluidic cell culture assays have been reported to better mimic the in vivo interactions between extracellular matrix (ECM) and the cells. In addition, they provide opportunities for high-resolution in situ cell imaging techniques [140, 141]. The dimensions of microfluidic structures are quite compatible with the size of single cells and can be adapted to a number of cell types with long cellular projections, such as neurons [142]. These desired dimensions not only increase diffusive mixing, but also improve the speed and reproducibility of reactions [143]. Microfluidic cell culture has provided opportunities for a variety of in vitro diagnostic applications in biomedical research, whereby basic biological processes such as cell signaling and dynamic cell-to-cell interactions can be reliably reproduced in physiological cell culture situations, and by recapitulating the complex 3D structures of tissues and organs [144]. For example, recent reports have demonstrated that microfluidic devices are able to enhance the yield of cDNA produced from mRNA transcripts, and reduce the technical variability due to the lower reaction volumes [145]. Single-cell level quantification of cellular responses to both internal and external stimuli was facilitated with a good temporal resolution over a long-time cell culture span. Microfluidic cell culture also enables the exact regulation of cell numbers and density within a distinct area or volume and allows precise cellular location in multiplex geometries [146].

By integrating microfluidic devices with conventional imaging techniques, these systems can provide a means of following cellular trajectories over time, although improved experimental platforms are crucial to bridge the gap between imaging results and downstream single-cell gene expression profiles [147]. Yeo et al. developed a promising microfluidic device that could successfully separate very scarce CTCs in blood samples (only present as 1 in 20,000 white blood cells).

They used a novel microfluidic device capable of high throughput specific selection and isolation of single rare cells from a mixed population, which could track variations of acquired T790M mutations. They found that isolated single CTCs possessed dominant EGFR mutations such as T790M and L858R that were found in the primary tumor [148]. Microfluidic devices were also used in the study of chemotaxis (the movement of an organism in response to a chemical stimulus) because chemokine gradients could be precisely designed and controlled [149]. Nevertheless, the low throughput levels of capturing single cells [150], poor gene recovery, and cross-contamination issues are problems that microfluidic approaches have not yet overcome [145].

1.5 Biosensors

Biosensors are analytical devices, used for integrating a biological recognition element that produces a signal upon binding in direct spatial contact with a transduction element [151, 152]. Biosensors now play an indispensable role in multiple fields such as the food industry [153], bioanalytical and clinical analysis [152], metabolic engineering [154], POC studies [155], and environmental monitoring [156]. A critical look at the technological innovations made in microfluidics shows a variety of sophisticated applications using electronic fluidics, as a consequence, countless bioassays have claimed benefits like rapid analysis, good compatibility, and adaptability with the need for only small sample volumes in addition to higher sensitivity [157]. The integration between biosensors and microfluidics to provide miniaturized systems with beneficial properties has captured the attention of both scientists and manufacturers. Microfluidic-based biosensors not only display reduced reagent consumption and shorter processing times, but also have laminar flow, limited production of toxic compounds, multiplex sample detection, and are portable and versatile [94]. For example, Jang et al. reported a versatile approach for integrating microfluidic devices as biosensors in μTASs for a variety of biomedical applications, and particularly the simultaneous detection of glucose and alcohol [157].

Magnetic biosensors have also been investigated as quantification techniques for biological species, and can be coupled with microfluidics in order to generate assays with high simplicity, sensitivity, and portability providing rapid results [20]. Recently, Duarte and colleagues developed a microfluidic device for the magnetic detection of *Streptococcus agalactiae* (a Group B streptococci bacteria) and *Streptococcus uberis* in raw milk samples. They showed a low detection limit of 100 cfu/mL of both bacteria using antibodies. Milk samples were combined with a solution mixing specific antibodies and magnetic nanoparticles, before the analysis. This experiment reported a 73% positive diagnosis of streptococci species using an anti-*S. agalactiae* antibody and 41% using a more general anti-GB streptococcal antibody. Additionally, this system could be used in different applications such as the integration of a milk pretreatment step with the microfluidic platform, and electronics could be introduced to allow multiplex analysis of many samples simultaneously [158].

In addition to the described applications of microfluidics in chemical synthesis, drug delivery, cell biology, and biosensors, the microfluidic approach can be applied in many other fields. Microfluidic systems may replace many traditional approaches due to their low consumption of reagents and samples, ability to manipulate small volumes, and rapid reactions and separations. Microfluidics have been gaining popularity owing to the number and the improved quality of articles and books that have recently been published on this topic. Despite all the benefits of microfluidic platforms developed for various applications, some major obstacles could still be delaying the advancement. Furthermore, because the development of new microfluidic devices needs big budget technologies as well as dedicated training courses, the number of commercial products on the market is still limited. In fact, the incompatibility of many microfluidic systems with large-volume sample-processing equipment systems has become a serious issue that requires more experiments to reconcile. Moving forward, we believe that new high-impact applications of microfluidic devices could drive much more investment in the LoC field among others.

References

[1] O.J. Dressler, R.M. Maceiczyk, S.-I. Chang, A.J. de Mello, Droplet-based microfluidics: enabling impact on drug discovery, J Biomol Screen 19 (4) (2014) 483–496.

[2] Y. Song, D. Cheng, L. Zhao, Microfluidics: fundamentals, devices, and applications, John Wiley & Sons, 2018.

[3] W.-L. Chou, P.-Y. Lee, C.-L. Yang, W.-Y. Huang, Y.-S. Lin, Recent advances in applications of droplet microfluidics, Micromachines 6 (9) (2015) 1249–1271.

[4] G.M. Whitesides, The origins and the future of microfluidics, Nature 442 (7101) (2006) 368.

[5] N.-T. Nguyen, S.T. Wereley, S.A.M. Shaegh, Fundamentals and applications of microfluidics, Artech House, 2019.

[6] F.A. Gomez, Biological applications of microfluidics, John Wiley & Sons, 2008.

[7] O. Ki, K. Tachikawa, A. Manz, Microfluidics: applications for analytical purposes in chemistry and biochemistry, Electrophoresis 29 (22) (2008) 4443–4453.

[8] Y.J. Juang, J.S. Chang, Applications of microfluidics in microalgae biotechnology: a review, Biotechnol J 11 (3) (2016) 327–335.

[9] Y. Jun, E. Kang, S. Chae, S.-H. Lee, Microfluidic spinning of micro-and nano-scale fibers for tissue engineering, Lab Chip 14 (13) (2014) 2145–2160.

[10] S. Tasoglu, U.A. Gurkan, S. Wang, U. Demirci, Manipulating biological agents and cells in micro-scale volumes for applications in medicine, Chem Soc Rev 42 (13) (2013) 5788–5808.

[11] G.A. Cooksey, J.T. Elliott, A.L. Plant, Reproducibility and robustness of a real-time microfluidic cell toxicity assay, Anal Chem 83 (10) (2011) 3890–3896.

[12] N.M. Oliveira, S. Vilabril, M.B. Oliveira, R.L. Reis, J.F. Mano, Recent advances on open fluidic systems for biomedical applications: a review, Mater Sci Eng C 97 (2018) 851–863.

[13] A. Bohr, S. Colombo, H. Jensen, Future of microfluidics in research and in the market. Microfluidics for pharmaceutical applications, Elsevier, 2019, pp. 425–465.

[14] C.H. Chen, Y. Lu, M.L. Sin, K.E. Mach, D.D. Zhang, V. Gau, et al., Antimicrobial susceptibility testing using high surface-to-volume ratio microchannels, Anal Chem 82 (3) (2010) 1012–1019.

[15] H. Feng, T. Zheng, M. Li, J. Wu, H. Ji, J. Zhang, et al., Droplet-based microfluidics systems in biomedical applications, Electrophoresis 40 (11) (2019) 1580–1590.

[16] S. Marre, Y. Roig, C. Aymonier, Supercritical microfluidics: opportunities in flow-through chemistry and materials science, J Supercrit Fluids 66 (2012) 251–264.

[17] W.-C. Tian, E. Finehout, Microfluidics for biological applications, Springer Science & Business Media, 2009.

[18] S. Haeberle, R. Zengerle, Microfluidic platforms for lab-on-a-chip applications, Lab Chip 7 (9) (2007) 1094–1110.

[19] D.G. Rackus, M.H. Shamsi, A.R. Wheeler, Electrochemistry, biosensors and microfluidics: a convergence of fields, Chem Soc Rev 44 (15) (2015) 5320–5340.

[20] I. Giouroudi, G. Kokkinis, Recent advances in magnetic microfluidic biosensors, Nanomaterials 7 (7) (2017) 171.

[21] M. Shayan, S. Bhattacharjee, J. Tang, K. Chakrabarty, R. Karri, Bio-protocol watermarking on digital microfluidic biochips, IEEE Trans Inf Forensics Secur 14 (11) (2019) 2901–2915.

[22] C.M.B. Ho, S.H. Ng, K.H.H. Li, Y.-J. Yoon, 3D printed microfluidics for biological applications, Lab Chip 15 (18) (2015) 3627–3637.

[23] D. Erickson, D. Li, Integrated microfluidic devices, Anal Chim Acta 507 (1) (2004) 11–26.

[24] S. Marre, K.F. Jensen, Synthesis of micro and nanostructures in microfluidic systems, Chem Soc Rev 39 (3) (2010) 1183–1202.

[25] S. Marre, J. Baek, J. Park, M.G. Bawendi, K.F. Jensen, High-pressure/high-temperature microreactors for nanostructure synthesis, J Assoc Lab Autom 14 (6) (2009) 367–373.

[26] M. Björnmalm, Y. Yan, F. Caruso, Engineering and evaluating drug delivery particles in microfluidic devices, J Control Release 190 (2014) 139–149.

[27] L.R. Volpatti, A.K. Yetisen, Commercialization of microfluidic devices, Trends Biotechnol 32 (7) (2014) 347–350.

[28] T.A. Duncombe, A.M. Tentori, A.E. Herr, Microfluidics: reframing biological enquiry, Nat Rev Mol Cell Biol 16 (9) (2015) 554.

[29] F. Li, Z. Zheng, B. Yang, X. Zhang, Z. Li, L. Lei, A laminar-flow based microfluidic microbial three-electrode cell for biosensing, Electrochim Acta 199 (2016) 45–50.

[30] M.A. Modestino, D.F. Rivas, S.M.H. Hashemi, J.G. Gardeniers, D. Psaltis, The potential for microfluidics in electrochemical energy systems, Energy Environ Sci 9 (11) (2016) 3381–3391.

[31] C. Chen, B.T. Mehl, A.S. Munshi, A.D. Townsend, D.M. Spence, R.S. Martin, 3D-printed microfluidic devices: fabrication, advantages and limitations—a mini review, Anal Methods 8 (31) (2016) 6005–6012.

[32] N. Pamme, Magnetism and microfluidics, Lab Chip 6 (1) (2006) 24–38.

[33] Y. Ding, J. Choo, A.J. Demello, From single-molecule detection to next-generation sequencing: microfluidic droplets for high-throughput nucleic acid analysis, Microfluid Nanofluid 21 (3) (2017) 58.

[34] F. Eduati, R. Utharala, D. Madhavan, U.P. Neumann, T. Longerich, T. Cramer, et al., A microfluidics platform for combinatorial drug screening on cancer biopsies, Nat Commun 9 (1) (2018) 2434.

[35] V. Solis-Tinoco, S. Marquez, T. Quesada-Lopez, F. Villarroya, A. Homs-Corbera, L.M. Lechuga, Building of a flexible microfluidic plasmo-nanomechanical biosensor for live cell analysis, Sensors Actuators B Chem 291 (2019) 48–57.
[36] S. Fang, H. Tian, X. Li, D. Jin, X. Li, J. Kong, et al., Clinical application of a microfluidic chip for immunocapture and quantification of circulating exosomes to assist breast cancer diagnosis and molecular classification, PLoS One 12 (4) (2017), e0175050.
[37] C. Furlan, R.A. Dirks, P.C. Thomas, R.C. Jones, J. Wang, M. Lynch, et al., Miniaturised interaction proteomics on a microfluidic platform with ultra-low input requirements, Nat Commun 10 (1) (2019) 1525.
[38] R. Pol, F. Céspedes, D. Gabriel, M. Baeza, Microfluidic lab-on-a-chip platforms for environmental monitoring, TrAC Trends Anal Chem 95 (2017) 62–68.
[39] K. Kant, M.-A. Shahbazi, V.P. Dave, T.A. Ngo, V.A. Chidambara, L.Q. Than, et al., Microfluidic devices for sample preparation and rapid detection of foodborne pathogens, Biotechnol Adv 36 (4) (2018) 1003–1024.
[40] K.L. Chen, M.M. Crane, M. Kaeberlein, Microfluidic technologies for yeast replicative lifespan studies, Mech Ageing Dev 161 (2017) 262–269.
[41] A.S. Nezhad, Microfluidic platforms for plant cells studies, Lab Chip 14 (17) (2014) 3262–3274.
[42] I. Barbulovic-Nad, S.H. Au, A.R. Wheeler, A microfluidic platform for complete mammalian cell culture, Lab Chip 10 (12) (2010) 1536–1542.
[43] H. Becker, L.E. Locascio, Polymer microfluidic devices, Talanta 56 (2) (2002) 267–287.
[44] C. Iliescu, H. Taylor, M. Avram, J. Miao, S. Franssila, A practical guide for the fabrication of microfluidic devices using glass and silicon, Biomicrofluidics 6 (1) (2012), 016505.
[45] S. Vyawahare, A.D. Griffiths, C.A. Merten, Miniaturization and parallelization of biological and chemical assays in microfluidic devices, Chem Biol 17 (10) (2010) 1052–1065.
[46] C.-W. Tsao, Polymer microfluidics: simple, low-cost fabrication process bridging academic lab research to commercialized production, Micromachines 7 (12) (2016) 225.
[47] A.K. Au, N. Bhattacharjee, L.F. Horowitz, T.C. Chang, A. Folch, 3D-printed microfluidic automation, Lab Chip 15 (8) (2015) 1934–1941.
[48] Z. Liu, X. Han, L. Qin, Recent progress of microfluidics in translational applications, Adv Healthc Mater 5 (8) (2016) 871–888.
[49] M.A. Eddings, M.A. Johnson, B.K. Gale, Determining the optimal PDMS–PDMS bonding technique for microfluidic devices, J Micromech Microeng 18 (6) (2008), 067001.
[50] J. Zhou, A.V. Ellis, N.H. Voelcker, Recent developments in PDMS surface modification for microfluidic devices, Electrophoresis 31 (1) (2010) 2–16.
[51] J.R. Lake, K.C. Heyde, W.C. Ruder, Low-cost feedback-controlled syringe pressure pumps for microfluidics applications, PLoS One 12 (4) (2017), e0175089.
[52] Y. Wang, S. Chen, H. Sun, W. Li, C. Hu, K. Ren, Recent progresses in microfabricating perfluorinated polymers (Teflons) and the associated new applications in microfluidics, Microphysiol Syst 2 (2018).
[53] E. Berthier, J. Warrick, H. Yu, D.J. Beebe, Managing evaporation for more robust microscale assays part 1. Volume loss in high throughput assays, Lab Chip 8 (6) (2008) 852–859.
[54] F.A. Gomez, Paper microfluidics in bioanalysis, Bioanalysis 6 (21) (2014) 2911–2914.

[55] T. Akyazi, L. Basabe-Desmonts, F. Benito-Lopez, Review on microfluidic paper-based analytical devices towards commercialisation, Anal Chim Acta 1001 (2018) 1–17.
[56] Y. Xia, J. Si, Z. Li, Fabrication techniques for microfluidic paper-based analytical devices and their applications for biological testing: a review, Biosens Bioelectron 77 (2016) 774–789.
[57] M.I.G. Almeida, B.M. Jayawardane, S.D. Kolev, I.D. McKelvie, Developments of microfluidic paper-based analytical devices (μPADs) for water analysis: A review, Talanta 177 (2018) 176–190.
[58] E.K. Sackmann, A.L. Fulton, D.J. Beebe, The present and future role of microfluidics in biomedical research, Nature 507 (7491) (2014) 181.
[59] M.I. Mohammed, S. Haswell, I. Gibson, Lab-on-a-chip or Chip-in-a-lab: challenges of commercialization lost in translation, Procedia Technol 20 (2015) 54–59.
[60] T. Akyazi, J. Saez, J. Elizalde, F. Benito-Lopez, Fluidic flow delay by ionogel passive pumps in microfluidic paper-based analytical devices, Sensors Actuators B Chem 233 (2016) 402–408.
[61] Š. Selimović, H. Kaji, H. Bae, A. Khademhosseini, Microfluidic systems for controlling stem cell microenvironments. Microfluidic cell culture systems, Elsevier, 2019, pp. 31–63.
[62] X.C. i Solvas, A. DeMello, Droplet microfluidics: recent developments and future applications, Chem Commun 47 (7) (2011) 1936–1942.
[63] A.J. Demello, Control and detection of chemical reactions in microfluidic systems, Nature 442 (7101) (2006) 394.
[64] I.U. Khan, C.A. Serra, N. Anton, T.F. Vandamme, Production of nanoparticle drug delivery systems with microfluidics tools, Expert Opin Drug Deliv 12 (4) (2015) 547–562.
[65] E. Samiei, M. Tabrizian, M. Hoorfar, A review of digital microfluidics as portable platforms for lab-on a-chip applications, Lab Chip 16 (13) (2016) 2376–2396.
[66] C.-K. Chung, W.-J. Chang, C.-L. Hsiao, K.-Y. Weng, Microfluid driving device, Google Patents, 2004.
[67] R. Gorkin, J. Park, J. Siegrist, M. Amasia, B.S. Lee, J.-M. Park, et al., Centrifugal microfluidics for biomedical applications, Lab Chip 10 (14) (2010) 1758–1773.
[68] S.-K. Hoi, C. Udalagama, C.-H. Sow, F. Watt, A. Bettiol, Microfluidic sorting system based on optical force switching, Appl Phys B 97 (4) (2009) 859.
[69] D. Beebe, M. Wheeler, H. Zeringue, E. Walters, S. Raty, Microfluidic technology for assisted reproduction, Theriogenology 57 (1) (2002) 125–135.
[70] E. Mirowski, J. Moreland, A. Zhang, S.E. Russek, M.J. Donahue, Manipulation and sorting of magnetic particles by a magnetic force microscope on a microfluidic magnetic trap platform, Appl Phys Lett 86 (24) (2005) 243901.
[71] C.G. Cooney, C.-Y. Chen, M.R. Emerling, A. Nadim, J.D. Sterling, Electrowetting droplet microfluidics on a single planar surface, Microfluid Nanofluid 2 (5) (2006) 435–446.
[72] A. Suea-Ngam, P. Rattanarat, O. Chailapakul, M. Srisa-Art, Electrochemical droplet-based microfluidics using chip-based carbon paste electrodes for high-throughput analysis in pharmaceutical applications, Anal Chim Acta 883 (2015) 45–54.
[73] Y. Bai, M. Gao, L. Wen, C. He, Y. Chen, C. Liu, et al., Applications of microfluidics in quantitative biology, Biotechnol J 13 (5) (2018) 1700170.
[74] G.T. Vladisavljević, N. Khalid, M.A. Neves, T. Kuroiwa, M. Nakajima, K. Uemura, et al., Industrial lab-on-a-chip: design, applications and scale-up for drug discovery and delivery, Adv Drug Deliv Rev 65 (11–12) (2013) 1626–1663.

[75] Y. Zhang, H.F. Chan, K.W. Leong, Advanced materials and processing for drug delivery: the past and the future, Adv Drug Deliv Rev 65 (1) (2013) 104–120.
[76] W. Li, L. Zhang, X. Ge, B. Xu, W. Zhang, L. Qu, et al., Microfluidic fabrication of microparticles for biomedical applications, Chem Soc Rev 47 (15) (2018) 5646–5683.
[77] D. Liu, H. Zhang, F. Fontana, J.T. Hirvonen, H.A. Santos, Microfluidic-assisted fabrication of carriers for controlled drug delivery, Lab Chip 17 (11) (2017) 1856–1883.
[78] E. Samiei, G.S. Luka, H. Najjaran, M. Hoorfar, Integration of biosensors into digital microfluidics: impact of hydrophilic surface of biosensors on droplet manipulation, Biosens Bioelectron 81 (2016) 480–486.
[79] B. Seale, C. Lam, D.G. Rackus, M.D. Chamberlain, C. Liu, A.R. Wheeler, Digital microfluidics for immunoprecipitation, Anal Chem 88 (20) (2016) 10223–10230.
[80] S.L. Freire, Perspectives on digital microfluidics, Sensors Actuators A Phys 250 (2016) 15–28.
[81] L. Pang, J. Ding, X.-X. Liu, S.-K. Fan, Digital microfluidics for cell manipulation, TrAC Trends Anal Chem 117 (2019) 291–299.
[82] U. Sen, S. Chatterjee, S. Sen, M.K. Tiwari, A. Mukhopadhyay, R. Ganguly, Dynamics of magnetic modulation of ferrofluid droplets for digital microfluidic applications, J Magn Magn Mater 421 (2017) 165–176.
[83] B. Coelho, B. Veigas, E. Fortunato, R. Martins, H. Águas, R. Igreja, et al., Digital microfluidics for nucleic acid amplification, Sensors 17 (7) (2017) 1495.
[84] R.P. de Campos, D.G. Rackus, R. Shih, C. Zhao, X. Liu, A.R. Wheeler, "Plug-n-play" sensing with digital microfluidics, Anal Chem 91 (3) (2019) 2506–2515.
[85] P.Q. Vo, M.C. Husser, F. Ahmadi, H. Sinha, S.C. Shih, Image-based feedback and analysis system for digital microfluidics, Lab Chip 17 (20) (2017) 3437–3446.
[86] M. Sonker, V. Sahore, A.T. Woolley, Recent advances in microfluidic sample preparation and separation techniques for molecular biomarker analysis: a critical review, Anal Chim Acta 986 (2017) 1–11.
[87] K. Choi, E. Boyacı, J. Kim, B. Seale, L. Barrera-Arbelaez, J. Pawliszyn, et al., A digital microfluidic interface between solid-phase microextraction and liquid chromatography–mass spectrometry, J Chromatogr A 1444 (2016) 1–7.
[88] J. Cheng, Y. Jun, J. Qin, S.-H. Lee, Electrospinning versus microfluidic spinning of functional fibers for biomedical applications, Biomaterials 114 (2017) 121–143.
[89] C.M. Pandey, S. Augustine, S. Kumar, S. Kumar, S. Nara, S. Srivastava, et al., Microfluidics based point-of-care diagnostics, Biotechnol J 13 (1) (2018) 1700047.
[90] L.Y. Yeo, H.C. Chang, P.P. Chan, J.R. Friend, Microfluidic devices for bioapplications, Small 7 (1) (2011) 12–48.
[91] S.K. Sia, L.J. Kricka, Microfluidics and point-of-care testing, Lab Chip 8 (12) (2008) 1982–1983.
[92] C.D. Chin, T. Laksanasopin, Y.K. Cheung, D. Steinmiller, V. Linder, H. Parsa, et al., Microfluidics-based diagnostics of infectious diseases in the developing world, Nat Med 17 (8) (2011) 1015.
[93] P. Yager, T. Edwards, E. Fu, K. Helton, K. Nelson, M.R. Tam, et al., Microfluidic diagnostic technologies for global public health, Nature 442 (7101) (2006) 412.
[94] S. Kumar, S. Kumar, M.A. Ali, P. Anand, V.V. Agrawal, R. John, et al., Microfluidic-integrated biosensors: prospects for point-of-care diagnostics, Biotechnol J 8 (11) (2013) 1267–1279.
[95] S. Sharma, J. Zapatero-Rodríguez, P. Estrela, R. O'Kennedy, Point-of-care diagnostics in low resource settings: present status and future role of microfluidics, Biosensors 5 (3) (2015) 577–601.

[96] C.D. Chin, V. Linder, S.K. Sia, Commercialization of microfluidic point-of-care diagnostic devices, Lab Chip 12 (12) (2012) 2118–2134.
[97] B. Nasseri, N. Soleimani, N. Rabiee, A. Kalbasi, M. Karimi, M.R. Hamblin, Point-of-care microfluidic devices for pathogen detection, Biosens Bioelectron 117 (2018) 112–128.
[98] A. Naderi, N. Bhattacharjee, A. Folch, Digital manufacturing for microfluidics, Annu Rev Biomed Eng 21 (2019) 325–364.
[99] V. Silverio, S.C. de Freitas, Microfabrication techniques for microfluidic devices. Complex fluid-flows in microfluidics, Springer, 2018, pp. 25–51.
[100] N.P. Macdonald, J.M. Cabot, P. Smejkal, R.M. Guijt, B. Paull, M.C. Breadmore, Comparing microfluidic performance of three-dimensional (3D) printing platforms, Anal Chem 89 (7) (2017) 3858–3866.
[101] C.I. Rogers, K. Qaderi, A.T. Woolley, G.P. Nordin, 3D printed microfluidic devices with integrated valves, Biomicrofluidics 9 (1) (2015), 016501.
[102] Y. He, Y. Wu, J.Z. Fu, Q. Gao, J.J. Qiu, Developments of 3D printing microfluidics and applications in chemistry and biology: a review, Electroanalysis 28 (8) (2016) 1658–1678.
[103] A.K. Au, W. Huynh, L.F. Horowitz, A. Folch, 3D-printed microfluidics, Angew Chem Int Ed 55 (12) (2016) 3862–3881.
[104] S. Waheed, J.M. Cabot, N.P. Macdonald, T. Lewis, R.M. Guijt, B. Paull, et al., 3D printed microfluidic devices: enablers and barriers, Lab Chip 16 (11) (2016) 1993–2013.
[105] M. Beauchamp, H. Gong, A. Woolley, G. Nordin, 3D printed microfluidic features using dose control in X, Y, and Z dimensions, Micromachines 9 (7) (2018) 326.
[106] X. Cheng, R.J. Lee, The role of helper lipids in lipid nanoparticles (LNPs) designed for oligonucleotide delivery, Adv Drug Deliv Rev 99 (2016) 129–137.
[107] A.A. Yazdi, A. Popma, W. Wong, T. Nguyen, Y. Pan, J. Xu, 3D printing: an emerging tool for novel microfluidics and lab-on-a-chip applications, Microfluid Nanofluid 20 (3) (2016) 50.
[108] R. Amin, S. Knowlton, A. Hart, B. Yenilmez, F. Ghaderinezhad, S. Katebifar, et al., 3D-printed microfluidic devices, Biofabrication 8 (2) (2016), 022001.
[109] I.M. Hutchings, G.D. Martin, Inkjet technology for digital fabrication, John Wiley & Sons, 2012.
[110] N. Bhattacharjee, A. Urrios, S. Kang, A. Folch, The upcoming 3D-printing revolution in microfluidics, Lab Chip 16 (10) (2016) 1720–1742.
[111] S.A. Gowers, V.F. Curto, C.A. Seneci, C. Wang, S. Anastasova, P. Vadgama, et al., 3D printed microfluidic device with integrated biosensors for online analysis of subcutaneous human microdialysate, Anal Chem 87 (15) (2015) 7763–7770.
[112] V. Bertana, C. Potrich, G. Scordo, L. Scaltrito, S. Ferrero, A. Lamberti, et al., 3D-printed microfluidics on thin poly (methyl methacrylate) substrates for genetic applications, J Vac Sci Technol, B: Nanotechnol Microelectron: Mater, Process, Meas, Phenom 36 (1) (2018) 01A106.
[113] D. Dendukuri, P.S. Doyle, The synthesis and assembly of polymeric microparticles using microfluidics, Adv Mater 21 (41) (2009) 4071–4086.
[114] H. Kim, K.-I. Min, K. Inoue, D.-P. Kim, J.-I. Yoshida, Submillisecond organic synthesis: outpacing fries rearrangement through microfluidic rapid mixing, Science 352 (6286) (2016) 691–694.
[115] K.S. Elvira, X.C. i Solvas, R.C. Wootton, A.J. Demello, The past, present and potential for microfluidic reactor technology in chemical synthesis, Nat Chem 5 (11) (2013) 905.
[116] Y. Liu, X. Jiang, Why microfluidics? Merits and trends in chemical synthesis, Lab Chip 17 (23) (2017) 3960–3978.

[117] Y. Song, D. Cheng, Perspective for microfluidics, in: Microfluidics: Fundamental, Devices and Applications: Fundamentals and Applications, Wiley, USA, 2018, pp. 517–540.
[118] A. Günther, K.F. Jensen, Multiphase microfluidics: from flow characteristics to chemical and materials synthesis, Lab Chip 6 (12) (2006) 1487–1503.
[119] C.-C. Lee, G. Sui, A. Elizarov, C.J. Shu, Y.-S. Shin, A.N. Dooley, et al., Multistep synthesis of a radiolabeled imaging probe using integrated microfluidics, Science 310 (5755) (2005) 1793–1796.
[120] N. Hao, Y. Nie, J.X. Zhang, Microfluidic synthesis of functional inorganic micro–/nanoparticles and applications in biomedical engineering, Int Mater Rev 63 (8) (2018) 461–487.
[121] N. Hao, Y. Nie, J.X. Zhang, Microfluidic flow synthesis of functional mesoporous silica nanofibers with tunable aspect ratios, ACS Sustain Chem Eng 6 (2) (2018) 1522–1526.
[122] N. Hao, Y. Nie, A. Tadimety, T. Shen, J.X. Zhang, Microfluidics-enabled rapid manufacturing of hierarchical silica-magnetic microflower toward enhanced circulating tumor cell screening, Biomater Sci 6 (12) (2018) 3121–3125.
[123] N. Hao, Y. Nie, Z. Xu, J.X. Zhang, Ultrafast microfluidic synthesis of hierarchical triangular silver core-silica shell nanoplatelet toward enhanced cellular internalization, J Colloid Interface Sci 542 (2019) 370–378.
[124] R.L. Hartman, J.P. McMullen, K.F. Jensen, Deciding whether to go with the flow: evaluating the merits of flow reactors for synthesis, Angew Chem Int Ed 50 (33) (2011) 7502–7519.
[125] S. Yadavali, H.-H. Jeong, D. Lee, D. Issadore, Silicon and glass very large scale microfluidic droplet integration for terascale generation of polymer microparticles, Nat Commun 9 (1) (2018) 1222.
[126] J. Ahn, J. Ko, S. Lee, J. Yu, Y. Kim, N.L. Jeon, Microfluidics in nanoparticle drug delivery; from synthesis to pre-clinical screening, Adv Drug Deliv Rev 128 (2018) 29–53.
[127] D. Liu, S. Cito, Y. Zhang, C.F. Wang, T.M. Sikanen, H.A. Santos, A versatile and robust microfluidic platform toward high throughput synthesis of homogeneous nanoparticles with tunable properties, Adv Mater 27 (14) (2015) 2298–2304.
[128] S.S. Datta, A. Abbaspourrad, E. Amstad, J. Fan, S.H. Kim, M. Romanowsky, et al., 25th anniversary article: double emulsion templated solid microcapsules: mechanics and controlled release, Adv Mater 26 (14) (2014) 2205–2218.
[129] W.M. Saltzman, W.L. Olbricht, Building drug delivery into tissue engineering design, Nat Rev Drug Discov 1 (3) (2002) 177.
[130] F. Fontana, M.P. Ferreira, A. Correia, J. Hirvonen, H.A. Santos, Microfluidics as a cutting-edge technique for drug delivery applications, J Drug Delivery Sci Technol 34 (2016) 76–87.
[131] C.-X. Zhao, Multiphase flow microfluidics for the production of single or multiple emulsions for drug delivery, Adv Drug Deliv Rev 65 (11–12) (2013) 1420–1446.
[132] R. Vasiliauskas, D. Liu, S. Cito, H. Zhang, M.-A. Shahbazi, T. Sikanen, et al., Simple microfluidic approach to fabricate monodisperse hollow microparticles for multidrug delivery, ACS Appl Mater Interfaces 7 (27) (2015) 14822–14832.
[133] J. Wan, Microfluidic-based synthesis of hydrogel particles for cell microencapsulation and cell-based drug delivery, Polymers 4 (2) (2012) 1084–1108.
[134] P. Sundararajan, J. Wang, L.A. Rosen, A. Procopio, K. Rosenberg, Engineering polymeric Janus particles for drug delivery using microfluidic solvent dissolution approach, Chem Eng Sci 178 (2018) 199–210.

[135] W. Li, H. Dong, G. Tang, T. Ma, X. Cao, Controllable microfluidic fabrication of Janus and microcapsule particles for drug delivery applications, RSC Adv 5 (30) (2015) 23181–23188.

[136] A. Bains, Y. Cao, S. Kly, J.E. Wulff, M.G. Moffitt, Controlling structure and function of polymeric drug delivery nanoparticles using microfluidics, Mol Pharm 14 (8) (2017) 2595–2606.

[137] E.W. Young, D.J. Beebe, Fundamentals of microfluidic cell culture in controlled microenvironments, Chem Soc Rev 39 (3) (2010) 1036–1048.

[138] G. Du, Q. Fang, J.M. den Toonder, Microfluidics for cell-based high throughput screening platforms—A review, Anal Chim Acta 903 (2016) 36–50.

[139] S. Parlato, A. De Ninno, R. Molfetta, E. Toschi, D. Salerno, A. Mencattini, et al., 3D microfluidic model for evaluating immunotherapy efficacy by tracking dendritic cell behaviour toward tumor cells, Sci Rep 7 (1) (2017) 1093.

[140] M. Karimi, S. Bahrami, H. Mirshekari, S.M.M. Basri, A.B. Nik, A.R. Aref, et al., Microfluidic systems for stem cell-based neural tissue engineering, Lab Chip 16 (14) (2016) 2551–2571.

[141] Y. Shin, S. Han, J.S. Jeon, K. Yamamoto, I.K. Zervantonakis, R. Sudo, et al., Microfluidic assay for simultaneous culture of multiple cell types on surfaces or within hydrogels, Nat Protoc 7 (7) (2012) 1247.

[142] D.T. Chiu, A.J. de Mello, D. Di Carlo, P.S. Doyle, C. Hansen, R.M. Maceiczyk, et al., Small but perfectly formed? Successes, challenges, and opportunities for microfluidics in the chemical and biological sciences, Chem 2 (2) (2017) 201–223.

[143] G.A. Lopez, M.-C. Estevez, M. Soler, L.M. Lechuga, Recent advances in nanoplasmonic biosensors: applications and lab-on-a-chip integration, Nanophotonics 6 (1) (2017) 123.

[144] M. Rothbauer, H. Zirath, P. Ertl, Recent advances in microfluidic technologies for cell-to-cell interaction studies, Lab Chip 18 (2) (2018) 249–270.

[145] R. Zilionis, J. Nainys, A. Veres, V. Savova, D. Zemmour, A.M. Klein, et al., Single-cell barcoding and sequencing using droplet microfluidics, Nat Protoc 12 (1) (2017) 44.

[146] M. Mehling, S. Tay, Microfluidic cell culture, Curr Opin Biotechnol 25 (2014) 95–102.

[147] R.J. Kimmerling, G.L. Szeto, J.W. Li, A.S. Genshaft, S.W. Kazer, K.R. Payer, et al., A microfluidic platform enabling single-cell RNA-seq of multigenerational lineages, Nat Commun 7 (2016) 10220.

[148] T. Yeo, S.J. Tan, C.L. Lim, D.P.X. Lau, Y.W. Chua, S.S. Krisna, et al., Microfluidic enrichment for the single cell analysis of circulating tumor cells, Sci Rep 6 (2016) 22076.

[149] J. Sai, M. Rogers, K. Hockemeyer, J.P. Wikswo, A. Richmond, Study of chemotaxis and cell–cell interactions in cancer with microfluidic devices, Methods Enzymol 570 (2016) 19–45. Elsevier.

[150] H.C. Fan, G.K. Fu, S.P. Fodor, Combinatorial labeling of single cells for gene expression cytometry, Science 347 (6222) (2015) 1258367.

[151] S. Choi, M. Goryll, L.Y.M. Sin, P.K. Wong, J. Chae, Microfluidic-based biosensors toward point-of-care detection of nucleic acids and proteins, Microfluid Nanofluid 10 (2) (2011) 231–247.

[152] F. Arduini, L. Micheli, D. Moscone, G. Palleschi, S. Piermarini, F. Ricci, et al., Electrochemical biosensors based on nanomodified screen-printed electrodes: recent applications in clinical analysis, TrAC Trends Anal Chem 79 (2016) 114–126.

[153] P. Mehrotra, Biosensors and their applications—a review, J Oral Biol Craniofac Res 6 (2) (2016) 153–159.

[154] D. Liu, T. Evans, F. Zhang, Applications and advances of metabolite biosensors for metabolic engineering, Metab Eng 31 (2015) 35–43.
[155] H. Inan, M. Poyraz, F. Inci, M.A. Lifson, M. Baday, B.T. Cunningham, et al., Photonic crystals: emerging biosensors and their promise for point-of-care applications, Chem Soc Rev 46 (2) (2017) 366–388.
[156] G. Maduraiveeran, W. Jin, Nanomaterials based electrochemical sensor and biosensor platforms for environmental applications, Trends Environ Anal Chem 13 (2017) 10–23.
[157] M. Selmi, M.H. Gazzah, H. Belmabrouk, Optimization of microfluidic biosensor efficiency by means of fluid flow engineering, Sci Rep 7 (1) (2017) 5721.
[158] C. Duarte, T. Costa, C. Carneiro, R. Soares, A. Jitariu, S. Cardoso, et al., Semi-quantitative method for streptococci magnetic detection in raw milk, Biosensors 6 (2) (2016) 19.

CHAPTER

Microfluidic devices: Synthetic approaches

2

Shahin Aghamiri[a,b], Navid Rabiee[c,*], Sepideh Ahmadi[a,b], Mohammad Rabiee[d], Mojtaba Bagherzadeh[c], and Mahdi Karimi[e,f,g,h]

[a]*Student Research Committee, Department of Medical Biotechnology, School of Advanced Technologies in Medicine, Shahid Beheshti University of Medical Sciences, Tehran, Iran*
[b]*Cellular and Molecular Biology Research Center, Shahid Beheshti University of Medical Sciences, Tehran, Iran*
[c]*Department of Chemistry, Sharif University of Technology, Tehran, Iran*
[d]*Biomaterials Group, Department of Biomedical Engineering, Amirkabir University of Technology, Tehran, Iran*
[e]*Cellular and Molecular Research Center, Iran University of Medical Sciences, Tehran, Iran*
[f]*Department of Medical Nanotechnology, Faculty of Advanced Technologies in Medicine, Iran University of Medical Sciences, Tehran, Iran*
[g]*Oncopathology Research Center, Iran University of Medical Sciences, Tehran, Iran*
[h]*Research Center for Science and Technology in Medicine, Tehran University of Medical Sciences, Tehran, Iran*
Corresponding author. E-mail: nrabiee94@gmail.com

Microfluidics has now obtained many diverse applications in the fields of chemistry, biology, and engineering. The optimum fabrication of these devices is a central challenge in advancing their medical and industrial applications [1]. Fortunately, several innovative approaches have been designed over the past few years that could be applicable in both research and commercial fields [2]. In 1998, soft lithography (replica molding), especially using polydimethylsiloxane (PDMS), became a breakthrough approach in microfluidics fabrication after being introduced by Whitesides [3]. Despite soft lithography's good efficiency, its application has been somewhat restricted because of the crucial requirement for cleanroom manufacturing, which leads to high costs and a loss of time. To address these challenges and also to improve the overall functionality, several innovative microfluidic fabrication techniques have been described.

In this chapter, we first describe software tools such as AutoCAD, which are useful for the design of microfluidic devices. Next, we review techniques including replica molding, three-dimensional (3D) printing, polymer laminates, and some new

Biomedical Applications of Microfluidic Devices. https://doi.org/10.1016/B978-0-12-818791-3.00003-6

technologies that have been investigated in nanofabrication. Finally, we explain some methods for testing microfluidic devices.

2 Cleanroom

A cleanroom is an important laboratory facility used to control external contamination. The presence of any type of contamination could result in a disturbance of the production workflow, and could moreover inadvertently lead to infections in staff or patients. Hence, the elimination of contaminants such as dust, chemical agents, and microorganisms in cleanrooms is vital [4].

2.1 Classification

A cleanroom is able to control the level of pollutants and environmental factors (e.g., temperature, air circulation, humidity, etc.). The level of particulate matter contamination is governed by the maximum permissible amount of particles/unit volume at a specific particle size. A laser light-scattering instrument is applied for particle counting and can control the concentration of airborne particles in selected samples. ISO Class 1 to 9 according to ISO 14644-1 lays down standards for a cleanroom. In this standard, the decimal logarithm of the number of particles allowed per cubic meter of air is specified. In an ISO 5 cleanroom, the maximum is 10,000 particles/cubic meter. In an ISO 1 cleanroom, there can be only 10 particles in that size range. For biotechnology procedures, the number of nonparticulate pollutants such as bacteria, fungi, and viruses must be considered and restricted based on the principles of good manufacturing practice (GMP) [5].

In each defined cleanroom class, dust removal is accomplished by air filtration. High-efficiency particulate air (HEPA) filters are applied to continually recirculate the air inside and eliminate internally produced contaminants. Either laminar airflow or turbulent airflow systems can be used to keep any pollution away from the workspace [6].

Another major source of contaminating particles is from personnel working in cleanrooms. Therefore, special clothing that prevents the release of contaminants from garments and from the human body is necessary.

2.2 Cleanroom concepts

There are some concepts that must be considered when preparing a cleanroom. These factors depend on the size, acquisition costs, feasibility, and modifiability of the procedures. A specific room with a unique design that assures all the requirements of the intended ISO class is called a conventional cleanroom. This is the minimum, unchangeable requirement and simultaneously can be the most expensive design of a cleanroom. Many different parts of the infrastructure, including the walls, ceiling, and floor, have recently been specified. Properties such as resistance to solvents and other chemicals as well as abrasion-free surfaces are required. Moreover, cleanroom systems have to be efficient to reduce noise levels, vibration damping, and electrostatic charge. The essential components include air conditioning systems, changing rooms, and integrated air circulation. For instance, the Institute of Microtechnology cleanroom specifies 300 m^2 of working space [7].

2.3 Cleanroom equipment

The aforementioned guidelines are mostly used for microsystem/semiconductor preparation technology, but can also be applied for medical/pharmaceutical/biological cleanrooms. To decrease the number of particles using laminar flow in semiconductor/microsystem cleanrooms, the tables, workbenches, and other surfaces need to be perforated. Polymers such as polypropylene (PP) and melamine resin are common materials for the construction of semiconductor cleanroom equipment. On the other hand, the equipment surfaces of pharmaceutical cleanrooms are often constructed of stainless steel, which is an easy-to-sterilize material that is sealed [8].

2.4 Materials

2.4.1 Polydimethylsiloxane

The favorable physical properties, cost-effectiveness, and easy fabrication process make polydimethylsiloxane (PDMS) the most commonly employed material in the synthesis of microfluidic systems. Dow Corning and General Electric performed a revolutionary study on the use of silicones (and specifically PDMS) in the middle of the 20th century. A two-component kit with a specific mixture ratio of cross-linker and curing agent to siloxane was fixed at 1:10, and this formula remains to this day. PDMS can take several different geometric forms consisting of rods, thin films, tubes, etc. Extrusion, soft lithography, calendars, coating, and molding can convert PDMS into the required form [9]. PDMS is composed of an Si–O backbone and a repeating ($Si(CH_3)_2O$) unit. The $Si(CH_3)_2O$ units define the physical properties such as the molecular weight and viscoelastic features. Modifications to the viscoelastic properties can be performed to satisfy the specific requirements of the application. These modifications include cross-linking the polymer and the addition of fillers such as silicon dioxide to the polymer network [10].

2.4.2 SU-8

SU-8 is an epoxy-based photoresist intended for microelectronic applications where a thick image is thermally and chemically stable. SU-8 consists of Bisphenol A Novolac epoxy, which is dissolved in an organic solvent and up to 10 wt% of hexafluoroantimonate-triarylsulfonium salt. Depending on the amount of solvent, SU-8 exists with various viscosities, resulting in different layer thicknesses [11, 12].

2.4.3 Silicon

Silicon has unique properties. With the ability to integrate sensors and electronics into a single platform, it can play a key role in the production of MEMS. Two main methods can be used to produce silicon structures. The first is surface micromachining, which is the synthesis of micromechanical structures from deposited thin films. The second is bulk micromachining, in which the microstructure is synthesized by etching the substrate [13, 14].

2.4.4 Glass

The advantage of glass in the manufacture of microfluidic systems is its small coefficient of thermal expansion, α. Silica with boron trioxide and borosilicate glass can achieve this requirement with an α of around 3×10^{-6}/°C giving good resistance to thermal shock. Borosilicate glass contains boron trioxide and silica as the key glass-forming elements. Borosilicate glasses have low coefficients of thermal expansion ($\approx 3 \times 10^{-6} K^{-1}$ at 20°C), and high resistance to thermal shock. Optical transparency is the key benefit of glass in comparison with other materials. Furthermore, glass has a high Young's modulus of 64 kN/mm^2, and is resistant to many acids and bases.

Another interesting material used for microfluidics and MEMS is the photosensitive glass called Foturan. Foturan is the trade name for a lithium-aluminosilicate glass doped with silver oxides and cerium oxides. This material combines special glass features such as thermal and hardness resistance with the chance to obtain very good construction with high aspect ratios. The microstructures are transferred by 290 and 330 nm UV light; as a result, the exposed sections become crystalline. Either the mask-based exposure technique or the direct laser writing process can be used for exposure. Then, a 10% solution of hydrofluoric acid is used to etch Foturan. The etching is anisotropic, but the crystallized areas have a high etching rate. In order to increase the aspect ratio, ultrasound can be used to support the etch process. Thermal diffusion bonding makes a connection between different parts of Foturan (including structured or unstructured individual parts) [15, 16].

2.4.5 Nonmetal thin films

Silicon bulk micromachining is bonded with two thin layers (in the range of a few hundred nanometers) as well as silicon nitride (Si_3N_4) and silicon oxide (SiO_2) layers. These materials not only can be used in semiconductor devices (such as resistors, capacitors, and transistors), but also applied as masking layers for silicon etching. Both materials can be imaged by photolithography and then etched. Both materials can be patterned by photolithography, etched in phosphoric acid at 180°C (Si_3N_4), and buffered by a hydrofluoric acid solution (SiO_2) [17].

2.4.6 Metals

Metals are another central group of materials for the fabrication of MOEMS and MEMS consisting of microfluidic devices. Metallic conductor lines such as adhesion layers are photolithographically patterned and thin-film deposited (aluminum, copper, chrome, titanium, gold). Electromagnetic coils, microstamps, and magnetic field-conducting structures are thicker metallic components that are usually electroplated. Stainless steel is a much better choice than silicon or glass, especially in microdevice uses with enhanced working pressures bulk; however, stainless steel can be wet, but its etching is low [18].

2.5 Deposition methods

2.5.1 Deposition methods for Si_3N_4 and SiO_2

SiO_2 can be deposited with mostly two techniques, which lead to various layer properties. Thermal oxidation is the method used and requires a pure silicon substrate.

Heating the silicon wafer to temperatures between 1000°C and 1250°C results in the growth of SiO_2. The reaction of silicon with oxygen causes the resulting SiO_2 layer to grow not only on the substrate surface (45%) but also upward (55%). Dry oxidation occurs when oxidation occurs under pure oxygen atmospheres:

$$Si + O_2 \rightarrow SiO_2$$

The oxidation is known as "wet" if the reactions happen between silicon and water:

$$Si + 2H_2O \rightarrow SiO_2 + 2H_2$$

The rate of wet oxidation deposition may be higher than dry type, but it has lower dielectric strength.

Plasma increased chemical vapor deposition (PE CVD) is another method for the production of thin SiO_2 films at less significant temperatures and in near-arbitrary substrates. CVD approaches are categorized by ingredients of a vapor phase. It is often diluted with inert carrier gas and reacted on a hot surface to ventilate a solid film.

Thermal energy, ions, and electrons can be used to direct the surface reaction. According to the PE CVD method, ionized gas (plasma) is the key source of energy. The procedure temperature may hence be relatively small. In order to deposit SiO_2, the reactants are nitrous oxide (N_2O) and silane (SiH_4).

$$SiH_4 + 2N_2O \rightarrow SiO_2 + \text{Gases}$$

Two different methods can be used to deposit CVD silicon nitride Si_3N_4: low pressure (LP) and, like SiO_2, a plasma-increased CVD procedure [19]. The LP CVD procedure happens in a vertical diffusion furnace, and is shown in the following chemical reactions:

$$\text{LP CVD} \quad 3SiH_2Cl_2 + 4NH_3 \rightarrow Si_3N_4 + 6HCl + 6H_2$$

$$\text{PE CVD} \quad 3SiH_4 + 4NH_3 \rightarrow Si_3N_4 + 12H_2$$

2.5.2 Deposition methods for thin metal layers

Vapor deposition (PVD) is a generic term for the deposition of thin metal layers. Evaporation depends on the sublimation or boiling of the heated material and its condensation on a substrate. Thermal evaporation is the first PVD technique. The evaporation source, a vacuum chamber, a substrate holder, and an aperture to regulate the stream are the components of evaporation. Evaporation is a low-cost method, but these thin films are heterogeneous and the deposition rates differ. Another limitation is the lower melting point of the evaporated material compared to the tie and limit the range of film materials. Lower melting point of the evaporated material compared with the crucible; restrictive the range of film materials are another limitation. To address these limitations, alternatively an electron beam or laser radiation can be used to heat the material. However, these technologies are more complex and hence more costly. Aluminum, silver, nickel, chrome, gold, platinum, and titanium are proper metals for the evaporation process. Alloys are not very suitable, due to the fact that their stoichiometry is hard to control, mostly if the alloy ingredients have diverse melting points, thus diverse deposition rates. Sputtering is other common PVD vacuum-based method. The bombardment of materials targeted at one another is accomplished with positive argon ions. If the voltage is increased, the ions created in the plasma are accelerated to the target. The impulse of the ions is transported to the target atoms and then the noncharged target atoms are released. Sputtering with intermittent present voltage is also common, but not definitely essential with copper, gold, or platinum as the conducting material. Sputtering has some advantages because of a better step coverage, broader diversity of thin-film materials, and better adhesion to the substrate than evaporation [20].

2.5.3 Deposition methods for thick metal layers

In the field of microdevice fabrication, thick metal materials are not commonly applied. A microplasma reactor is one of the most important instances, which has been typically fabricated at the IMT. To decompose the waste gas, a nickel-made reactor could be used. Copper die is another instance employed for die-sinking electrical discharge machining. Electroplating, using electric current to decrease the soluble metal cations by getting electrons generating a metal coating on a cathode, is a popular method for the fabrication of microstructure thick metal layers. At first, a thin metal layer, also known as a seed layer, is used for the deposition of the substrate. In a second stage, depth lithography is usually used to fabricate a reverse template of the photoresist such as SU-8. For the second time, electroplating is used to plate nickel, copper, or gold at the top of the seed layer into the voids left by the photoresist. In order to ensure suitable plating, the structure is happening in an electrolytic cell, where all contributors such as the current density, temperature, and solution are sensibly tuned [21].

2.6 Lithography

2.6.1 Photolithography

Photolithography has been applied to create different patterns in microchips, MEMS devices, and IC manufacturing. It depends on the exposure of light-sensitive polymers (photoresists) that are reactive to UV light. The procedure of the pattern transfer can be parallel through a mask that contains astonishing features on a transparent substrate with a focused beam [22]. The photoresist changes occur due to exposure, so as a result, the showing areas either become soluble or insoluble [23]. The photoresist layer helps for a sample in a subsequent etch procedure. The resist keeps the subservient material in contrast to the etching; as a consequence, only the unprotected areas are etched. The lift-off process is another application for the photoresist layer [24]. There are three ways of printing, including (1) proximity printing (2) contact printing, and (3) projection printing. The mask aligner is an alignment instrument, adjusting the mask to a substrate (wafer) with high accuracy. Often, just the upper side of the wafer is visible. Hence, the wafer and mask are loaded into the mask aligner [25].

2.7 Etching techniques

2.7.1 Features of etching procedures

The anisotropy *A* and selectivity *S* are key parameters to describe the etching process. The etch rate relation between various materials is selectivity. A usual example of a treble etch method includes the substrate and layer to be etched. The layer to be etched has a higher etch rate, but a lower etch rate refers to both the mask layer and the substrate.

This means that the discrimination must be as high as possible. The anisotropy *A* can be the communication between the vertical and lateral etch rate [26]:

$$A = 1 - \frac{v_1}{v_2}$$

ν_l: lateral etch rate
ν_v: vertical etch rate

2.7.2 Wet etching of thin films

The most common SiO_2 thin film materials can be etched with chemical solutions. Usually, isotropic is a wet etching process. On the subjects of thin films with less than 1 μm, the undercutting of the mask layer decreases the resolution; however, this can be typically ignored [26].

2.7.3 Isotropic wet etching of silicon and glass

Hydrofluoric acid (HF) can be used to etch glass and silicon. The glass etching solution contains different concentrations of HF, HNO_3, and HCL to increase the etch rate. Gold, chrome, or a photographer can be used to synthesize the mask layer with less risk of adhesion. A solution consisting of HNO_3, NH_3COOH, and HF solution with a mask layer composed of SiO_2 is applied for isotropic etching of silicon. Both isotropic wet etching and glass can be applied to obtain large etch depths; therefore, the isotropic etching behavior in shaping the mask design should be considered [26].

2.7.4 Anisotropic wet etching of silicon

Single-crystalline silicon has anisotropic crystal plane behavior and is classified relating to the etch rates in precise etch solutions. Various etching rates of crystal planes can be brilliantly applied to create three-dimensional mechanical and fluid microliquids. The left SEM image displays a passive microvalve containing a lower and an upper part [27]. The valve is normally closed, but when the fluid pressure is opened, it closes when the fluid pressure falls below a defined limit.

The best recognized etch solution for anisotropic wet chemical etching of silicon is to use the KOH solution. In the current instance, anisotropy expresses the etch rate relation of various crystal planes, such as the {1 1 0},{1 0 0}, and {1 1 1} planes.

Ethylenediaminpyrocatechol (EDP, $C_2H_8N_2+C_6H_6O_2+H_2O$) and tetramethylammoniumhydroxide (TMAH $C_4H_{13}NO$) can be used as a further solution for anisotropic.

2.7.5 Dry etching methods

When the etch happens in a gaseous atmosphere without the use of liquids, it is commonly called "dry etching."

Deep silicon reactive ion etching (DRIE) is an important alternate to KOH etching of silicon. It depends on a silicon etching procedure, and was developed by Robert Bosch GmbH in the early 1990s. This procedure continually modifies between the deposition of a chemically inert passivation layer and a closely isotropic plasma etch step. The etch rate is approximately equal to KOH, and a photoresist is suitable as the mask layer.

The DRIE procedure can be applied for glass deep etching. Vias and fluid channels, although not useful in a conventional wet chemical etching procedure, can be produced in silicon dry etching machines. Currently, gases such as SF6 and CHF3 can be applied for etching.

The ionization of plasma gas into carbon radicals and fluorine is carried out; this is then moved to the glass substrate. Fluorine radicals react with carbon ions with the O_2 and Si atoms of the glass to unstable compounds to be pumped out of the chamber. Other gases such as Ar, H_2, and O_2 advance the constancy of the procedure. Materials such as SU-8, silicon, electroplated nickel, and resist can be used as masking materials [28].

2.8 Types of molding

Molding-based microfluidic fabrication can be divided into three different types including soft lithography, injection molding, and hot embossing.

2.8.1 Soft lithography

Soft lithography, or replica molding, is based on the use of photolithography in the creation of a photoresist and silicon model, over which a liquid polymer composition such as PDMS is decanted and cured [29]. SU-8 is the most commonly used epoxy-based negative, and it has many advantages such as mold durability and great resolution [11, 12]. The mold is filled with a liquid polymer and then the resulting cured polymer is peeled off the mold surface. Furthermore, channels can be formed when the mold bonds with a glass slide [30]. This method is derived from techniques that previously have been used in silicon-based fabrication procedures. This method has found many applications in biomedical microfluidics because of using a biodegradable polymer, known as PDMS, with high flexibility and resolution. To obtain high resolution, a cleanroom is needed for the fabrication of the mold. Providing these facilities requires a lot of time and money [31]. Nanoimprint lithography (NIL) is one of the most recent replica molding techniques with a sub-15 nm scale [32]. The advantages of soft lithography are high resolution in replicates, 3D geometries, and the capacity to stack multiple molded layers above each other.

In general, replica molding occurs in five steps: (1) spin-on photoresist film; (2) align and expose mask to UV light; (3) develop a pattern of the mold on the substrate (e.g., a silicon substrate); (4) pour the material (e.g., PDMS) into the mold; and (5) bonding to the substrate and punching access holes using a biopsy punch [33].

2.8.2 Injection molding

Microinjection molding is a well-documented technique that was developed in the 1980s. This molding method utilizes numerous different thermoplastics to create accurate, low-cost, and highly efficient microfluidic devices. As a result, injection molding has received much attention for commercial purposes over the last four decades. This technique consists of four fundamental steps. In this method, a high-pressure melted thermoplastic is injected into a mold. Then, a mold cavity is created by closing the two halves of the mold to shape the desired material into the required shape [34, 35]. At last, the mold is cooled and the cast part is removed from the mold. A significant drawback of this technique is the need for a sophisticated micromold insert. Several polymers have been employed, such as polycarbonate (PC), polymethylmethacrylate (PMMA), polystyrene (PS), polyoxymethylene (POM), and polyetheretherketone (PEEK) [36].

2.8.3 Hot embossing

Hot embossing is a procedure based on polymer melting by raising the temperature, then shaping into the desired shape using a high-temperature mold and compressing the polymer [37]. Polymethylmethacrylate, polycarbonate, polyethylene terephthalate, and cyclic olefin copolymer are the most common thermoplastic materials used in the hot embossing technique [38, 39]. It is noteworthy that this technique has several benefits such as precision, low cost, rapidity, easy set-up, and low lead times related to its implementation. In this method, a thermoplastic raw material is inserted into an HE machine. Next, the temperature is elevated to the embossing temperature of the mold. In the next step, the thermoplastic polymer is softened by the mold. To obtain full replication, the mold pressure should be continued. Finally, it is cooled down to the demolding temperature and then the cast is separated (Fig. 2.1) [40].

This promising high-throughput technique can offer cost-efficient and precise microscale devices for commercial purposes. In addition, after reduction of the fabrication costs of the molds, HE could seize a large part of microfluidics fabrication in research laboratory settings.

2.9 3D printing

3D printing is a recent new approach to microfluidics fabrication [42]. In this groundbreaking technique, a successive layer of raw materials is laid down to fabricate any desired objects or devices [43]. This technology has breathed new life into

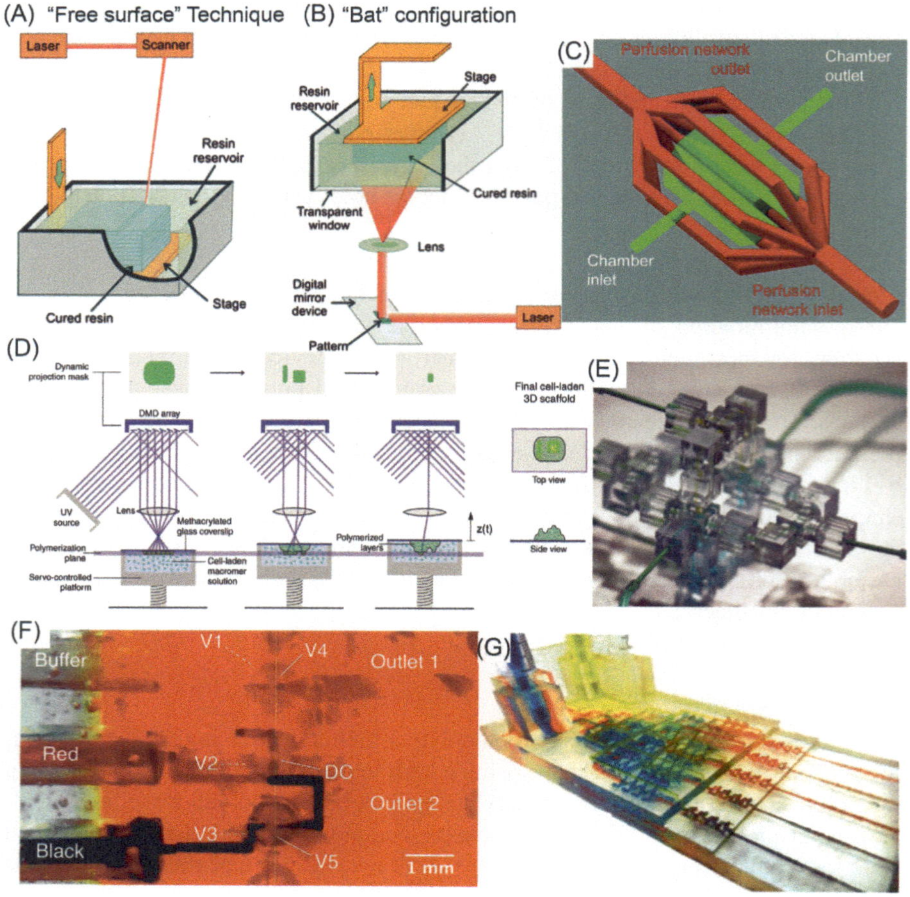

FIG. 2.1

(A) The resin surface is cured by free surface stereolithography. (B) Bat configuration, so called vat stereolithography. (C) Microfluidic perfusion network using weighted PEGDA resin. (D) Cell encapsulation at three different times by constant gelatin-methacrylic resin curing. (E) Regulatory microdevice elements prepared by stereolithography can be reused to meet the microdevice requirements. (F) PEGDA and Sudan I absorption are used to fabricate microfluidics with pumps and valves. (G) Fabrication of microfluidic gradient generator by stereolithography [41].

microfluidic device fabrication due to efficient and rapid prototyping, simplicity, and lack of any need for cleanrooms, photomasks, and photoresists [44]. In recent years, several novel 3D printing-based technologies have been developed, including stereolithography (SL), fused deposition modeling (FDM), two-photon polymerization, and multijet modeling [45]. In this section, we explain the capabilities of these novel technologies.

2.10 Stereolithography

Stereolithography (SLA) is a typical fast prototyping technology that was designed and created by Chuck Hull in 1986 [46, 47]. Numerous solid objects can be generated using this apparatus and method. These solid objects are fabricated in a layer-by-layer manner through spatially controlled photopolymerization of a melted photopolymerization resin that can be conducted by either a scanning laser or a digital light projector (DLP) [46, 48]. In the scanning laser apparatus, a scanning galvano-mirror and a focused light-emitting diode (LED) laser are applied for spot curing at the surface. Several commercial printers utilize this innovative technique. A DLP projector is another well-known method for photopolymer exposure to light. In this technique, the whole surface of the polymer is simultaneously exposed to the light by a digital micromirror display technology (DMD) [49].

Fig. 2.1A and B show the layering procedure can be achieved by two methods, including the free surface approach and the constrained surface approach (also known as "bat" configuration) [41].

The constrained surface approach is the most well-known and documented process due to the fact that no oxide formation or other potential contamination can be observed, and also less resin polymer is needed than the "free surface" configuration. Generally, in the constrained surface approach, the object is fabricated as a movable resin polymer in a hanging position. The main drawback of this method is surface distortion. To address this problem, some materials such as glass, PDMS, and FEP can be used because these materials can decrease the force experienced over the cured layer [42].

To fabricate microscale devices by the stereolithography technique, the use of biocompatible resins is essential. In recent years, several biocompatible resins such as Somos Watershed 11,122 XC (DSM, Netherlands), which can be classified as medical grade or class VI, have been developed. Many studies have been conducted on hydrogel-based biocompatible resins.

Various microscale devices such as cell separation chips, gradient generators, microneedles, multicellular devices, and micromixers have been generated using stereolithography. For example, to study spheroid cultures, a multicellular device was generated using SL and Polyjet printing [50].

Going forward, we believe that this technology can be improved to fabricate robust microfluidics devices.

2.11 Fused deposition molding

Fused filament fabrication (FFF), or fused deposition modeling (FDM), is the best documented extrusion-based 3D printing process, and it uses a continuous thermoplastic polymer filament [51, 52]. In order to print various layers of two-dimensional (2D) planes on top of each other, a nozzle is used in extrusion-based approaches. In FDM, a melted thermoplastic material is placed onto the previous layer, which binds together before cooling [53].

Since 2002, because of its cost efficiency, accessibility, and simplicity, the application of FDM in microfluidics has become increasingly popular. To assess the

ABS plus-P430 filament printing accuracy, resolution, biocompatibility, and surface roughness, many studies have been conducted by Lee and his colleagues. An FDM printer has been used to print microfluidic devices. High accuracy and surface roughness with the protruding filament strand have been observed [54].

FDM can also be applied for the generation of capillary valves. Valve channels fabricated by this printing process have a ridged pattern. An innovative 3D sugar printer was used by He et al. to design a cost-efficient and simple microfluidic device. They designed an extruder-modified desktop printer to extrude melted maltitol by pneumatic force. The printed structure was fabricated by printing lines of mannitol onto a PDMS base layer and then molding PDMS onto the sugar layer. It has been demonstrated that printing speed is the most critical element that affects the quality of the printed products. Furthermore, they showed that to fabricate micron-wide channels, a nozzle with a small size should be used [55].

References

[1] A. Mullard, Microfluidics platform lowers barrier to drug combination screening, Nat Rev Drug Discov 17 (10) (2018) 691–692.

[2] S.D. Minteer, Microfluidic techniques: reviews and protocols, Springer Science & Business Media, USA, 2006.

[3] Y. Xia, G.M. Whitesides, Soft lithography, Annu Rev Mater Sci 28 (1) (1998) 153–184.

[4] W. Den, H. Bai, Y. Kang, Organic airborne molecular contamination in semiconductor fabrication clean rooms, J Electrochem Soc 153 (2) (2006) G149.

[5] B. Liu, D. Pui, W. Kinstley, W.G. Fisher, Aerosol charging and neutralization and electrostatic discharge in clean rooms, J Environ Sci 30 (2) (1987) 42–46.

[6] D.I. Walsh, D.S. Kong, S.K. Murthy, P.A. Carr, Enabling microfluidics: from clean rooms to makerspaces, Trends Biotechnol 35 (5) (2017) 383–392.

[7] C.A. Jackson, D.A. Wilson, World at work: hospital pharmacy clean-rooms, Occup Environ Med 63 (1) (2006) 68.

[8] T. Xu, Considerations for efficient airflow design in cleanrooms, J IEST 47 (1) (2004) 24–28.

[9] B.J. Leyerle, M. LoBue, M.M. Shabot, The PDMS as a focal point for distributed patient data, Int J Clin Monit Comput 5 (3) (1988) 155–161.

[10] Y. Hwang, R.N. Candler, Non-planar PDMS microfluidic channels and actuators: a review, Lab Chip 17 (23) (2017) 3948–3959.

[11] C. Ad, C. Greiner, SU-8: a photoresist for high-aspect-ratio and 3D submicron lithography, J Micromech Microeng 17 (6) (2007) R81–R95.

[12] P. Abgrall, V. Conedera, H. Camon, A.-M. Gue, N.-T. Nguyen, SU-8 as a structural material for labs-on-chips and microelectromechanical systems, Electrophoresis 28 (24) (2007) 4539–4551.

[13] J.M. Ruano, V. Benoit, J.S. Aitchison, J.M. Cooper, Flame hydrolysis deposition of glass on silicon for the integration of optical and microfluidic devices, Anal Chem 72 (5) (2000) 1093–1097.

[14] E. Kjeang, N. Djilali, D. Sinton, Microfluidic fuel cells: a review, J Power Sources 186 (2) (2009) 353–369.
[15] B. Kuswandi, H.J. Nuriman, W. Verboom, Optical sensing systems for microfluidic devices: a review, Anal Chim Acta 601 (2) (2007) 141–155.
[16] P. Smejkal, D. Bottenus, M.C. Breadmore, R.M. Guijt, C.F. Ivory, F. Foret, et al., Microfluidic isotachophoresis: a review, Electrophoresis 34 (11) (2013) 1493–1509.
[17] K.F. Lei, Microfluidic systems for diagnostic applications: a review, J Lab Autom 17 (5) (2012) 330–347.
[18] C.-Y. Lee, C.-L. Chang, Y.-N. Wang, L.-M. Fu, Microfluidic mixing: a review, Int J Mol Sci 12 (2011) 5.
[19] J.A.N. Willem Erisman, C. Beier, G. Draaijers, S. Lindberg, Review of deposition monitoring methods, Tellus Ser B Chem Phys Meteorol 46 (2) (1994) 79–93.
[20] M.S. Ata, Y. Liu, I. Zhitomirsky, A review of new methods of surface chemical modification, dispersion and electrophoretic deposition of metal oxide particles, RSC Adv 4 (43) (2014) 22716–22732.
[21] A. Anders, Metal plasma immersion ion implantation and deposition: a review, Surf Coat Technol 93 (2) (1997) 158–167.
[22] Z. Zhang, C. Geng, Z. Hao, T. Wei, Q. Yan, Recent advancement on micro-/nano-spherical lens photolithography based on monolayer colloidal crystals, Adv Colloid Interf Sci 228 (2016) 105–122.
[23] C.C. Gerry, A. Benmoussa, Heisenberg-limited interferometry and photolithography with nonlinear four-wave mixing, Phys Rev A 65 (3) (2002) 033822.
[24] N.E. Kurland, T. Dey, S.C. Kundu, V.K. Yadavalli, Precise patterning of silk microstructures using photolithography, Adv Mater 25 (43) (2013) 6207–6212.
[25] L.L. Doskolovich, E.A. Kadomina, I.I. Kadomin, Nanoscale photolithography by means of surface plasmon interference, J Opt A Pure Appl Opt 9 (10) (2007) 854–857.
[26] N. Convery, N. Gadegaard, 30 years of microfluidics, Micro Nano Eng 2 (2019) 76–91.
[27] A. Dietzel, Microsystems for pharmatechnology, Springer, USA, 2016.
[28] Z. Huang, N. Geyer, P. Werner, J. de Boor, U. Gösele, Metal-assisted chemical etching of silicon: a review, Adv Mater 23 (2) (2011) 285–308.
[29] P. Kim, K.W. Kwon, M.C. Park, S.H. Lee, S.M. Kim, K.Y. Suh, Soft lithography for microfluidics: a review, Biochip .J 2 (1) (2008) 1–11.
[30] W. Jing, G. Min, Microfluidic sensing: state of the art fabrication and detection techniques, J Biomed Opt 16 (8) (2011) 1–13.
[31] V.C. Pinto, P.J. Sousa, V.F. Cardoso, G. Minas, Optimized SU-8 processing for low-cost microstructures fabrication without cleanroom facilities, Micromachines 5 (3) (2014) 738–755.
[32] Z. Li, Y. Gu, L. Wang, H. Ge, W. Wu, Q. Xia, et al., Hybrid nanoimprint–soft lithography with sub-15 nm resolution, Nano Lett 9 (6) (2009) 2306–2310.
[33] D. Qi, D.J. Hoelzle, A.C. Rowat, Probing single cells using flow in microfluidic devices, Eur Phys J Special Top 204 (1) (2012) 85–101.
[34] J. Giboz, T. Copponnex, P. Mélé, Microinjection molding of thermoplastic polymers: a review, J Micromech Microeng 17 (6) (2007) R96–R109.
[35] J. Giboz, T. Copponnex, P. Mélé, Microinjection molding of thermoplastic polymers: morphological comparison with conventional injection molding, J Micromech Microeng 19 (2) (2009) 025023.
[36] C. Yang, X.-H. Yin, G.-M. Cheng, Microinjection molding of microsystem components: new aspects in improving performance, J Micromech Microeng 23 (9) (2013) 093001.

[37] H. Becker, U. Heim, Hot embossing as a method for the fabrication of polymer high aspect ratio structures, Sensors Actuators A Phys 83 (1) (2000) 130–135.

[38] M. Heckele, W. Bacher, K.D. Müller, Hot embossing-the molding technique for plastic microstructures, Microsyst Technol 4 (3) (1998) 122–124.

[39] J. Wang, P. Yi, Y. Deng, L. Peng, X. Lai, J. Ni, Recovery behavior of thermoplastic polymers in micro hot embossing process, J Mater Process Technol 243 (2017) 205–216.

[40] T.-Y. Lin, T. Do, P. Kwon, P.B. Lillehoj, 3D printed metal molds for hot embossing plastic microfluidic devices, Lab Chip 17 (2) (2017) 241–247.

[41] B.K. Gale, A.R. Jafek, C.J. Lambert, B.L. Goenner, H. Moghimifam, U.C. Nze, et al., A review of current methods in microfluidic device fabrication and future commercialization prospects, Inventions 3 (3) (2018) 60–85.

[42] A. Urrios, C. Parra-Cabrera, N. Bhattacharjee, A.M. Gonzalez-Suarez, L.G. Rigat-Brugarolas, U. Nallapatti, et al., 3D-printing of transparent bio-microfluidic devices in PEG-DA, Lab Chip 16 (12) (2016) 2287–2294.

[43] F. Rengier, A. Mehndiratta, H. von Tengg-Kobligk, C.M. Zechmann, R. Unterhinninghofen, H.U. Kauczor, et al., 3D printing based on imaging data: review of medical applications, Int J Comput Assist Radiol Surg 5 (4) (2010) 335–341.

[44] H. Lipson, M. Kurman, Fabricated: the new world of 3D printing, John Wiley & Sons, USA, 2013.

[45] B.G. Compton, J.A. Lewis, 3D-printing of lightweight cellular composites, Adv Mater 26 (34) (2014) 5930–5935.

[46] F.P.W. Melchels, J. Feijen, D.W. Grijpma, A review on stereolithography and its applications in biomedical engineering, Biomaterials 31 (24) (2010) 6121–6130.

[47] Y. He, Y. Wu, J.-Z. Fu, Q. Gao, J.-J. Qiu, Developments of 3D printing microfluidics and applications in chemistry and biology: a review, Electroanalysis 28 (8) (2016) 1658–1678.

[48] O. Packer, L.C. Diller, J. Verweij, B.B. Lee, J. Pokorny, D.R. Williams, et al., Characterization and use of a digital light projector for vision research, Vis Res 41 (4) (2001) 427–439.

[49] P.J. Bártolo, Stereolithography: materials, processes and applications, Springer Science & Business Media, USA, 2011.

[50] L.J.Y. Ong, A. Islam, R. DasGupta, N.G. Iyer, H.L. Leo, Y.-C. Toh, A 3D printed microfluidic perfusion device for multicellular spheroid cultures, Biofabrication 9 (4) (2017) 045005.

[51] S.H. Ahn, M. Montero, D. Odell, S. Roundy, K. Wright Paul, Anisotropic material properties of fused deposition modeling ABS, Rapid Prototyp J 8 (4) (2002) 248–257.

[52] I. Zein, D.W. Hutmacher, K.C. Tan, S.H. Teoh, Fused deposition modeling of novel scaffold architectures for tissue engineering applications, Biomaterials 23 (4) (2002) 1169–1185.

[53] D.T. Pham, R.S. Gault, A comparison of rapid prototyping technologies, Int J Mach Tools Manuf 38 (10) (1998) 1257–1287.

[54] J.M. Lee, M. Zhang, W.Y. Yeong, Characterization and evaluation of 3D printed microfluidic chip for cell processing, Microfluid Nanofluid 20 (1) (2016) 5.

[55] Y. He, J. Qiu, J. Fu, J. Zhang, Y. Ren, A. Liu, Printing 3D microfluidic chips with a 3D sugar printer, Microfluid Nanofluid 19 (2) (2015) 447–456.

CHAPTER 3

Microchannels for microfluidic systems

Behzad Nasseri[a,*], Samet Akar[b], and Erdinc Naseri[c]

[a]*Drug Applied Research Center, Department of Medical Biotechnology, Faculty of Advanced Medical Sciences, Tabriz University of Medical Sciences, Tabriz, Iran*

[b]*Department of Mechanical Engineering, Çankaya University, Ankara, Turkey*

[c]*Department of Cardiovascular Surgery, Park Hayat Hospital, Afyon, Turkey*

**Corresponding author: bnaseri2000@googlemail.com*

3.1 Introduction

Microfluidic systems (which are also known as microchannel devices) are an important and versatile practical apparatus applicable in different areas of science and technology. The appropriate design of the microfluidic system demands the accurate calculation of the parameters of the microfluidic devices. The channels used in microfluidic systems are critical compartments of the device, which affect the efficiency of the system. The purpose of this chapter is to survey the microchannels and their characteristics in microfluidic systems. After a detailed discussion of microchannels, their applications for nonliving phantoms for cardiovascular, neuroscience, and respiratory studies will be discussed [1]. In the biomedical applications of microchannels, the areas such as cell studies, e.g., cytoskeleton behavior, cell-to-cell interaction [2], detecting cell-derived moieties [3] are important. Also, cellular level tissue engineering, such as cell vaso-occlusion in tissue biomimicking [4,5] is described. The other applications of microfluidic devices are material science and chemical reaction studies related to biological studies, and also biophysics and bio-optic fields. In this chapter we provide a comprehensive study of the following aspects of microchannels for microfluidic systems:

- The channel geometry and microchannel arrangement of the microfluidic devices
- The flow regime evaluation in microchannels
- The phase study in the microfluidic systems and the microchannel patterns
- The specifications of fluid flow inside the microchannels
- Physical and mechanical characteristics of microchannels.
- Multientrance microfluidic systems for microdroplet production
- Flow characteristics in the microfluidic devices
- Channel design for flow regimes (Turbulent and Laminar flow)
- The mass, momentum, and energy transport evaluation in the microchannels

Biomedical Applications of Microfluidic Devices. https://doi.org/10.1016/B978-0-12-818791-3.00002-4

- Reusable microchannels for microfluidic devices
- The applications of soft microchannels

There are many physical parameters, which dictate the differences between macroscale and microscale phenomena. A few mechanisms, which are impossible to implement on a large scale can be effectively used in microdevices for sensing purposes. The microscale fluid mechanics, cell studies used in biomedical research, and many other applications can be considered in this category. Therefore, the physical rules and different characteristics of microdevices need to be appropriately considered. Different studies have been published regarding microfluidics. Nasseri et al. presented a comprehensive study of the detection of pathogens using microfluidic systems [6]. Besides, many applications of microchannels have been known in different disciplines, such as chemistry, biology, material science, and medicine [7]. A wide-range of material-based processes such as separation, mixing, detection of biomolecules have used microfluidic devices. Many improvements in the field of continuous-flow microfluidics and biomolecule separation methods, recent diagnostic techniques for pathogens, molecular biology, and medicine have been developed. These examples exhibit a promising outlook for microchannel devices compared to conventional techniques in the aforementioned fields. Compared to newer generations of microfluidic devices, the conventional PDMS microfluidic devices based on glass or silicon microarrays, and even the simple paper-based microchannel systems are still used by many scientists. Separation techniques are one of the most important processes in all of science. There are different approaches for separation processes in the analysis of biomolecules, such as resin packed membranes [8] used in industry, and recent microscale and nanoscale techniques such as nanowires (NWs). The separation of microorganisms and cells using hydrogels [9] is a recent technique in microchannel-based processes. This method can be used in regenerative medicine. In 2010, Kachouie et al. reported a tissue engineering study based on the hydrogels for the separation of cells in microchannels. The hydrogel blocks were used for harvesting the desired cells. This technique was different from other cell collection techniques used in tissue engineering. The microchannels used for the mentioned procedure had one, two, or ten input gates with packed glass beads.

3.2 Cross-section geometry in microchannels in microfluidic systems

The different applications of microfluidic systems require the design of specific geometries and patterns inside the microfluidic devices [10]. The different channel configurations such as straight, T-shape, Y-shaped, and multigate modules are particularly beneficial for different applications of microfluidic devices [11]. However, many studies have addressed the shapes and arrangement of microchannels regarding different applications of microfluidic devices. The rectangular arrangement [12] is a common cross-sectional geometry of microchannels. The geometry of microchannels is the crucial factor in microfluidic devices used in fields, such as flow hydrodynamics, biology, and fluid mechanics. The conical, tubular, and triangular geometries are more complex shapes for the microchannels. Generally, the biochemical applications of microfluidic devices encompassing multiphase flow, transporting,

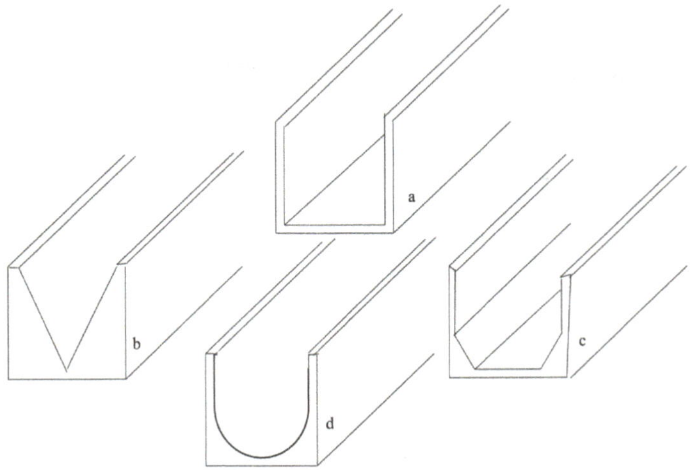

FIG. 3.1

Microchannel patterns of microfluidic devices, rectangular (A), triangular (B), circular (C), and tapered (D).

mixing, and separation bioprocesses, cell biology biosynthesis processes in the liquid-liquid phase are all influenced by channel shape. Fig. 3.1 is a schematic illustration of the different cross-sectional shapes of channels in microfluidic devices. The half-tubular pattern is applied to increase the dynamic flow velocity along the microchannels to avoid obstructions as can happen in the blood circulation capillaries. The circular cross-sectional shape is a potential flow dynamic geometry to optimize the flow regime and fluid velocity. The other cross-sectional shapes can be compared to the tubular geometry of microchannels. In circular geometry, the diameter (D) and length (L) of the channel can influence the flow regime and the Reynolds number that are the main design parameters. In biomedical applications, circular microchannels are designed to mimic body vessels in different research areas such as drug-delivery and investigation of cardiovascular and pulmonary thrombosis diseases. Choi and colleagues reported a mimicking pattern of smooth muscle cells in perpendicular structures to the blood vessels. In their study, layer by layer cell growth was carried out to investigate the behavior of cells in the tubular shape of vascular microcapillaries [13]. In another study, Vecchione et al. reported a novel spin-coating technique to fabricate microchannels. They reported that the circular microchannels had higher cell adhesion and more homogeneity compared to nontubular channels in microfluidic systems [14]. In the rectangular cross-sectional shape of microchannels, the performance of devices is related to the length (L), width (w), and depth (h) of the channels. The application of rectangular and square-shaped channels can be used in cell separation for biology researches. For immiscible liquid-liquid systems, rectangular and square-shaped microchannels are two different geometries, where the flow pattern can be related to the hydrophilicity/hydrophobicity of the drug delivery systems used to model the blood-brain barrier [15]. Yagodnitsyna and colleagues investigated the flow behavior in immiscible water-oil emulsions in rectangular microchannel patterns. They followed the superficial velocity profile through three sets of samples, and triggered flow behavior in the interface layer. In biomedical studies, the combination of microparticles and cells has been studied by biologists. In this field, a homogenous particle-cell combination is highly important for investigations. A research group at University of Naples Federico II, investigated the behavior of microparticles and the focal shear gradient on the microchannel walls for square geometry microchannels [16]. Del Giudice and colleagues reported that the shear stress on the square-shaped microchannel walls depends on the particle arrangement. The microfunnel shaped microchannels have been fabricated for specific purposes such as stochastic sensing applications (Fig. 3.1B).

The fluid behavior in the channels can be described by a detailed discussion of the cross-sectional geometry of the microchannels. The fluid behavior is a key parameter for the efficiency of microfluidic devices in different fields of science. The fluid flow behavior in the capillaries is highly influenced by the actual application of the microdevice.

In addition to the geometry of the channels, other different dimensions can affect the behavior of the flow. In microchannels with y shaped patterns, the inlet and outlet lengths and junction angle are also important. In passive mixing or separation processes, the proper design of channels for achieving sufficient performance of the microfluidic device is considered crucial. The setting-up of the length, microchannel diameter, and junction points require to be calculated besides other dimensions for accurate modeling of microdevices before their manufacture. Therefore, the design optimization procedure should be run several times to achieve the best dimensions. The flow-3D software is one of the simulation programs that can be used to calculate the optimum design of micropatterns, where more than 150 calculations can be run in less than 0.05 s for each run. This program is equipped to deal with nine variables, which can be changed during geometry optimization. The variables which need to be considered are shown in Fig. 3.2.

The junction angle and junction length are factors that influence the flow regime and are important in different applications such as biomimetics (biofluids behavior within the body), biology studies (cancer cell separation), and in industry. In addition,

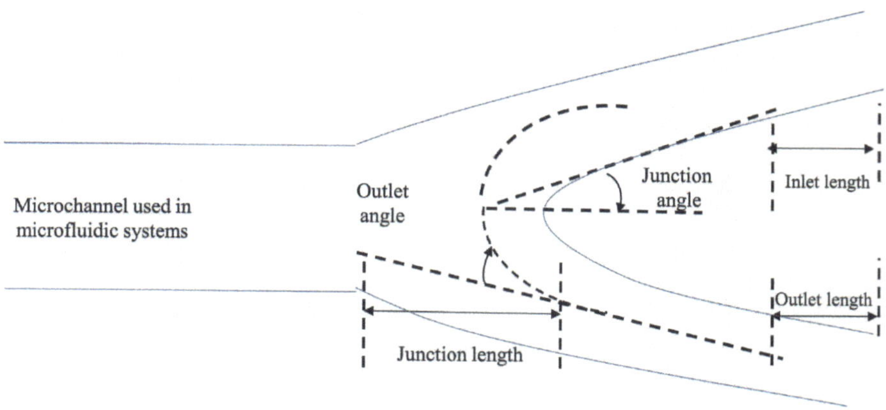

FIG. 3.2

Schematic illustration of junction characteristics in microchannel design.

the mimicking of biological mixing (heart valves) is another aspect of this study. The lengths of the inlet and outlet of microchannels are crucial for the design of microfluidic systems. These parameters are particularly important in fluid mechanics studies. The input length can influence the optimum velocity profile development of the flow in microchannels. This factor also can influence the flow regime in the primary stage of the liquid entrance. The efficiency of microchannels can be affected by the outlet angle of the flow. In 2016, Lee and his research team studied microchannel modeling and performance evaluation in passive rapid mixing processes [17]. In 2014, Parsa and colleagues published a study on parameter definition in rapid mixing processes [18]. The results of the mentioned study showed that the output angle in the microchannels influenced the yield of the mixing process. A satisfactory mixing rate was obtained with lower output angles. Fig. 3.3 demonstrates the modeling of channels in mixing processes by focusing on the output angles of the microchannel. As shown in Fig. 3.3 (top image), the most complete mixing occurred at the lowest outlet angle, whereas a poor mixing was found at the highest output angle in this model.

In addition to the main factors mentioned above, there are several complementary components such as buffers, separators; flow circulation units which are capable of increasing the performance of microfluidic systems. Separators with suitable lengths have been shown to provide satisfactory results in mixing processes in biological studies. Fang et al. reported a study about mixing enhancement by applying the proper periodic separators along the length of the microchannels [19]. In this study, by applying periodic buffers inside the microchannels, an appropriate mixing rate was achieved. The mixing of biofluids (especially for laminar flow) is one interesting area of biomedical research, which can be used for optimizing therapeutic techniques and drug administration (Fig. 3.4).

In addition, there are several studies about complementary design components in the microchannels, such as the groove depth of the internal structure of the microchannels, and directions of the internal patterns. These factors affect the efficiency of microchannel devices in biomedical, chemical, and industrial applications. The depth of microchannels in microfluidic systems was a research topic of Du et al. [20]. In 2013, Carrier and colleagues reported a study in the field of microchannels for Newtonian and nonNewtonian fluids with caterpillar micromixing equipment [21]. They investigated the pressure drop created by the micromixer platforms along with the microchannel system. The results showed that the split-combined buffer micromixer structures provided a large friction coefficient and a very low Reynolds number in the viscoelastic fluids.

The micromixer device is a simplified type of agitator, which is used in the production of hydrogels for tissue engineering, which is necessary for cell adherence. The hydrogels used as blocking agents in cardiovascular hemostasis are in the non-Newtonian category of fluids. It is necessary to have an active agitation of the polymeric material mixture to produce hydrogels. Active micromixing is a process requiring external energy, such as mechanical, ultrasound, etc., needed for the agitation of the materials. The concept is seen when a highly viscous material such as a polymeric or mineral mixture is required to be mixed. In microfluidic devices equipped with active micromixing devices, high amounts of external energy can

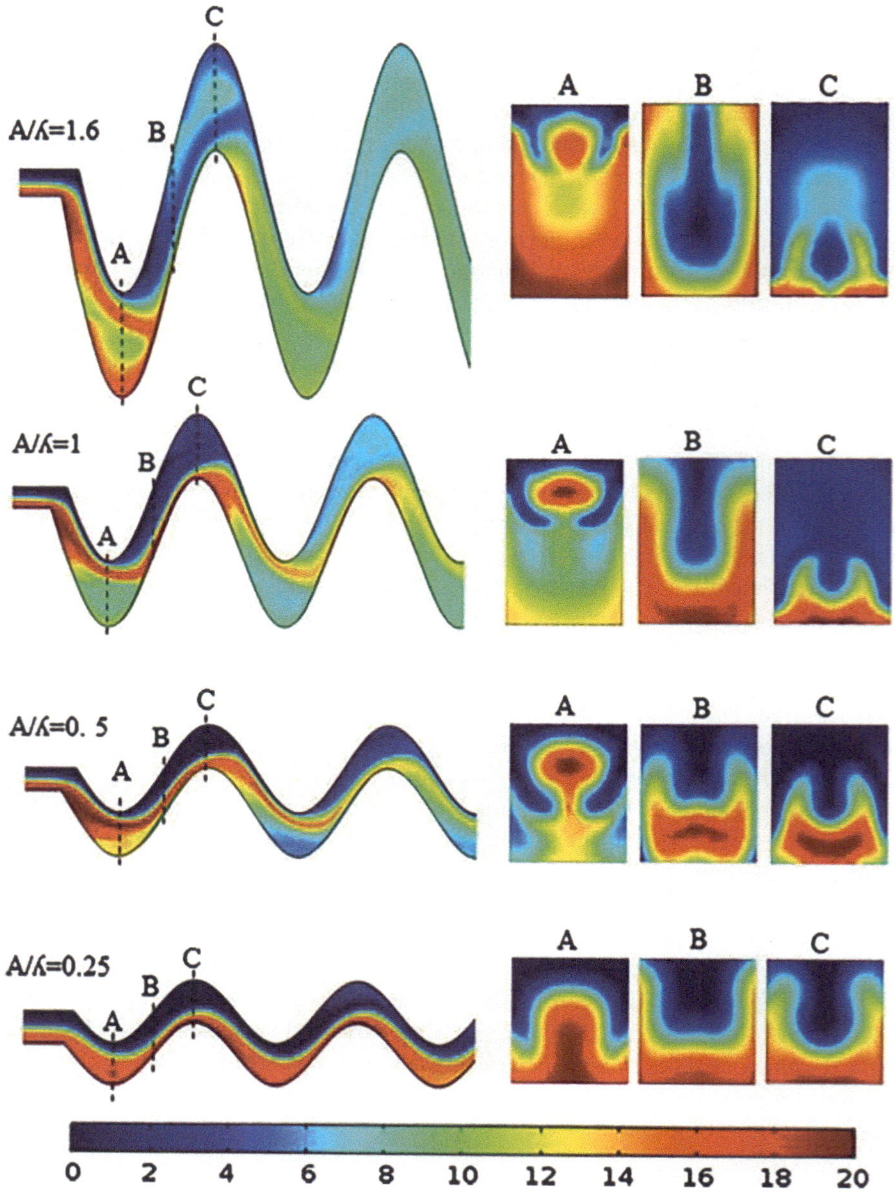

FIG. 3.3

The simulation of flow in the microchannels at different output angles.

Reprinted with permission from Parsa MK, Hormozi F, Jafari D. Mixing enhancement in a passive micromixer with convergent–divergent sinusoidal microchannels and different ratio of amplitude to wave length. Comput Fluids 2014;105:82–90.

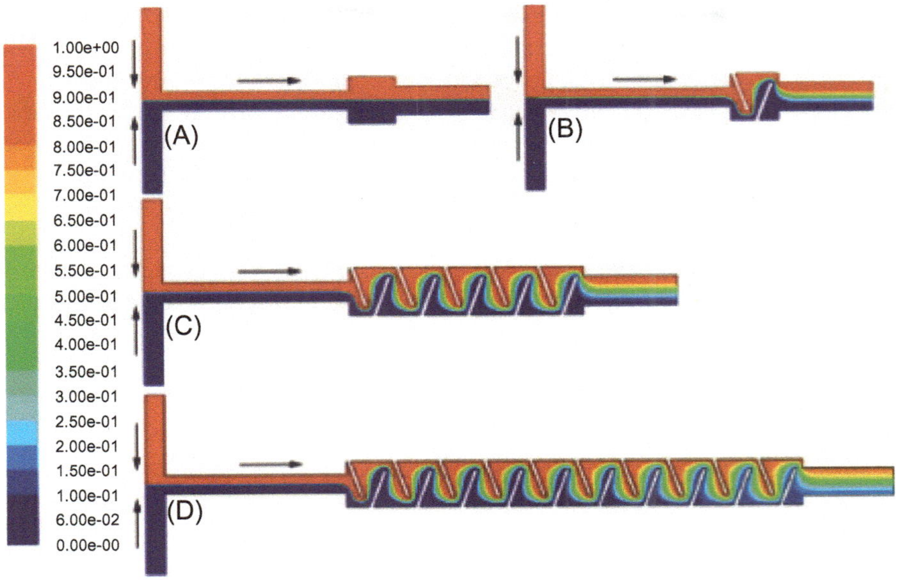

FIG. 3.4

Mixing profile simulation in the microchannels at different mixing period of (A) 0, (B) 1, (C) 5, (D) 10 U at a flow rate of 20 μL/s.

Reprinted with permission from Fang Y, et al. Mixing enhancement by simple periodic geometric features in microchannels. Chem Eng J 2012;187:306–310.

damage the medium, which contains biological objects such as cells or living microorganisms. Hence, the system needs to apply the proper amount of force by the correct equipment without any harmful effects.

The arrangement of microchannels is another study in the field of microfluidic devices. The time-dependent process of passive micromixing has critical parameters, which affect the performance of the microfluidic device. In the primary stages of passive mixing, the phases show resistance against the phase-fusion phenomenon. Other parameters such as flow rate, flow regime in the channels, phase-type (W/O), density, viscosity, and the dynamic properties of the fluid regarding Newtonian or non-Newtonian physics need to be considered carefully to achieve sufficient performance. One of the most common applications of microfluidic devices is the production of microdroplets used in drug delivery and cell interaction studies. Besides the above-mentioned applications, other uses such as electrohydrodynamic, acoustic, electrokinetic, and many other areas can be mentioned. Fig. 3.6 shows the microchannel types used in passive processes such as separation and mixing. The microchannel lengths, angles, inlet, and outlet diameters in the T-shaped, Y-shaped, and other patterns need to be properly designed for optimum performance. As can be seen in Fig. 3.6, the most common arrangement of the micromixing process and microdroplet fabrication in microfluidic devices is a T-shaped pattern. The mixing process gradually develops until a fully mixed profile is achieved [22]. The multientrance microfluidic systems (such as multi entrance T-shaped patterns) are a more complex design of microchannels used for a high rate of fluid flow and specific microdroplet morphology which need to be optimized. The bifurcated (Y-shaped) microchannels are among the most investigated microchannel types which are similar to T-shaped patterns. T-shaped and Y-shaped microchannels are two useful techniques to produce particles with a concentrically laminated structure. In the T- and Y-shaped patterns, mixing can be achieved by breaking the main upstream flow into some substreams and then collecting them in the downstream flow [23]. For these additional devices such as agitators will be needed. Fig. 3.5 (middle) demonstrates the different phase entrances in the

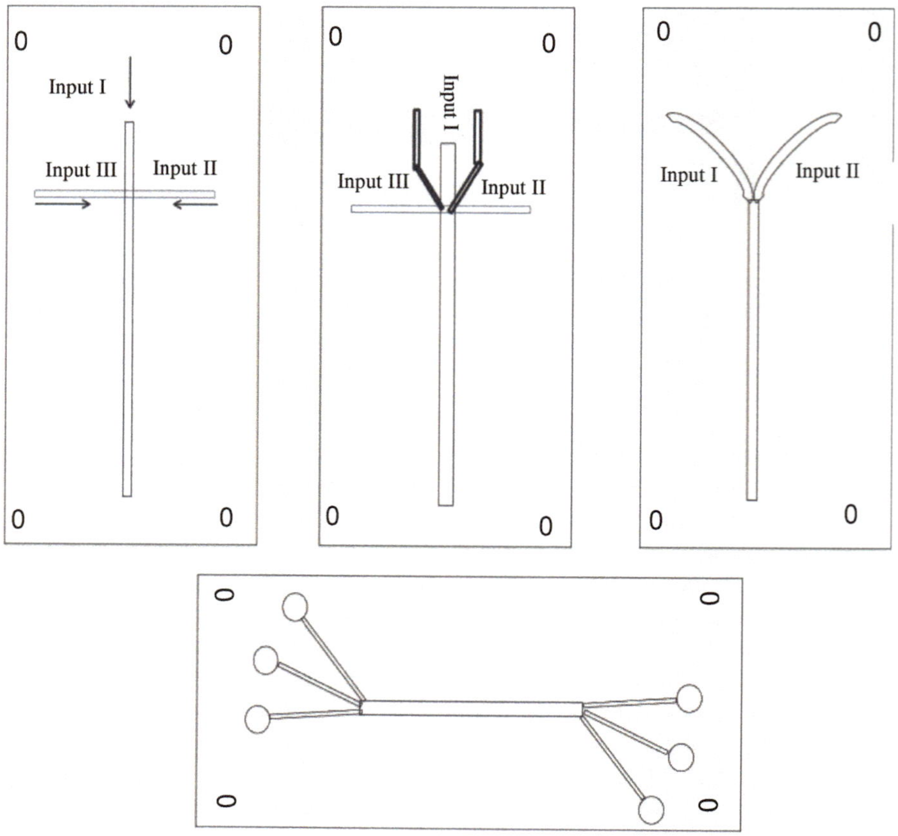

FIG. 3.5

A schematic illustration of microchannel arrangements in microfluidic devices, T-shaped *(left)*, multientrance microchannels *(middle)*, Y-shaped *(right)*, and multicavity microfluidic systems *(bottom)*.

Reprinted (adapted) with permission from Kashid N, Renken MA, Kiwi-Minsker L. Influence of flow regime on mass transfer in different types of microchannels. Ind Eng Chem Res 2011;50(11):6906–14. Copyright (2020) American Chemical Society.

microchannel device. Multicavity patterns in microfluidic devices (Fig. 3.5, bottom) are generally applied in biological studies, where it is necessary to have positive and negative control groups simultaneously for comparison purposes [24].

Fig. 3.6, is a schematic representation of the chemical reactions, which can be implemented by microscale reactors. In these microreactors, the accurately designed channels play important roles in the chemical reactions. Generally, the T- shaped multiple microchannels are selected for multiphase reactions and microparticle fabrication. The presence of multiple T junctions along the channels can lead to different reactions for producing or laminating the microparticles.

The increase of the flow rate requires the design of appropriate channels with a sufficient number of inlets along with the microfluidic device. In the case of

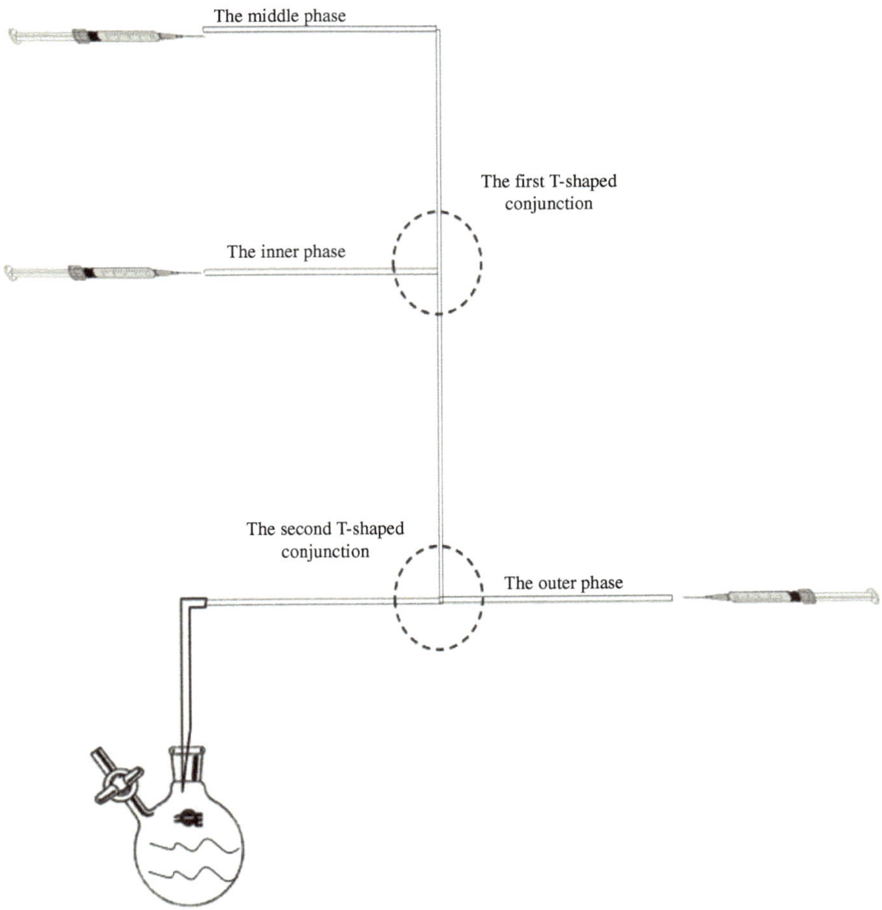

FIG. 3.6

A sophisticated T-shaped, two-phase, multientrance chemical reaction in microfluidic devices.

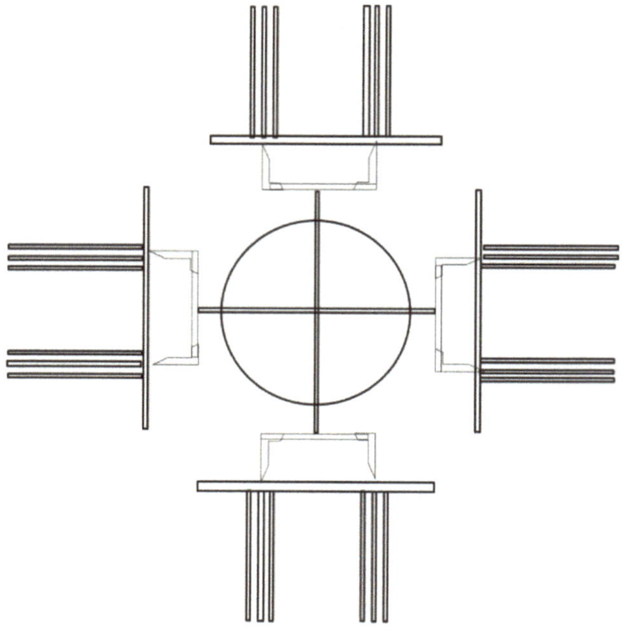

FIG. 3.7

Complex tree-shaped microchannel arrangement for concentration gradients in biomedical and chemical studies.

microdevices for examining the concentration gradient of the chemical process used in biochemistry, tree shape structures with T-junctions are commonly applied [25]. Wang and colleagues reported a study, which addressed the design of complex tree-shaped flow patterns. Their microchannel system allowed upstream to downstream flow to supply a concentration gradient for chemical reactions and biological assays. The main streamflow in the larger channel led into capillary microchannels in the downstream. In the complex tree-shaped microfluidic device which is shown in Fig. 3.7, the geometry and channel sizes of the microfluidic devices were designed to provide a cell separation ability. Furthermore, tree-shaped microchannels can be used in blood circulation studies, cell studies (separation of cells contained in bio-fluids), toxic effects of chemical and drugs on cells (in vitro assessment), and nanoparticle synthesis in microfluidic platforms.

A serpentine-type pattern of microfluidic channels can play a role in the development of micromixing protocols [26], biomolecule assay methods [27], and other biomedical uses. A simple schematic illustration of serpentine patterns of microchannels is shown in Fig. 3.8. The geometry, symmetry, size and number of microchannels and the conditions needed for the experiments are factors that affect the serpentine design of microchannels. The presence of transverse vortices, and the pressure drop along the microchannels are other key factors that need to be considered for the design of serpentine microfluidic devices. The diameter of the channels is shown

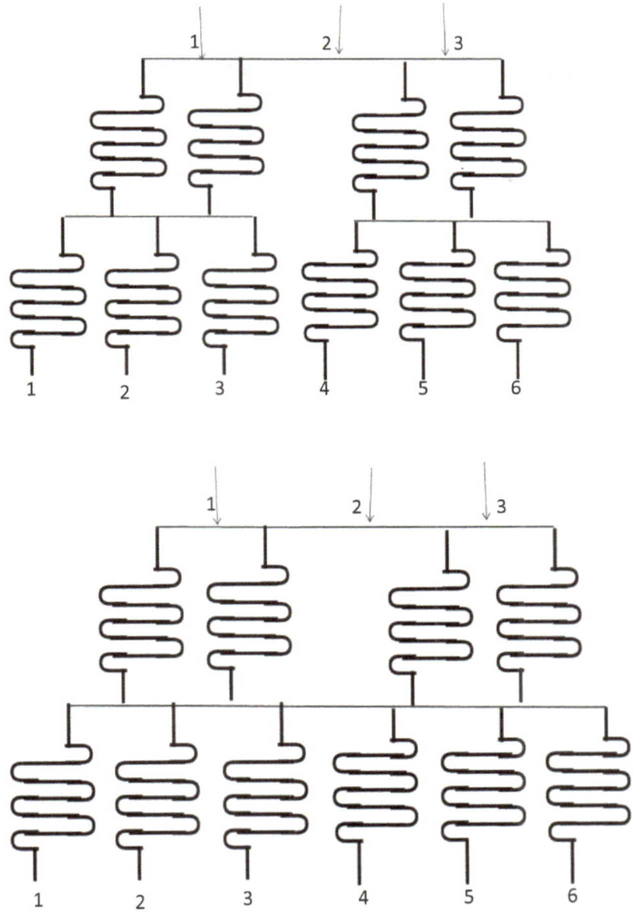

FIG. 3.8

Comparison of microchannel configuration for serpentine type patterns (concentration gradient studies).

in Fig. 3.8 (top and bottom), which depends on the fluid flow rates occurring both upstream and downstream. There are different studies involving numerical modeling efforts concerning both rectangular and nonrectangular cross-sectional geometries in serpentine microchannels. The microchannel diameter needs to be calculated carefully to provide sufficient velocity, fluid flow rate, appropriate flow regime, and other factors. A larger microchannel diameter in the upstream which reduces to a smaller diameter in the downstream, completely changes the flow regime, flow velocity, and flow rate. Separation techniques use tailored hydrodynamic behavior due to the smaller diameter of the downstream capillaries compared to the upstream.

Multientrance microchannel devices have been discussed briefly above. Multientrance microchannel devices can be used for microdroplet formation in the biomedical arena [28]. Microdroplets are commonly used in the bio-nanotechnology field and drug delivery, biotechnology, and molecular medicine. The polymer types for the preparation of microdroplets are selected according to the particular application. Collagen, polycaprolactone (PCL), polylactic acid (PLA) and polyethylene glycol (PEG) are the most common biocompatible polymers, which have been used for these purposes. These polymers are used in biomaterials due to their good biocompatibility and low toxicity. The outer layer of the biomaterials provides an appropriate surface for bio-conjugation of various biomolecules and ligands. The structure of microdroplets contains a single-core as the inner phase and is surrounded by a concentric polymer layer as the shell. The immiscibility difference between the inner and outer layer determines the final structure of the droplets. The two layers (double emulsion), three layers (triple emulsion), four layers (quadruple emulsion) [29] and even five layers (quintuple emulsion) [29] are new generations of droplets that can be used in more sophisticated applications. These multilayered microdroplets are generally known as onion structures [30]. These microdroplets have found widespread applications for drug delivery [31], medical imaging contrast agents [32], in pharmaceutical biotechnology [33], and regenerative medicine. Microdroplets can be used in theranostics, which combines imaging and therapy into a single agent for simultaneous use. Drugs can be loaded into the core while contrast agents can be conjugated via biomolecular linkers onto the shell surfaces. Multilaminar particles using different materials in the form of core-shell structures is an area of increasing interest. Microfluidics assisted multivesicular structures, such as multisomes and vesosomes are other types of microdroplets with different cores inside a single shell [30].

Fig. 3.9 describes the fabrication of microdroplets with Janus (or two-faced) morphology. The Janus type of microdroplets is best prepared by using microfluidic systems. The specific design of microchannels in multiphase emulsions (W/O/O) resulted in different properties in double-sided particles with unique core structures.

Janus type microparticles can be used in different research areas such as physiochemical approaches (biphasic catalyst) [34] nanomotor applications [35], polymeric material research, in biomedical applications such as gene delivery and imaging [36], and industry for microscale phenomena. In Janus microdroplets, there is an anisotropic structure between the two sides of the droplets [37]. There are several studies reporting the preparation of Janus-type beads. Yuet and colleagues reported a protocol for the fabrication of a chain-like suprastructure of magnetic microbeads [38]. Due to the controlled alignment of the suprastructure of the magnetic particles, they were able to use these microparticles in tissue engineering applications. In another study, Ling developed a controllable patching procedure for the chemical preparation of bifunctionalized Janus type particles [39]. The fabricated microbeads were prepared by a chemical masking/unmasking technique. An applied host-guest biphasic interaction protocol was used after the microfabrication. In another study, Ju and co-workers synthesized a new generation of theranostics (Janus type structures) and applied them for simultaneous imaging and therapy [36].

Other types of microchannels have been used for biomedical purposes [40]. The design of separation techniques for isolating bacteria and other microorganisms is

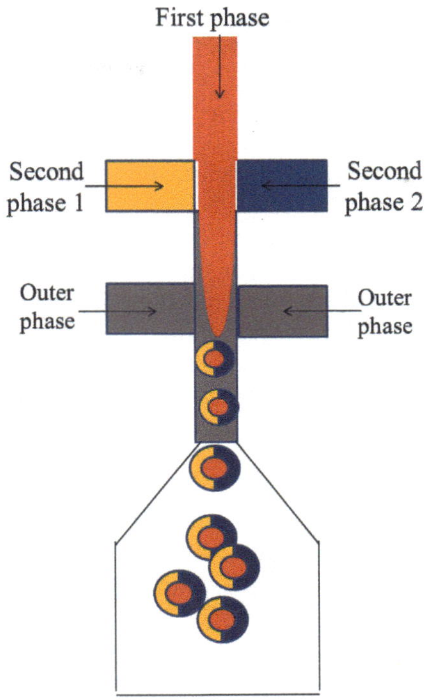

FIG. 3.9

Schematic illustration of Janus shaped (two-faced) microdroplets using microchannels.

a growing area in medicine. In recent designs for cell separation processes, nanotechnology and biology principles and engineering methods are combined to design a more efficient protocol. In the biological approaches, the flow characteristics are very important. In the following sections, nanotechnology assisted protocols for cell separation will be discussed.

Spiral microchannels with an inertial effect are well-known nanotechnology-based microfluidic systems for the separation of microorganisms in a cost-effective and rapid manner [41]. In microfluidics detection techniques, the safe, easy, and rapid capture of bacterial cells or cancer cells is important. In addition to factors such as the cross-sectional geometry of the channels, other factors such as flow velocity, particle density, deformation, and viscosity need to be considered. The above-mentioned factors determine the position of particles in the circular channel of the microfluidic device [42]. In the circular movement of particles, multimodal core nanoparticles, and the attached bio-conjugated linkers, a specific antibody, and the biofluid sample are the main components (Fig. 3.12). The migration of bound nanoparticle- microorganism pairs through the fluid which moves toward the outer walls of the microchannels, and in a circular motion is crucial. The path of the nanoparticles depends on different parameters such as the inertial effect in the curved microchannel route.

The migration of particles in the curved channels was reported for first time by Dean [43,44]. Berger offered an equation for the Dean coefficient as follows (Eq. 3.1).

$$D_e = R_e\sqrt{\frac{H}{2R}} \tag{3.1}$$

In the Dean theory, R is the curved radius in the microchannel, and H is the hydraulic diameter. By e increasing the Reynolds (Re) number, the Dean number (and related Dean flow is also improved. Eddies created by turbulent flow are directly proportional to the Dean coefficient. The flight of particles and their migration depends on the mass of the particles. More massive microparticles in the circular path remain nondisturbed, whereas the smaller particles move away from the central line of the curve and toward the outer borders of the curve. The Ookawara simulation e was created according to the Dean Vortex model where number was implemented in all steps of the calculation [45]. This vortex flow can be considered in different areas of science. The turbulent blood flow in the healthy and diseased aortic valve is an interesting topic in cardiovascular disease of the ascending aorta. The turbulent blood flow combined with defects in the aorta can lead to degenerative pathophysiological changes with a serious risk of death [46]. As a result of the Ookawara numerical model, the Dean flow and eddies equation is as follows.

$$U_D = 1.8\times10^{-4} D_e^{1.63} \tag{3.2}$$

e number means that no Dean flow exists in the straight channels.

The mass of the particles, and the velocity and viscosity of the flow define the trapping efficiency in spiral microfluidic devices. The higher the distance to be traversed means a better separation performance. The conjugated nanoparticles and microorganisms are trapped within the circular microchannels where the smaller particles flow.

3.3 Channel design for different flow regimes (turbulent and laminar flow)

The geometry specification of the microchannels was discussed in the previous sections. In this section, the influence of the dynamic properties of flow will be studied [47]. In straight channels, the mixing efficiency, the conversion rate of liquid-liquid interaction, and the mass transfer efficiency are highly dependent on the flow regime, which is the main factor determining the efficiency of the mechanism. The flow regime can be divided into turbulent or laminar flows [48]. There are many factors that influence the flow regime, such as viscosity, the velocity of flow, hydrophilicity property, and friction coefficient of the inner surface of the channels. Factors such as the cross-sectional geometry of the microchannels, and their dimensions also affect the flow regime in the fluid dynamics.

In the modeling of microchannels it is necessary to include information about the flow regime that influences the performance of the microfluidic device. In the microchannels, the fluid regime, sizes of microdroplets, components, and enormous parameters alter the performance of the applied mechanism. The Reynolds number (*Re*) determines the flow regime in the case of laminar or turbulent flow. In microfluidics, the value of *Re* is obviously small (on the order of 1.0 or lower) whereas in macroscale fluid *Re* can be within a range of 1–1000 [49].

The Re number in Eq. (3.3) depends on the dimensions of the microchannels, fluid viscosity (μ). The *Re* number can be determined in circular and rectangular shaped channels as follows;

$$Re = \frac{12\mu L}{h^2 w} \quad \text{Rectangular shape} \tag{3.3}$$

$$Re = \frac{128\mu L}{\pi d^2} \quad \text{Circular shape} \tag{3.4}$$

As can be seen in Eqs. (3.3), (3.4), the *Re* number depends on the length, width, height of the channel in rectangular channels and it depends on the diameter and length for circular channels. The viscosity is another factor that influences the flow regime in the channel. In biological studies, the flow in the vessels is generally laminar. Mimicking the blood circulation in the capillaries of the human body can be achieved by modeling the laminar flow regime. In turbulent flow, due to eddy formation and increased material transfer, the mass transfer rate is increased. In order to provide a complete summary of fluid mechanics in the microchannels, the friction-Reynolds number for a fully developed flow regime should be considered. The simplified expression is presented in Eq. (3.5).

$$C* = \frac{(fRe)_{Exp}}{(fRe)_{Theory}} \tag{3.5}$$

where $(fRe)_{Exp}$ is the value obtained by experiments, and $(fRe)_{Theory}$ is the parameter obtained by theoretical calculation [50]. The $C*$ ratio is a factor which depends on the geometry of the microchannel. In all fluid mechanic studies, the graphical data of $C*$ ratio vs. *Re* number are given in the form of tabulated data. The flow regime factor in the case of the laminar or turbulent flow is important in the study of microfluidic systems. The ideal value for $C*$ ratio can be considered to be $C* = 1.0$ whereas the values for $C*$ ratio is generally achievable in the range of $0.6 < C* < 1.4$.

3.4 Phase study in microfluidic devices and microchannel patterns

Starting from early 1990, microfluidics underwent many advancements in order to reduce research costs. The invention of a new generation of miniaturized reactors promised the new opportunities in the scientific research at the microscale and nanoscale, which even extends to the femto-scale for different material phases (gas, liquid or solid) [51]. The "phase study" is the study of the physicochemical properties of fluids in the different states of the matter, which are involved in physics, chemistry, biology, and medicine. The mentioned fields can be considered as interphase reactions, microscale physical events, mass transport, cell-material interactions in biology, and many other processes that can occur in microchannels. The liquid phase with liquid-liquid interactions deals with the polar and nonpolar properties of different phases. Liquid-gas multiphase systems are an integration of liquid and gas which can be seen in the dry etching process using microchannels. In these systems, an accurate phase study will be mandatory in the case of reaction types and conversion ratio of reactions in the microchannels. In addition to the phase differences between the liquid-liquid and liquid-gas systems, another challenging field is the mass and heat transfer and the types of microparticles involved. In the liquid-liquid systems, they are microdroplets, and in the liquid-gas systems, they are microbubbles [52–54]. In 2016, Yang and colleagues studied the mass transfer in Taylor microbubbles using microchannels. They investigated the total gas-liquid mass transfer in the microbubble-forming stages of the process. The results showed that the mass transfer progressed via microbubbles was obviously higher compared to the next stages [54].

In gas-liquid phase experiments, the gas fraction of the microbubbles is the main factor, which affects the performance of the device. The highest conversion rate of gas-liquid interactions occurs when the microbubbles carry a saturated amount of the incorporated gas. In this type of microchannel, the length and diameter of microchannels, and also the friction coefficient of the channels (surface roughness) will be important [55]. Microbubbles are the main way that oxygen can deliver for cell experiments. Different studies cover the use of microbubbles as microvehicles for biological applications in microfluidic systems. The deformation of microbubbles within the pulmonary microvessels of an aspiration mimicking system is a challenging area of microfluidics in the biomedical area. Bento et al. reported a study about the contraction (deformation) phenomenon in red blood cells, bubbles, and droplets during flowing through blood vessels and micron-sized vessels in the pulmonary system [56]. Their results revealed that this method could be appropriate to evaluate healthy and diseased cells by using a cell flexibility factor. The principle of their technique was the contraction of cells, which could be considered in the evaluation of different cells in blood flow.

One common application area of aqueous multiphase microchannels and microdroplet systems is encapsulation processes, such as occur in drug delivery and pharmacokinetics [57], biochemical reactions, and cell biology [58–60]. The advantages of microfluidic-incorporated microdroplet-based studies are that the parameters of water-oil (W/O) reactions can be controlled, rapid assessment, low consumption of reagents, and the use of simplified microchannel devices. Tissue engineering is a general concept that often uses modified hydrogels and microdroplets in biomedical research. Drug delivery protocols and cell transport using microcarriers are other applications of microdroplets in microfluidic systems. In 2016, Avery and colleagues studied a combination of gelatin and nanoclay for stopping bleeding (hemostasis) using microchannel platforms [61]. They used the gelatin/nanoclay (GNC) material in order to cause endovascular embolization and block the vessels. The GNC was synthesized via a cross-linking reaction of the matrix (gelatin) and a reinforcement agent (nanoclay) at the optimized ratio. They assessed the blocking results in a 2D embolization model and designed a suitable ex-vivo model for mimicking the virtual aneurysm. The system showed actual occlusion occurring in the whole channels of the microfluidic platform as shown in Fig. 3.10. The aneurysm model was mimicked, and the phase study between nanoclay and gelatin, as well as blocking of blood flow, coagulation time, and percent of blocking were analyzed.

In droplet (microgel formation) in a microfluidic chip, an immersion vehicle fluid (continuous phase) flows along a main channel. The size optimization is a desirable feature in the microgel formation, which is specified by two factors; good dispersion of the different phases within the microgel, and the use of the proper device.

In order to prepare a microgel in a two-phase pattern (Fig. 3.11), the continuous phase (solidified core flow) passes along the inner channel, while the other phase flows across the channel. In biomedical applications of hydrogels, which are often used for tissue regeneration, the cell growth occurs on the hydrophilic biopolymer surface. A conventional type of microdroplets for hydrogel infusion and microparticle incorporation is shown in Fig. 3.11.

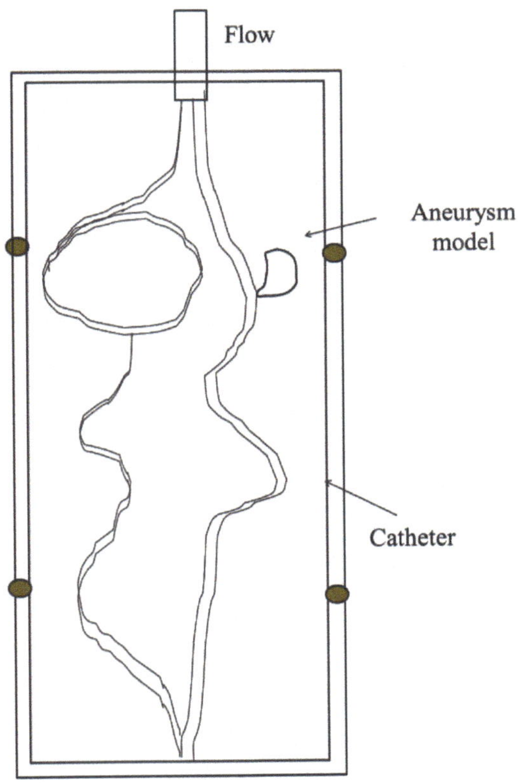

FIG. 3.10

The blood flow blocking mechanism in a microchannel system.

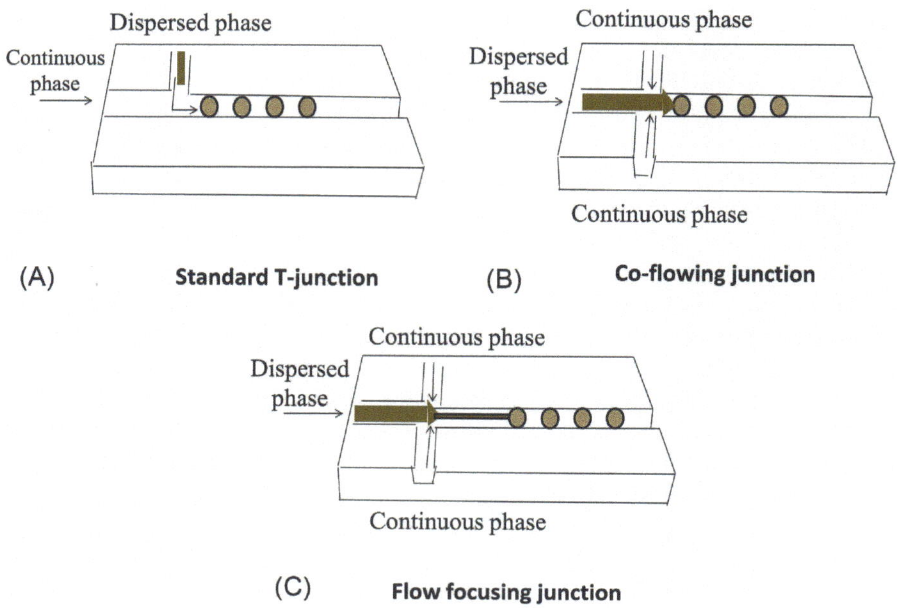

FIG. 3.11

Droplet formation in microfluidic devices for drug embedded microparticles: (A) Simple droplet formation inner core and outer shell, (B) double inlet at the outer part to increase droplet formation density, and (C) flow focusing junction (double entrance for the continuous phase).

One of the promising applications of microfluidics in the biomedical arena is the neuroscience field. The blood-brain barrier is an impermeable membrane lining the brain blood vessels that prevent hydrophobic drugs from reaching the brain. The fluid viscosity, surface tension, and velocity profile in the microchannels are completely different, compared to these parameters in scales other than micrometer. In a microdroplet-mediated hydrogel preparation, the virtual viscosity of the fluid is quite challenging [62].

3.5 Hydrodynamic behavior of the flow in microfluidic systems

The flow velocity is another factor that determines the performance of microfluidic devices. The development of hydrodynamic flow is a useful concept in the design of the microchannels. Due to the limited length of the microchannels, the improved hydrodynamic behavior of the channel is important and can be categorized as follows:

Non-developed regime
Semi-developed regime
Fully developed regime

The circular geometry of microchannels is the simplest shape in the flow behavior studies. In the flow velocity and hydrodynamic development studies, the flow distance coefficient will be accomplished in Eq. (3.6) given as follows;

$$x^{+} = \frac{x}{D_h.R_e} \tag{3.6}$$

where the x^+ can be assumed as dimensionless flow distance coefficient, x is the axial direction of flow, Re is the Reynold number and D_h is the hydraulic diameter of the microchannel. For $x^+ = 0.5$ the flow is assumed as a fully developed regime. In the flow development concept, the pressure drop can be related to the apparent friction coefficient which is given in Eq. (3.7) as follows;

$$\Delta p = \frac{2(f_{app}\,\mathrm{Re})\mu\bar{V}^2}{D_h^2} \tag{3.7}$$

where f_{app} is apparent friction factor, μ is viscosity, x is the axial direction in fluid flow, and D_h is the hydraulic diameter. In cases that microchannels have the same length of the microfluidic device, where x can take values from zero the total length of the channel.

The apparent friction coefficient is the combination of two components as friction coefficient taken from fully developed flow theory and the pressure defect (Hagenbach factor), as it can be seen in Eq. (3.8);

$$\Delta p = \frac{2(fR_e)\mu L}{D_h^2} + \frac{k(x)\rho\bar{V}^2}{2} \tag{3.8}$$

In Eq. (3.9), the k (kappa) is presented as

$$k(x) = (f_{app} - f_{FD})\frac{4x}{D_h} \tag{3.9}$$

The Hagenbach coefficient, $k(x)$ owns the zero (for nondeveloped flow) stretches to the semi-developed flow and finally fully developed flow with a value of 1. The $k(\infty)$ coefficient in the rectangular geometry of channels represents Hagenbach factor, $k(\infty)$ with 0.04% deviation in the term of the flow behavior.

$$k(\infty) = (0.6796 + 1.2197\alpha_c + 3.3089\alpha_c^2 - 9.5921\alpha_c^3 + 8.9089\alpha_c^4 - 2.9959\alpha_c^5) \tag{3.10}$$

3.6 The velocity development in the microchannels

In the conventional hydrodynamic theory in the term of single-phase fluids, the nature of fluid flow and its properties and related characteristics play the main role in the performance of the microfluidic systems [63]. The factors such as viscosity, flow rate, shear stress, and intermolecular force can influence the efficiency of the flow behavior into the microchannel [64]. The well-known fully developed flow concept introduces the shear stress between fluid particles and microchannel walls (boundary layer) for expressing the velocity profile. The shear rate affects the velocity profile which differs in the Newtonian and non-Newtonian flows. As given in the Fig. 3.17, in the inner surface of the channel which is in contact with the flow, the shear stress is the highest, where the velocity is in the lowest amount (velocity ≈ 0) while in the center of the microchannel, the velocity has the highest value and shear stress is in its lowest amount ($\tau \approx 0$). The viscosity of the fluids is highly related to the intermolecular forces of fluid which influences the flow velocity behavior. The entrance length is the distance the flow needs to travel undisturbed to achieve the fully developed profile. The *Re* number dependent entrance length is directly related to the viscosity of the fluid. The flow regime (*Re* number) and related factors such as fluid viscosity, friction coefficient in channel surfaces, and dimensions of the microchannel are the main parameters in defining the entrance lengths as follows;

$$\frac{L}{D} = 0.06.R_e \tag{3.11}$$

$$\frac{L}{D} = 4.4\left(R_e\right)^{1.6} \tag{3.12}$$

where *L* is the entrance length, *D* is the microchannel diameter and *Re* is the Reynolds number. The Eq. (3.11) reveals the entrance lengths for laminar flow (biological phenomenon in the healthy vascular systems of the human body) and Eq. (3.12) represents the entrance length for turbulent flow in case of the diseased vessels of the body such as an aortic aneurysm.

The schematic illustration of Fig. 3.12 reveals the velocity developed profile in two different fluids regarding the viscosity. The top image presents the entrance lengths (L_1) in the term of low viscous fluid and the bottom image with specific

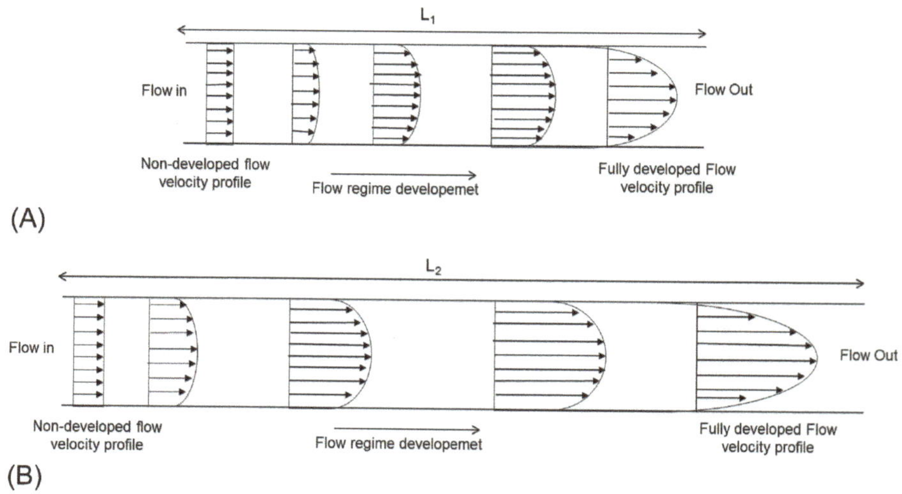

FIG. 3.12

Schematic illustrating of flow velocity development profile related to fluid viscosity. (A) Low viscose fluid. (B) High viscose fluid.

entrance lengths (L_2) is related to the higher viscous fluid. The entrance lengths are completely different ($L_2 \gg L_1$). Unlike, as seen in the Eqs. (3.11), (3.12) the velocity profile development is inversely proportional to the microchannel diameter. As it has been described in the previous parts, the flow behavior in the biomedical research area is important. Nagrath and colleagues studied the separating of CTC (circulating tumor cells) from the blood sample. They investigated many parameters related to the efficiency of a microfluidic device for the proper application of microfluidic systems [65].

In addition to the developed velocity of flow in the microchannels, the maximum velocity that can be reached is important. The simplified formula in which expresses the relation between the maximum velocity of flow (V_c) and flow rate as a function of the diameter of the microchannels is presented in the Eq. (3.13).

$$v_c = \frac{2Q}{\pi R^2} \tag{3.13}$$

where v_c is the maximum velocity, Q is the flow rate and R reveals the microchannel radius.

Hayat and his colleagues studied the formation of microdroplets in microfluidic platforms to identify the factors that affect the efficiency of the microdevices [66]. The study was based on the measurement of the size of the microdroplets using optical methods. The flow rate, T-junction configuration, flow-focusing, and co-flow arrangements of microchannels were considered in their study. The dimensional specifications of the microchannels were the main factors in the microdroplet production efficiency. Parameters such as velocity, length of the channel, and the diameter need to be considered. The velocity optimization of the flow phase was highly important. The high and low velocities of the fluids alter the final shape of the microdroplets, and high velocity can even cause a rupture in the microdroplets.

Fig. 3.13 is an illustration of these effects on the microdroplet shape. The shape deformation of microdroplets is related to the flow velocity (shear tension) at the droplet boundary. As shown in Fig. 3.13, the microdroplets adopt an oval shape in the higher velocity, and return to their spherical shape after the tension has been removed. The stretching of the spherical shape of the microdroplets and the adoption of a dual-core morphology seen in Fig. 3.13 (bottom) occur gradually as the velocity rises. This research was similar to a study by Bento and colleagues who studied red blood cells, air bubbles, and microdroplet deformation [56]. In biomedical applications, the process of cell fractionation can be realized by several microfluidic techniques. The most well-known are size-dependent microfluidic separation and microchannel-assisted bioaffinity based flow fractionation of cells [67].

In size-dependent cell separation, in addition to the velocity and shear stress, other factors such as the dimensional specification of the microchannels influence the form of the droplets (especially in the two-phase systems) and the separation yield. The channel diameter is inversely correlated with the flow velocity and spherical shape of the microdroplets in biomedical applications. A schematic demonstration of cell separation in serpentine microchannels is given in Fig. 3.14. Large cells (e.g., cancer

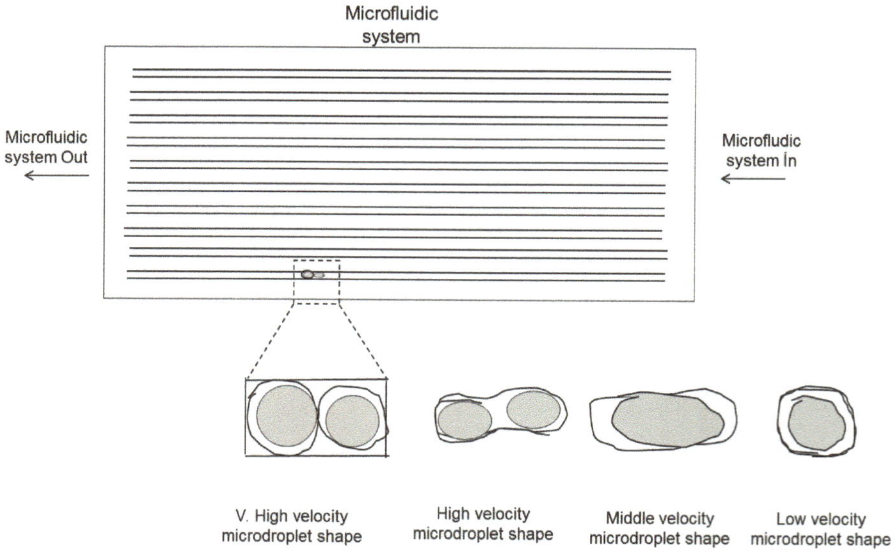

FIG. 3.13

Schematic illustration of the effect of flow velocity on the microdroplet shape.

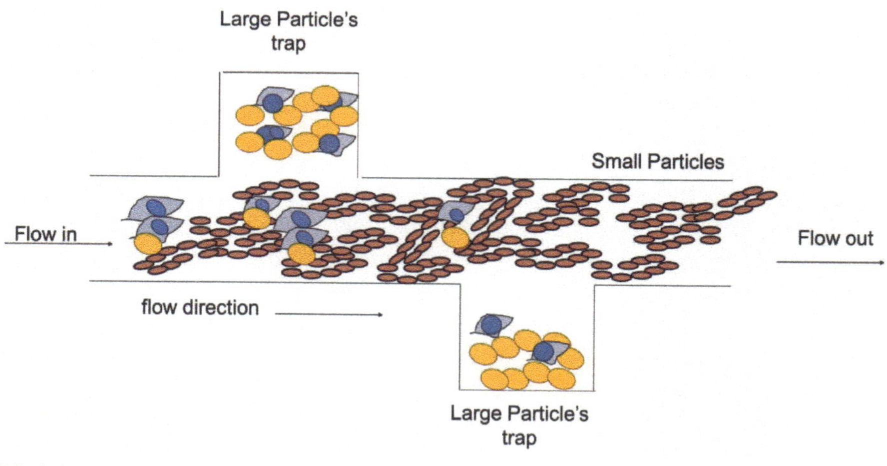

FIG. 3.14

Schematic illustration of the size-based separation of cells in symmetrical serpentine microfluidic devices.

cells) can be trapped when the lower velocity of flow inside the narrow channels causes the efficient separation via shape deformation of desired cells [65,68,69].

The channel size and the existence of binding sites along the microchannel, together with the rate of fluid flow (blood for example) determine the bioseparation efficiency. Different external forces can affect the cells, including electromagnetic force, gravity, eccentricity in the spiral route of the microfluidic device, and bioaffinity mechanisms. A novel technique to bind cancer cells can be provided by the attachment of antibody molecules that recognize epitopes, which are expressed on the surface of cancer cells. By using a cancer cell capture mechanism, cancer cells can be separated from healthy cells (brown particles in Fig. 3.14).

3.7 Hydrophilicity and hydrophobicity effects in microfluidic systems

Hydrophilicity and hydrophobicity of surfaces are important concepts in different fields of science and biomedicine. The efficiency of microfluidic devices for cell attachment and cell proliferation are influenced by the hydrophobicity of the surface. Also in the microbiology field such as the detection of infectious microbes, the modification of the device surface with proper techniques is critical [70]. Biomimicking is a very interesting area of science that uses biological phenomena to design inanimate devices. Roundberg designed an ultrahydrophobic surface by biomimicking a naturally-occurring Lotus leaf in a microfluidic system [71]. Processes such as bioseparation, lab-on-a-chip microarrays in biology, protein synthesis from DNA, or bioaffinity [72] and biosensors [73] are all applications in which hydrophilicity and hydrophobicity are important. The surface treatment is generally achieved by well-designed chemical, physical or optical methods. In recent years, nanotechnology has been used for surface coating techniques for different biomedical applications. Electrohydrodynamic techniques can be used to fabricate polymeric nanofibers, for instance in electrospinning, spin coating, or electro-spraying methods to produce hydrophobic nanofibers for microarrays and microchannel-assisted biomedical applications [74]. The polymers include both naturally occurring materials such as polysaccharide polymers, and synthetic polymers such as Polycaprolactone (PCL) or Polylactic acid (PLA) [75]. By using hydrophobic polymers in the microchannel biosensors, the objects to be analyzed such as cells or microorganisms, and their immobilization can be achieved on the platforms of microchannels or microarrays. Laser direct-writing (LDW) is another technique, where a laser beam is delivered to the photosensitive polymer to provide a hydrophobic pattern within the microchannel [76]. Atmospheric RF plasma treatment is another physical procedure for surface etching and modification of PDMS microchannels [77]. Oxygen mediated (CF_4/O_2, 50:50%) plasma is used for hydrophilic modification, where the PDMS alone has a hydrophobic property [78]. Physical vapor deposition can be used as a method of surface modification in microdevices to create hydrophobic surfaces. Another protocol for creating a water-repellent surfaces is the film (barrier) formation of waxes on the surface of microchannels in the microfluidic device. The advantages of water-repellent surfaces are lower absorption of analyte through the film, minimum loss of biofluid, and low cost. A recent technique, the chemical coating of repellent minerals such as perovskite microparticles can provide a superhydrophobic surface in the microdevice. Chan and his colleagues reported a microfluidic device with micron-sized silica beads in the form of a packed platform as the separation unit in pressure-driven liquid chromatography [79]. They evaluated the separation efficiency of dextran and bovine serum albumin (BSA) beads that had higher hydrophobicity than bare dextran, in the microchannels. In another study for cell separation, Bhattacharyya et al. designed a microfluidic system using monolith embedded Oligo particles [80]. They isolated the mRNA from various cell lysates, such as breast cancer cells (MCF-7) and fibroblast cells which were harvested from the human liver. The results showed the importance of hydrophobicity, which was the main factor determining the adhesion of particles in separation processes. Paper-based microfluidic devices are conventional types of detection devices that are used in biomedical applications [70,81]. A review article published by Yang and his colleagues discussed paper-based microfluidic systems, applications, and future directions [70]. Jiang et al. reported the hydrophobic to hydrophilic property conversion and vice versa by using octadecyltrichlorosilane (OTS) and a corona generator [82].

3.8 Physical specifications of channels in microfluidic systems

Developments in microfluidic devices have driven the growth of specific applications. This chapter gives a brief description of the main physical properties of the microchannels that influence the fluid flow. In addition to the dimensional and cross-sectional properties of the microchannels described above, other physical properties such as surface roughness and friction coefficient can affect the flow behavior. These factors are discussed in the following subsections.

3.8.1 Effect of friction coefficient of the microchannels in microfluidic devices

In addition to the cross-sectional parameters, mass and volumetric flow rates (which were discussed above), other specifications such as the surface roughness and the friction coefficient need to be considered in the design of microchannels [83]. There have been numerous articles about the effect of the friction coefficient on the performance of flow in the microchannels. A correct understanding about flow behavior in the microchannels necessitates a careful consideration of the parameters involved, such as the friction coefficient and related effects on the performance of the microfluidic device. On the macroscale, Bernoulli's law can describe the pressure drop, the kinetic energy of flow, and related parameters. The friction coefficient. Keener's research group studied the mathematical modeling of pressure regimes in normal and Fontan blood flow regimes [84]. Their investigation concerned the boundary conditions in the cardiovascular system and blood pressure distribution. The Fontan blood flow occurs in children with univentricular hearts. In another study, Mouza and colleagues reported a simplified model to estimate the friction coefficient in blood vessels [85]. It is clear that the flow pressure is one of the most critical factors in microfluidic systems. To mimic the clinical situation, Mouza and his research team prepared a model of healthy vessels constructed of stainless steel with varying diameter. The capillaries (300–1800 μm) in diameter and 35%–55% hematocrit were considered for modeling. Their model results showed a sufficient accuracy (10%) in the case of the pressure drop in laminar blood flow. In the clinical situation the downstream pressure drops, and in narrow capillaries needs to be carefully observed. This concept encouraged scientists to investigate the pressure drop in the microchannels, which are related to cardiovascular diseases. In order to evaluate the friction coefficient in microchannels (such as happens in the vascular capillaries), it is important to understand diabatic and adiabatic processes that occur in microchannel devices. More than 50% of the studies used channels with diameters between 100 and 200 μm, which are important in the pressure drop caused by the friction coefficient. In this section, we discuss the two different definitions of *f* (Darcy and Fanning definitions of *f*). The Fanning definition of the friction coefficient has more conformity with diabatic studies. The Fanning friction coefficient is more or less the same as the Colburn *j* factor equation. Here, the pressure drop efficiency depends on the *f* or *j* factors. The Fanning friction coefficient describes the ratio between the microchannel wall shear stress and the kinetic energy (per unit volume) by Eq. (3.14) as follows:

$$f = \frac{\tau_w}{{}^1\!/\!{}_2 \rho V_{mean}^{\,2}} \tag{3.14}$$

where f is the friction factor, τ_w is the shear stress between fluid and the microchannel wall, ρ is the fluid density and V_{mean} is the mean velocity. The Fanning factor in the case of bulk flux and pressure drop is shown by Eq. (3.15) as follows:

$$f = \frac{\rho \Delta_p D_h}{2LG^2} \tag{3.15}$$

where, f is the friction coefficient, Δ_p is the pressure drop, D_h is the hydraulic diameter, L is the length of the microchannel, and G is the bulk flux. The Poiseuille number is defined as:

$$Po = f.Re \tag{3.16}$$

Po (for laminar flow) is the friction-related constant in a circular passage according to Eq. (3.16). The friction coefficient (derived from the Poiseuille number) can be considered as a function of the rectangular channel aspect ratio. The friction factor, Reynolds number, and dimensional aspect ratio relation is given in the Shah and London formula in Eq. (3.17) as follows:

$$f\,Re = 24\left(1 - 1.3553\alpha_c + 1.9467\alpha_c^2 - 1.7012\alpha_c^3 + 0.9564\alpha_c^4 - 0.2537\alpha_c^5\right) \tag{3.17}$$

where α_c is the channel dimensional aspect ratio. In Eq. (3.7), the aspect ratio is always < 1. For the turbulent flow regime, different correlations can be considered in the Blasius equation. For smooth tubular microchannels this is given in Eq. (3.18).

$$f = \frac{0.0791}{Re^{1/4}} \tag{3.18}$$

The correlation given in Eq. (3.18) specifies fluid flow with a Re number around 2.

Also in systems with temperature gradients, the temperature-dependent parameters, such as viscosity can be altered. The friction coefficient of microchannels can be calculated according to Eq. (3.19) as follows:

$$\frac{f}{f_{cp}} = \left(\frac{\mu_b}{\mu_w}\right)^m \tag{3.19}$$

3.8.2 Roughness effects in channels of microfluidic devices

The friction coefficient described in the previous section, is a parameter which depends on the surface roughness of the microchannel. The roughness of the side walls of the channels influences the flow regime in the blood circulation [86,87], flow resistance in branched microchannels [88], cell biology [89] and transfer of mass and energy [86]. Johann Nikuradse demonstrated the relation between the roughness and the friction coefficient which is given in Eq. (3.20). Eq. (3.20) is applicable to microfluidic devices with d and for e/D ratios $< 1 \times 10^{-6}$.

$$\frac{1}{\sqrt{f}} = 3.48 - 1.737 \ln\left(\frac{e}{D}\right) \tag{3.20}$$

where e is the average surface roughness. For situations with $\frac{e}{D}$ ratio $> 1 \times 10^{-6}$, the friction coefficient can be calculated according to the implicit Colebrook equation, Eq. (3.21) as follows;

$$\frac{1}{\sqrt{f}} = 3..48 - 1.737 \ln\left(\frac{e}{D} + \frac{9.35}{\mathrm{Re}\sqrt{f}}\right) \tag{3.21}$$

The most accurate correlations of the phenomena are given by the Colebrook equation Eq. (3.21).

The roughness factor and its effects on the flow of the microchannels, depend on the microporous or nanoporous nature of the inner surface of the microchannels. The roughness of the microchannels also plays a major role in both pressure-driven and osmotic flow [90]. In biomedical applications using microfluidic devices, the attachment of biological moieties inside the microchannels is another important concept requiring an in-depth investigation. This trapping is due to physical barriers occurring along the channel in the microfluidic device. In some biomedical applications, surfaces with higher degrees of smoothness are more useful to reduce the physical adhesion of microorganisms on the surface.

3.9 Biomedical applications of transport phenomena in microfluidic systems

In biomedical applications, the mimicking of the blood circulation is an interesting field of medicine. The continuum concept describes a transfer phenomenon that is involved in different fields, such as physics, chemistry, biology, and nanotechnology. Practical approaches can model the mass transport [91], heat transfer, and the momentum [92]. In all of these models, the transported mass is influenced by the flow regime [48], and the hydrodynamic driving force as occurs in human blood vessels [93]. The mass transport can be provided by droplets, lipid vesicles, or microfluidic chambers [91]. Although the energy and momentum are other transport factors that are related to the mass, however, they should each be studied individually.

In this part of the chapter, an attempt has been made to provide a survey of transportation phenomena in microfluidic systems, and especially in the case of mass transfer. The transfer phenomena can be more sophisticated in different fields, such as biomedical, biotechnology, and nanotechnology, and can be combined to form a multipurpose system. Therefore, simultaneous mass and energy transportation is presented in the following equations. The mass amount displaced by the flow between the inlet and outlet is the main concept of mass transportation in microfluidic systems. According to the miniaturization theory, the mass, momentum, and heat transfer can be calculated using the following equations:

$$\frac{\partial P}{\partial t}+\frac{\partial \rho}{\partial x_i}(\rho U_i)=0 \tag{3.22}$$

$$\frac{\partial}{\partial t}(\rho U_i)+\frac{\partial}{\partial x_i}(\rho U_j U_i)=\rho F_i-\frac{\partial p}{\partial x_i}+\frac{\partial}{\partial x_j}\tau_{ji} \tag{3.23}$$

$$\frac{\partial}{\partial t}(\rho e)+\frac{\partial}{\partial t}(\rho U_i e)=p\frac{\partial U_i}{\partial x_i}-\frac{\tau_{ji}}{\partial x_j}\tau_{ji}+\frac{\partial q_i}{\partial x_i} \tag{3.24}$$

In the above equations (Eqs. 3.22, 3.23, and 3.24) the U_i is the flow velocity, ρ is the density of the fluid, and p is the pressure within the microchannel. Also, τ is the shear stress on the sidewalls applied to the fluid, and e is the internal energy, F is the body force and q is the heat flux [49]. The eddy patterns of flow increase the shear forces between the fluid layers. The shear motion improves the mixing efficiency which causes an increase in the mass transfer [94–96]. These microsegments have different applications such as colloidal nanoparticle synthesis [97] and quantitative analysis which can be affected by the rate of mass transfer [98]. The droplets within microchannel devices affect the mass transfer efficiency factor by different mechanisms. One of the mechanisms that is related to mass transfer is the immiscible liquid-liquid process in microchannel models. The time required for the system to achieve a steady-state in terms of mass transfer is highly important. The mass transfer rate in the liquid-liquid phase interaction depends on the length of the passage. In the microdroplets used in pharmaceutical drug delivery, the channel diameter influences the mass transfer rate. The equilibrium in dual-phase interactions is inversely correlated to the droplet diameter. This fact shows that the mass transfer is also inversely proportional to the droplet size. Droplets with radii on the micrometer and nanometer scale have thousand-fold higher mass transfer than millimeter dimension particles.

In human biology, the physiological and mechanical properties of blood vessels and blood flow are interesting areas for scientists. The heat transfer process for stabilizing the physiological temperature about 37°C is an important mechanism for body homeostasis. Blood circulation is governed by control of the tension within the vascular network, deformation of circulating blood compartments, blockages within vessels, and other factors that can be simulated in microfluidic systems [99,100]. The mass, momentum, and heat transport are referred to in the Eqs. (3.22)–(3.24) have been studied in microfluidic systems and are given by the Navier-stocks continuity equations [101]. The continuum concept requires taking into account the steady-state condition (such as constant temperature) of the microchannels in the microfluidic devices and relating it to human biology. The categorization of fluid behavior as Newtonian or non-Newtonian (such as blood flow) is crucial [102]. Compressible and incompressible fluids are other factors that must be considered. Signal propagation (which is essential for cell to cell communication [103]) is important in neuroscience studies, especially in the field of regenerative medicine for neural diseases [104], and cardiac abnormalities [105]. The microvoltage electrical signals of the body can be investigated in microfluidic platforms. Nano-transporters are objects that boost electrical signal transport through the neural network of the body [49]. Signal enhancement is achieved by the use of highly conductive materials. Lovat et al. studied the robust effect of carbon nanotubes on electrical signaling in the neural system [106]. In another study, Tang and his colleagues reported a significant boost in electrical signaling using graphene films [104].

3.10 Pathogen detection by microchannel devices using nanotechnology

According to the World Health Organization (WHO) 2016 report, infections are still in the top ten global causes of death. Therefore the detection of infectious pathogens remains an important area. Microdevices are useful in most scientific fields and particularly in the diagnosis of infections. Application of microfluidic devices in the detection of pathogens may provide more accurate, safe, and rapid detection methods. A color-change based, simple cell detection protocol would be desirable, as well as more sophisticated optical and electrical techniques, using nanotechnology for greater sensitivity and specificity.

In optical microarrays, nanoparticles and antibodies are combined via linker molecules as a surface modification of the optically-sensitive surface of the microchannel or microarray. Fig. 3.15 illustrates the trapping of target microorganisms such as pathogens (virus or bacterial cells) or cancer cells onto the surface of the microdevice that can be analyzed using the appropriate detection method. As shown in Fig. 3.15, the use of a specific antibody recognizing the target moiety, provides the capture mechanism. The binding of antibody to antigen can be evaluated by colorimetric, optical, or other analytical techniques.

As can be seen in Fig. 3.16, nanoparticles can act as platforms for the detection of microorganisms in microfluidic systems. Unlike microarrays (lab-on-a-chip), in microchannel devices, the inner surface of the channels acts as a substrate for

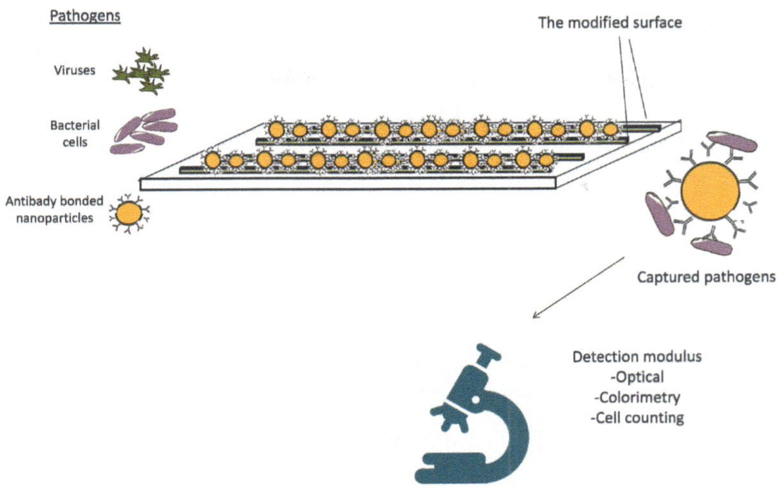

FIG. 3.15

Schematic illustration of lab-on-a-chip microarrays for the detection of pathogens using nanoparticles and specific antibodies.

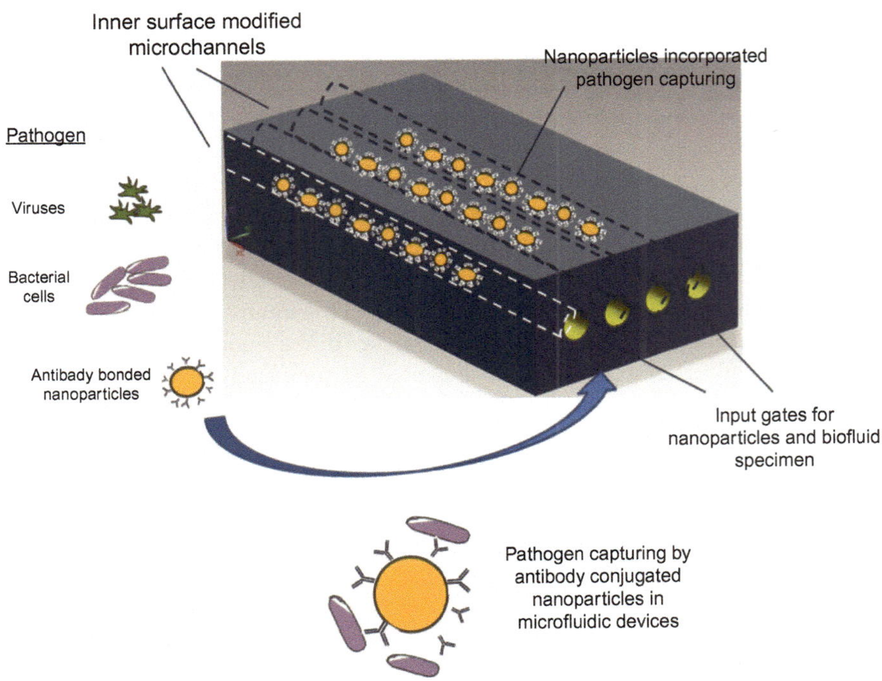

FIG. 3.16

A simplified schematic of nanoparticle-based diagnosis using microchannel devices.

the bio-conjugation reactions. The nanoparticles are bonded to the side-walls of the microchannels, that have been modified with functional groups. Afterward, the nanoparticles on the surface of the microchannels will be ready to bind to microorganisms in the biofluid samples obtained from the patient. Pathogen detection can be reported by conventional analytical methods, optical, colorimetric, or by more recent methods such as Raman spectroscopy.

3.11 Soft microchannels in biomedical applications

PDMS is a common material used in the fabrication of microchannels. In addition to PDMS, a new generation of soft elastomers as alternative materials for the fabrication of microchannels will be discussed. Biocompatible elastomers have biomedical applications for tissue modeling, artificial tissue fabrication, and also are used in biomedical studies, for the fabrication of microchannels and related components. Xi and colleagues reported a study on soft tubular microchannels for 2D and 3D applications [107]. This research group used a new elastomer to fabricate sophisticated geometries of microchannels, which would be impossible with thermosetting PDMS. The above-mentioned inexpensive and highly efficient fabrication method presented several benefits in the modeling of tissue. The flexural modulus of the elastomer used in the fabrication of the soft microchannels, rendered the inner surface of the microchannels suitable for studying the epithelization and endothelization required for tissue regeneration.

Soft microchannels can be used in cardiovascular studies, and for regenerative methods in tissue engineering of muscles, connective tissue, and neural structures (Fig. 3.17).

Microfluidic systems used for neuronal regeneration within 2D microchannels is an interesting field of study [108]. Regenerative medicine also involves tissue engineering for the repair of neuronal channels in neuroscience. Due to the appropriate flexibility of microchannels fabricated with soft biomaterials, it may be possible to implant laboratory-produced tissue constructions in the future.

Fig. 3.18A illustrates the structure of a nerve. In the traumatic neural injuries, the myelin shell of the nerve is often impaired or completely destroyed. The soft microchannels could function as cell scaffolds for the growth of tubular sections of new nerves, which could be implanted to repair the damage as seen in Fig. 3.18B.

3.12 Reusable microchannels in biomedical applications

The concept of reusable microchannels in microfluidic devices is promising and is of importance for different areas of science. In conventional microfluidic systems, the PDMS structure of the microchannels is disposed of after use. Developments in the manufacture of microfluidic devices has made them more precise tools. A research group in Spain investigated the design and manufacture of microchannels according to the ES 2626263B1 EU patent entitled "Reusable platform for assembling glass

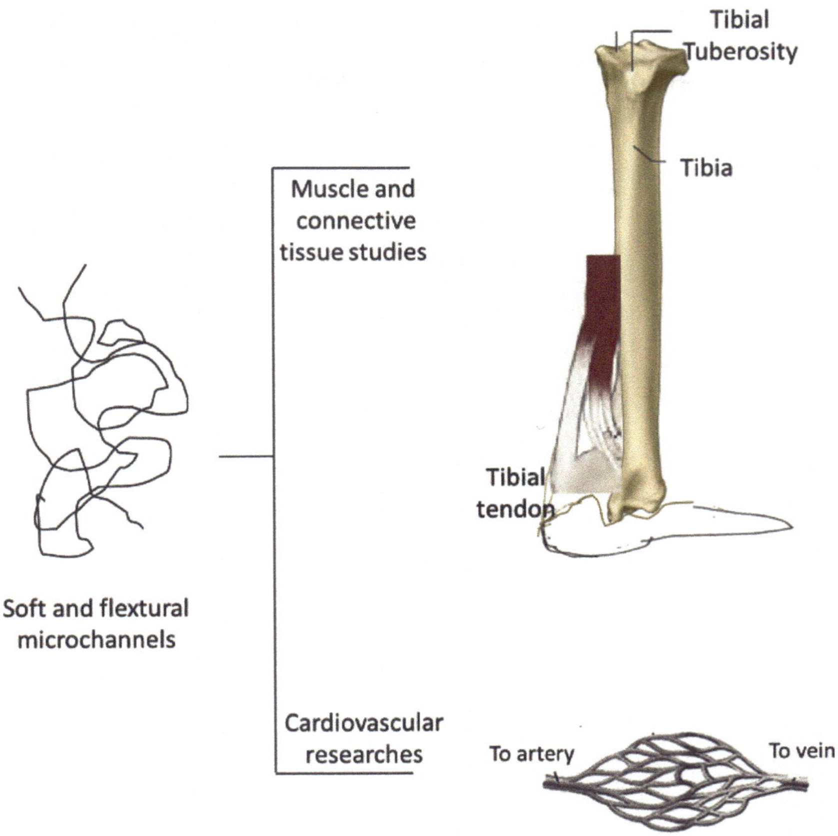

FIG. 3.17

Schematic of flexible microchannels in tissue engineering applications.

capillaries for microfluidics". Eloy and colleagues [109] assembled a new version of a reusable microfluidic system, in which replaceable glass capillaries were embedded within the body of the microfluidic device [110]. The holes for assembling the glass capillaries were constructed inside the PDMS body.

Impurities which are produced during the experimental procedures need to be removed from the inner surface of the microchannels. It has been stated that "This is a huge handicap of microfluidic devices fabricated with expensive materials, man-hours and machinery costs as well". Generally, the channels of the microfluidic devices need to be cleaned after each single experimental run. A new design was proposed for the generation of reusable microchannels for biological experiments. Molded PDMS microfluidic platform were used as the core body. The insertion of replaceable microchannels into the holes of the microfluidic device (glass microchannels) was the critical step (Fig. 3.19).

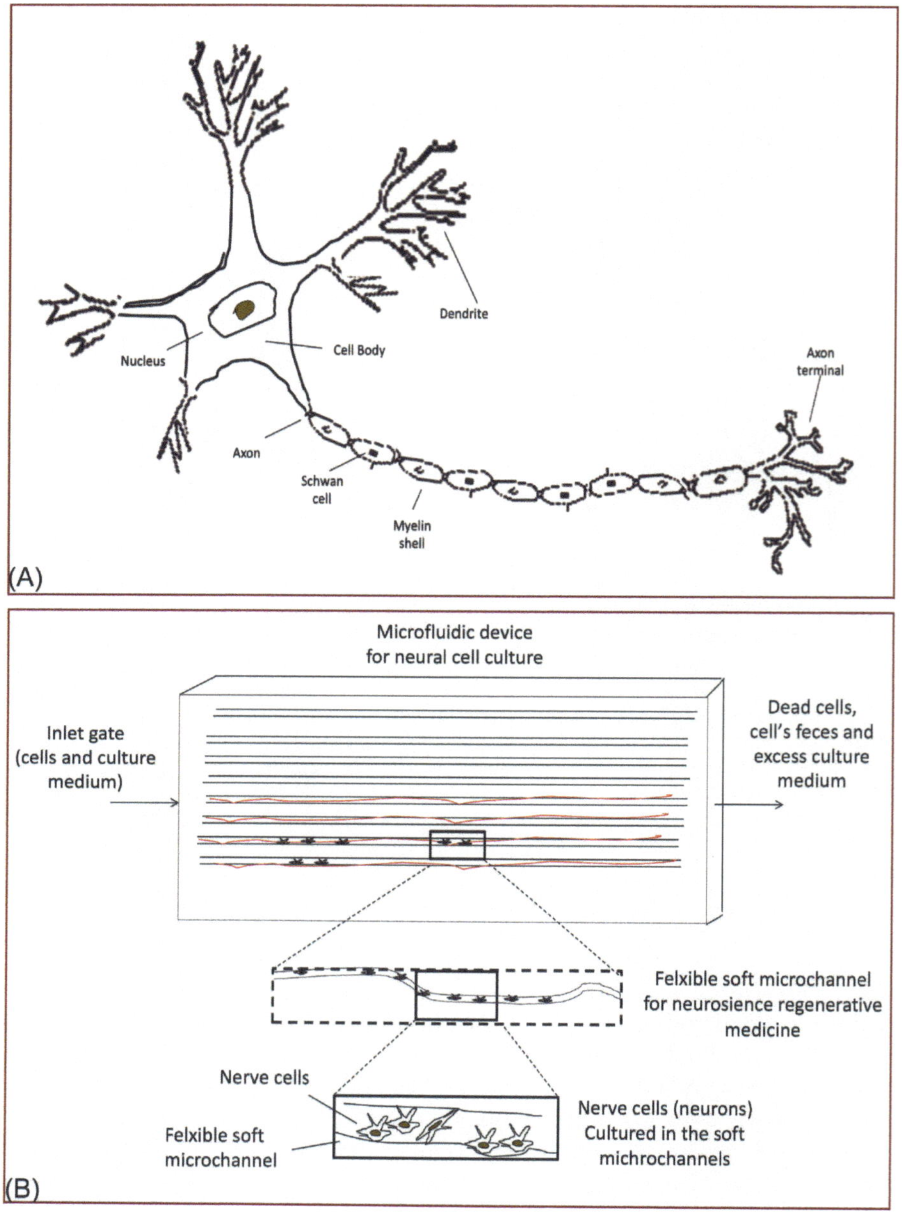

FIG. 3.18

Schematic demonstration of flexible microchannels for nerve repair. (A) Neural system biologic structure; (B) soft flexible microchannels in the regenerative medicine for neural regeneration.

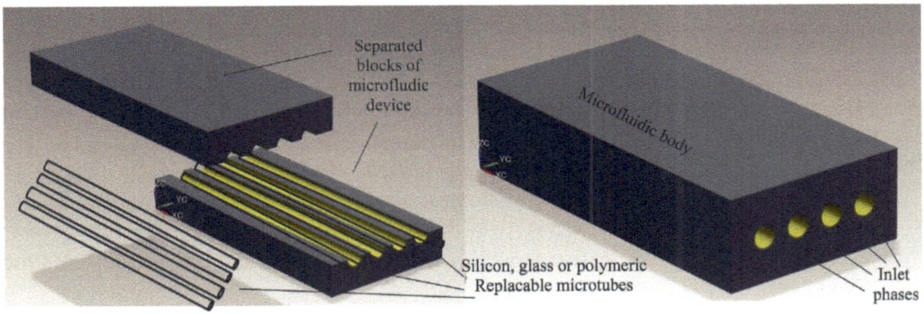

FIG. 3.19

Reusable microchannels in novel microfluidic devices.

For the detection of microorganisms using fixed-channel structures, the cleaning of the nanoparticles, the use of solvents, removal of surface-attached linker molecules, and microorganisms from the inner surface of the microchannels are important. The impurities accumulating inside the channels can cause a performance reduction in microfluidic devices. The device safety is even more important when high-risk pathogens, such as Zika, HIV, or TB are to be detected with microfluidics-based kits. In 2016, Song and his colleagues investigated the molecular detection of the Zika virus. The team designed a suitable colorimetric diagnotic microfluidic cassette for detection of the Zika virus [111]. They used a cassette with suitable microchannels designed for interaction with the virus. The kit had advantages such as cost-effectiveness, highly accurate rapid detection, and user safety.

3.13 Conclusions

This chapter has provided an overview of the factors that affect the performance of microfluidic systems. Three separate concepts concerning microfluidic devices were highlighted; (a) microchannel properties; (b) fluid flow in the device, and (c) dimensional dependent characteristics. The dimensions of the microchannels are the main parameters that affect the desired performance. The applications can be categorized as, microscale reactions, separation processes, flow dynamics studies, biology studies using cells, nanotechnology studies, etc. The flow regime in the case of turbulent or laminar flow must be considered in the microchannels. It has been found that the general flow regime in microchannels is laminar. The hydrophilicity and hydrophobicity of the surface is another property of the channels, which affects cell investigations. The friction coefficient resulting from the roughness of the inner surface of the microchannels is another factor that affects the microfluidic system performance.

References

[1] N.-T. Nguyen, et al., Design, fabrication and characterization of drug delivery systems based on lab-on-a-chip technology, Adv Drug Deliv Rev 65 (11-12) (2013) 1403–1419.
[2] M. Rothbauer, H. Zirath, P. Ertl, Recent advances in microfluidic technologies for cell-to-cell interaction studies, Lab Chip 18 (2) (2018) 249–270.
[3] I.L. Colao, et al., Manufacturing exosomes: a promising therapeutic platform, Trends Mol Med 24 (3) (2018) 242–256.
[4] J. Higgins, et al., Sickle cell vasoocclusion and rescue in a microfluidic device, Proc Natl Acad Sci 104 (51) (2007) 20496–20500.
[5] Y.I. Wang, H.E. Abaci, M.L. Shuler, Microfluidic blood–brain barrier model provides in vivo-like barrier properties for drug permeability screening, Biotechnol Bioeng 114 (1) (2017) 184–194.
[6] B. Nasseri, et al., Point-of-care microfluidic devices for pathogen detection, Biosens Bioelectron 117 (2018) 112–128.
[7] N.-T. Nguyen, et al., Recent advances and future perspectives on microfluidic liquid handling, Micromachines 8 (6) (2017) 186.
[8] R. Ghosh, Protein separation using membrane chromatography: opportunities and challenges, J Chromatogr A 953 (2002) 25.
[9] N.N. Kachouie, et al., Directed assembly of cell-laden hydrogels for engineering functional tissues, Organogenesis 6 (4) (2010) 234–244.
[10] M.I. Hasan, A.J.F. Ali, R.S. Tufah, Numerical study of the effect of channel geometry on the performance of magnetohydrodynamic micro pump, Eng Sci Technol 20 (3) (2017) 982–989.
[11] B.E. Rapp, Microfluidics: modeling, mechanics and mathematics, William Andrew, 2016.
[12] J.-A. Kim, et al., Inertial focusing in non-rectangular cross-section microchannels and manipulation of accessible focusing positions, Lab Chip 16 (6) (2016) 992–1001.
[13] J.S. Choi, Y. Piao, T.S. Seo, Circumferential alignment of vascular smooth muscle cells in a circular microfluidic channel, Biomaterials 35 (1) (2014) 63–70.
[14] R. Vecchione, et al., From square to circular polymeric microchannels by spin coating technology: a low cost platform for endothelial cell culture, Biofabrication 8 (2) (2016) 025005.
[15] A.A. Yagodnitsyna, A.V. Kovalev, A.V. Bilsky, Flow patterns of immiscible liquid-liquid flow in a rectangular microchannel with T-junction, Chem Eng J 303 (2016) 547–554.
[16] F. Del Giudice, et al., Fluid viscoelasticity drives self-assembly of particle trains in a straight microfluidic channel, Phys Rev Appl 10 (6) (2018) 064058.
[17] C.-Y. Lee, et al., Passive mixers in microfluidic systems: a review, Chem Eng J 288 (2016) 146–160.
[18] M.K. Parsa, F. Hormozi, D. Jafari, Mixing enhancement in a passive micromixer with convergent–divergent sinusoidal microchannels and different ratio of amplitude to wave length, Comput Fluids 105 (2014) 82–90.
[19] Y. Fang, et al., Mixing enhancement by simple periodic geometric features in microchannels, Chem Eng J 187 (2012) 306–310.
[20] Y. Du, et al., Evaluation of floor-grooved micromixers using concentration-channel length profiles, Micromachines 1 (1) (2010) 19–33.
[21] O. Carrier, et al., Pressure drop in a split-and-recombine caterpillar micromixer in case of newtonian and non-newtonian fluids, AIChE J 59 (7) (2013) 2679–2685.

[22] P. Vatankhah, A. Shamloo, Parametric study on mixing process in an in-plane spiral micromixer utilizing chaotic advection, Anal Chim Acta 1022 (2018) 96–105.
[23] A. Soleymani, E. Kolehmainen, I. Turunen, Numerical and experimental investigations of liquid mixing in T-type micromixers, Chem Eng J 135 (2008) S219–S228.
[24] R. Lopes, et al., Low cost microfluidic device for partial cell separation: micromilling approach, in: 2015 IEEE international conference on industrial technology (ICIT), IEEE, 2015.
[25] X. Wang, Z. Liu, Y. Pang, Concentration gradient generation methods based on microfluidic systems, RSC Adv 7 (48) (2017) 29966–29984.
[26] J. Clark, M. Kaufman, P. Fodor, Mixing enhancement in serpentine micromixers with a non-rectangular cross-section, Micromachines 9 (3) (2018) 107.
[27] E. Remiszewska, et al., Enzymatic method of urea determination in LTCC microfluidic system based on absorption photometry, Sensors Actuators B Chem (2019).
[28] G. Vladisavljević, R. Al Nuumani, S. Nabavi, Microfluidic production of multiple emulsions, Micromachines 8 (3) (2017) 75.
[29] A. Abate, D. Weitz, High-order multiple emulsions formed in poly (dimethylsiloxane) microfluidics, Small 5 (18) (2009) 2030–2032.
[30] T. Trantidou, et al., Droplet microfluidics for the construction of compartmentalised model membranes, Lab Chip 18 (17) (2018) 2488–2509.
[31] S. Fokong, et al., Image-guided, targeted and triggered drug delivery to tumors using polymer-based microbubbles, J Control Release 163 (1) (2012) 75–81.
[32] P. Koczera, et al., PBCA-based polymeric microbubbles for molecular imaging and drug delivery, J Control Release 259 (2017) 128–135.
[33] A. Burgess, et al., Alzheimer disease in a mouse model: MR imaging–guided focused ultrasound targeted to the hippocampus opens the blood-brain barrier and improves pathologic abnormalities and behavior, Radiology 273 (3) (2014) 736–745.
[34] T. Yang, et al., Dumbbell-shaped bi-component mesoporous janus solid nanoparticles for biphasic interface catalysis, Angew Chem 129 (29) (2017) 8579–8583.
[35] Y. Wang, et al., Bipolar electrochemical mechanism for the propulsion of catalytic nanomotors in hydrogen peroxide solutions, Langmuir 22 (25) (2006) 10451–10456.
[36] Y. Ju, et al., Monodisperse Au–Fe2C Janus nanoparticles: an attractive multifunctional material for triple-modal imaging-guided tumor photothermal therapy, ACS Nano 11 (9) (2017) 9239–9248.
[37] S. Seiffert, M.B. Romanowsky, D.A. Weitz, Janus microgels produced from functional precursor polymers, Langmuir 26 (18) (2010) 14842–14847.
[38] K.P. Yuet, et al., Multifunctional superparamagnetic Janus particles, Langmuir 26 (6) (2009) 4281–4287.
[39] X.Y. Ling, et al., Janus particles with controllable patchiness and their chemical functionalization and supramolecular assembly, Angew Chem Int Ed 48 (41) (2009) 7677–7682.
[40] Y. Gou, et al., Progress of inertial microfluidics in principle and application, Sensors 18 (6) (2018) 1762.
[41] S.C. Hur, et al., Deformability-based cell classification and enrichment using inertial microfluidics, Lab Chip 11 (5) (2011) 912–920.
[42] N. Xiang, et al., Fundamentals of elasto-inertial particle focusing in curved microfluidic channels, Lab Chip 16 (14) (2016) 2626–2635.
[43] W.R. Dean, XVI. Note on the motion of fluid in a curved pipe, London Edinburgh Dublin Philos Mag J Sci 4 (20) (1927) 208–223.

[44] W. Dean, LXXII. The stream-line motion of fluid in a curved pipe (second paper), London Edinburgh Dublin Philos Mag J Sci 5 (30) (1928) 673–695.
[45] S. Ookawara, et al., Feasibility study on concentration of slurry and classification of contained particles by microchannel, Chem Eng J 101 (1–3) (2004) 171–178.
[46] P.D. Stein, H.N. Sabbah, Turbulent blood flow in the ascending aorta of humans with normal and diseased aortic valves, Circ Res 39 (1) (1976) 58–65.
[47] M.E. Steinke, S.G. Kandlikar, Single-phase liquid friction factors in microchannels, in: ASME 3rd international conference on microchannels and minichannels, American Society of Mechanical Engineers, 2005.
[48] N. Kashid, M.A. Renken, L. Kiwi-Minsker, Influence of flow regime on mass transfer in different types of microchannels, Ind Eng Chem Res 50 (11) (2011) 6906–6914.
[49] T. Bayraktar, S.B. Pidugu, Characterization of liquid flows in microfluidic systems, Int J Heat Mass Transf 49 (5-6) (2006) 815–824.
[50] I. Papautsky, et al., Laminar fluid behavior in microchannels using micropolar fluid theory, Sensors Actuators A Phys 73 (1-2) (1999) 101–108.
[51] H. Feng, et al., High-performance gas-liquid-solid microreactor with polydopamine functionalized surface coated by Pd nanocatalyst for nitrobenzene hydrogenation, Chem Eng J 306 (2016) 1017–1025.
[52] S. Tanzi, et al., Fabrication of combined-scale nano-and microfluidic polymer systems using a multilevel dry etching, electroplating and molding process, J Micromech Microeng 22 (11) (2012) 115008.
[53] M. Akbar, D. Plummer, S.M. Ghiaasiaan, Gas-liquid two-phase flow regimes in microchannels, in: ASME 2002 international mechanical engineering congress and exposition, American Society of Mechanical Engineers, 2002.
[54] L. Yang, et al., Visualization and characterization of gas–liquid mass transfer around a Taylor bubble right after the formation stage in microreactors, Chem Eng Sci 143 (2016) 364–368.
[55] R. Xiong, J. Chung, An experimental study of the size effect on adiabatic gas-liquid two-phase flow patterns and void fraction in microchannels, Phys Fluids 19 (3) (2007) 033301.
[56] D. Bento, et al., Deformation of red blood cells, air bubbles, and droplets in microfluidic devices: Flow visualizations and measurements, Micromachines 9 (4) (2018) 151.
[57] X. Niu, Building droplet-based microfluidic systems for biological analysis, Portland Press Limited, 2012.
[58] T. Kaminski, P. Garstecki, Controlled droplet microfluidic systems for multistep chemical and biological assays, Chem Soc Rev 46 (20) (2017) 6210–6226.
[59] A.L. Paguirigan, D.J. Beebe, Protocol for the fabrication of enzymatically crosslinked gelatin microchannels for microfluidic cell culture, Nat Protoc 2 (7) (2007) 1782.
[60] Y. Zheng, et al., Recent advances in microfluidic techniques for single-cell biophysical characterization, Lab Chip 13 (13) (2013) 2464–2483.
[61] R.K. Avery, et al., An injectable shear-thinning biomaterial for endovascular embolization, Sci Transl Med 8 (365) (2016) 365ra156.
[62] C.-M. Ho, Y.-C. Tai, Micro-electro-mechanical-systems (MEMS) and fluid flows, Annu Rev Fluid Mech 30 (1) (1998) 579–612.
[63] Y. Su, G. Chen, Q. Yuan, Effect of viscosity on the hydrodynamics of liquid processes in microchannels, Chem Eng Technol 37 (3) (2014) 427–434.
[64] Z. Che, Y.F. Yap, T. Wang, Flow structure of compound droplets moving in microchannels, Phys Fluids 30 (1) (2018) 012114.

[65] S. Nagrath, et al., Isolation of rare circulating tumour cells in cancer patients by microchip technology, Nature 450 (7173) (2007) 1235.
[66] Z. Hayat, A. El Abed, High-throughput optofluidic acquisition of microdroplets in microfluidic systems, Micromachines 9 (4) (2018) 183.
[67] S. Bose, et al., Affinity flow fractionation of cells via transient interactions with asymmetric molecular patterns, Sci Rep 3 (2013) 2329.
[68] M. Abdelgawad, et al., Microfluidic platform with circular microchannels for facile cell trapping and single cell analysis, in: Proceedings of 14th international conference on miniaturized systems for chemistry and life science, 2010.
[69] S.C. Hur, A.J. Mach, D. Di Carlo, High-throughput size-based rare cell enrichment using microscale vortices, Biomicrofluidics 5 (2) (2011) 022206.
[70] Y. Yang, et al., paper-based microfluidic devices: emerging themes and applications, Anal Chem 89 (1) (2016) 71–91.
[71] A. Rundberg, Superhydrophobic surfaces for microfluidic applications, 2018.
[72] J.P. Lafleur, et al., Recent advances in lab-on-a-chip for biosensing applications, Biosens Bioelectron 76 (2016) 213–233.
[73] J. Liu, et al., An integrated impedance biosensor platform for detection of pathogens in poultry products, Sci Rep 8 (1) (2018) 16109.
[74] A. López-Córdoba, J.M. Lagarón, S. Goyanes, Fabrication of electrospun and electrosprayed carriers for the delivery of bioactive food ingredients, in: G.W. Smithers (Ed.), Reference module in food science, Elsevier, Amsterdam, The Netherlands, 2018.
[75] S. Jahanshahi-Anbuhi, et al., Design rules for fluorocarbon-free omniphobic solvent barriers in paper-based devices, ACS Appl Mater Interfaces 7 (45) (2015) 25434–25440.
[76] P. He, et al., Engineering fluidic delays in paper-based devices using laser direct-writing, Lab Chip 15 (20) (2015) 4054–4061.
[77] S.M. Hong, et al., Hydrophilic surface modification of PDMS using atmospheric RF plasma, J Phys Conf Ser 34 (2006) 108.
[78] A. Tropmann, et al., Completely superhydrophobic PDMS surfaces for microfluidics, Langmuir 28 (22) (2012) 8292–8295.
[79] A.S. Chan, et al., A simple microfluidic chip design for fundamental bioseparation, J Anal Methods Chem 2014 (2014), https://doi.org/10.1155/2014/175457.
[80] A. Bhattacharyya, C.M. Klapperich, Differential gene expression using mRNA isolated on plastic microfluidic chips, in: Engineering in medicine and biology society, 2009. EMBC 2009. Annual international conference of the IEEE, IEEE, 2009.
[81] X. Li, D.R. Ballerini, W. Shen, A perspective on paper-based microfluidics: current status and future trends, Biomicrofluidics 6 (1) (2012) 011301.
[82] Y. Jiang, et al., A simple method for fabrication of microfluidic paper-based analytical devices and on-device fluid control with a portable corona generator, RSC Adv 6 (4) (2016) 2888–2894.
[83] A. Malvandi, S. Moshizi, D. Ganji, Two-component heterogeneous mixed convection of alumina/water nanofluid in microchannels with heat source/sink, Adv Powder Technol 27 (1) (2016) 245–254.
[84] J. Keener, et al., Use of mathematical modeling to study pressure regimes in normal and Fontan blood flow circulations, arXiv preprint arXiv:1806.02416, 2018.
[85] A. Mouza, et al., A simplified model for predicting friction factors of laminar blood flow in small-caliber vessels, Fluids 3 (4) (2018) 75.
[86] S. Waheed, et al., 3D printed microfluidic devices: enablers and barriers, Lab Chip 16 (11) (2016) 1993–2013.

[87] S. Prentner, et al., Effects of channel surface finish on blood flow in microfluidic devices, Microsyst Technol 16 (7) (2010) 1091–1096.
[88] S. Yang, H. Fu, B. Yu, Fractal analysis of flow resistance in tree-like branching networks with roughened microchannels, Fractals 25 (01) (2017) 1750008.
[89] B. Chen, F. Guo, H. Xiang, Visualization study of motion and deformation of red blood cells in a microchannel with straight, divergent and convergent sections, J Biol Phys 37 (4) (2011) 429–440.
[90] T. Bayraktar, S.B. Pidugu, Characterization of liquid flows in microfluidic systems, Int J Heat Mass Transf 49 (5-6) (2006) 815–824.
[91] J.S. Kuo, D.T. Chiu, Controlling mass transport in microfluidic devices, Annu Rev Anal Chem 4 (2011) 275–296.
[92] D. Tripathi, A. Sharma, O.A. Bég, Electrothermal transport of nanofluids via peristaltic pumping in a finite micro-channel: effects of Joule heating and Helmholtz-Smoluchowski velocity, Int J Heat Mass Transf 111 (2017) 138–149.
[93] S. Mashaghi, et al., Droplet microfluidics: a tool for biology, chemistry and nanotechnology, TrAC Trends Anal Chem 82 (2016) 118–125.
[94] J. Xu, et al., Enhancement of mass transfer performance of liquid–liquid system by droplet flow in microchannels, Chem Eng J 141 (1-3) (2008) 242–249.
[95] J. Burns, C. Ramshaw, The intensification of rapid reactions in multiphase systems using slug flow in capillaries, Lab Chip 1 (1) (2001) 10–15.
[96] M. Ueno, et al., Phase-transfer alkylation reactions using microreactors, Chem Commun (8) (2003) 936–937.
[97] S.A. Khan, et al., Microfluidic synthesis of colloidal silica, Langmuir 20 (20) (2004) 8604–8611.
[98] B. Zheng, J.D. Tice, R.F. Ismagilov, Formation of droplets of alternating composition in microfluidic channels and applications to indexing of concentrations in droplet-based assays, Anal Chem 76 (17) (2004) 4977–4982.
[99] L. Campo-Deaño, et al., Viscoelasticity of blood and viscoelastic blood analogues for use in polydymethylsiloxane in vitro models of the circulatory system, Biomicrofluidics 7 (3) (2013) 034102.
[100] R. Paul, et al., Shear stress related blood damage in laminar couette flow, Artif Organs 27 (6) (2003) 517–529.
[101] H. Bruus, Acoustofluidics 1: Governing equations in microfluidics, Lab Chip 11 (22) (2011) 3742–3751.
[102] D. Tripathi, et al., Study of microvascular non-Newtonian blood flow modulated by electroosmosis, Microvasc Res 117 (2018) 28–36.
[103] A. Prindle, et al., Ion channels enable electrical communication in bacterial communities, Nature 527 (7576) (2015) 59.
[104] M. Tang, et al., Enhancement of electrical signaling in neural networks on graphene films, Biomaterials 34 (27) (2013) 6402–6411.
[105] M.E. Spira, A. Hai, Multi-electrode array technologies for neuroscience and cardiology, Nat Nanotechnol 8 (2) (2013) 83.
[106] V. Lovat, et al., Carbon nanotube substrates boost neuronal electrical signaling, Nano Lett 5 (6) (2005) 1107–1110.
[107] W. Xi, et al., Soft tubular microfluidics for 2D and 3D applications, Proc Natl Acad Sci 114 (40) (2017) 10590–10595.
[108] A.B. Shrirao, et al., Microfluidic platforms for the study of neuronal injury in vitro, Biotechnol Bioeng 115 (4) (2018) 815–830.

[109] G.N. Eloy, H.B. Barbara, S. Helder, plataforma reusable de ensamblaje de capilares de vidrio para micro fluidos, ES 2 626 263 A1, OFICINA ESPANOLA DE PATENTES Y MARCAS, 2017.
[110] B. Herranz-Blanco, et al., Microfluidic assembly of multistage porous silicon–lipid vesicles for controlled drug release, Lab Chip 14 (6) (2014) 1083–1086.
[111] J. Song, et al., Instrument-free point-of-care molecular detection of Zika virus, Anal Chem 88 (14) (2016) 7289–7294.

CHAPTER

Microarray technologies

4

Mohammad Rabiee[a,*], Azin Rostami[a], Navid Rabiee[b], and Mojtaba Bagherzadeh[b]

[a]*Biomaterials Group, Department of Biomedical Engineering, Amirkabir University of Technology, Tehran, Iran*

[b]*Department of Chemistry, Sharif University of Technology, Tehran, Iran*

**Corresponding author. E-mail: mrabiee@aut.ac.ir*

4.1 Introduction

Diagnostic methods are of great importance in biochemistry and clinical research. In recent years, extensive research and rapid developments have occurred in this branch of science. One of the impressive achievements that have been made in biology and clinical laboratory science is the use of microarrays, which are rapidly becoming more widely used than traditional methods due to their sensitivity and ease of use.

Microarrays are now widely used in research and clinical laboratories around the world for applications such as disease detection, nutrigenomics, plant biology, genetically altered foods, drug discovery and development, profiling biochemical pathways, large scale genotyping, gene expression profiling, etc.

All of these capabilities are due to the ability of microarrays to provide rapid, in vitro, parallel, and accurate analysis of large numbers of samples, or to detect a large number of molecules simultaneously [1–3].

In general terms, microarrays can be defined as devices which are constructed of a solid substrate such as a glass slide or a silicon chip, on which biological elements or capture molecules (recognition agents) are immobilized in a regular pattern (or array) on their surface. The system is equipped with biological capture or recognition agents, such as cDNA fragments, oligonucleotides, proteins, antibodies, aptamers, whole cells, or tissue fragments. These microscopic spots in the pattern are the critical parts of the microarray. They act as diagnostic probes for identifying genetic or biochemical molecular interactions and the spatial encoding allows multiplexing [2, 4, 5].

Microfluidic technology is a novel method employing microscale structures, which can have many advantages when combined with other scientific technologies. By merging the concept of microfluidics with microarrays, a new field called microfluidic arrays was introduced. Microfluidic arrays can simultaneously take advantage of more efficient sample handling provided by the fluidic system, and the rapid and accurate detection provided by microarray technology.

Biomedical Applications of Microfluidic Devices. https://doi.org/10.1016/B978-0-12-818791-3.00012-7

Sample detection in microfluidic arrays starts with a question. The question is, whether the analyte in question is present, and if so in what amount? Every single detail about the nature and behavior of the analyte and the biological significance is important. The next topic to be considered is the experimental design. There are so many systematic or random errors that may play a part in the detection performance. Factors such as the constituent materials of the substrate, the microfluidics structure and pattern, the ability of the microfluidic system to deliver the sample and reagents accurately, the functional groups on the surface, the biological recognition elements to detect the analyte, proper labeling for final detection and readout, etc. It is important to identify and control the source of noise, normalize the values, and make them comparable. The final step is statistical analysis and interpretation of the obtained results [1].

The introduction of microfluidics to microarray systems, has led to many beneficial consequences, such as decreases in the experimental time, minimizing reagent and sample consumption, high throughput sample analysis, providing a proper environment for sensitive samples, and so on.

To provide an efficient microfluidic array system, different scientific expertise, including physics, chemistry, biochemistry, optics, microfabrication, and bioinformatics are required. Microfluidic arrays are typically made up of microscale objects that are used for clinical diagnosis and measurements [6–8].

In the following sections, the concept of microarray technology and the main types of microarrays are discussed, and an overview of the combination of microarrays and microfluidics and, its application to biology and clinical diagnosis is presented.

4.2 What are microarrays?

Microarrays are a powerful diagnostic technology, which has gathered widespread applications in clinical laboratories around the world. The main function of this analytical device is the rapid and simultaneous screening of biological materials for their detection and amount. One of the main features of this device is its high sensitivity and the accuracy of the analytical results. Another key point is the ability to analyze multiple samples in a single test chip. The obtained results from microarrays help understand complex biological systems, in drug discovery, and for elucidating the molecular basis of diseases [2, 9, 10].

Microarrays are a biosensing technology consisting of a solid substrate like a plastic or glass slide covered by molecular capture probes or biological elements that are spatially arrayed in a defined micropattern. For the analysis, a small amount of sample is exposed to the array under the correct conditions for hybridization and interaction between the capture probe and the analyte. For reporting the occurrence and quantification of the target binding, different methods have been employed [2, 5, 11].

An elementary semi-microarray was first produced in 1979 and called a "dotted blot." The density of the spots in this device was quite low due to the poor performance of the spotting equipment used at that time. For this reason, there was only a small number of capture probes in each specified area. Therefore, the device was incapable of gaining enough data for complex analyses. As one example, to measure the gene expression of 40,000 different mRNAs, 160 arrayed microscope slides were required, making the analysis highly inefficient in terms of time and money.

Another traditional approach used microtiter plates, called a "microtiter plate solid-phase assay." In this technique, different capture molecules were placed in each well of a microtiter plate by pouring 100–200 μL of a solution containing the capture molecules. After removing the excess capture molecules by washing the solution containing the analyte was added. After additional washing steps, the unhybridized sample was removed and the analysis was performed. The main disadvantage of this technique was the relatively large amount of capture molecules compared to the concentration of analyte molecules causing a low signal to noise ratio.

Advanced microarray technology has allowed rapid analysis of different biological molecules simultaneously, with high accuracy and sensitivity [3, 12].

Some steps are essential to be taken to use microarray technology: (1) sample preparation which could include labeling steps; (2) hybridization; (3) washing steps; (4) optical scanning (absorption or fluorescence); (5) data analysis [4, 9].

For an accurate diagnosis with a microarray, there must be an appropriate experimental design, which means correct selection of the substrate, capture molecules, labels, linkers, blocking procedures, etc. The selection and immobilization of capture molecules play a key role in designing a microarray. Capture molecules are responsible for the recognition of the analyte molecule in the sample by interacting with it. The main property of a capture molecule is selective recognition of the target molecule, which is achieved by the chemical affinity between the two molecules. The capture probes could be one of the several biological molecules, like PCR products (nucleic acid sequences), DNA/RNA aptamers, oligonucleotides, proteins, antibodies, small molecules, or carbohydrates depending on the goal of the microarray.

Immobilization of various kinds of capture probes on a single slide of a microarray provides a parallel analysis of different targets in the sample in a single test. On the surface of a microarray chip, there are a large number of spots each containing several copies of each single capture molecule. The spots are spatially coded to allow identification. As shown in Fig. 4.1 each spot is specified by its coordinates in a 2D array, for instance, in a particular array it is clear that the spot with the coordinates (X1/Y1) named A1, contains capture probes that interact with gene G [3].

Generally, the capture probes immobilized on the solid substrate are exposed to the labeled sample under conditions including, specific buffers, temperatures, or linkers to allow hybridization of these two complementary molecules. If the hybridization occurs, this means that the target molecules are immobilized in the same spot as the capture molecules. To remove unbound or cross-hybridized molecules, washing steps must be carried out. After the washing steps, only the hybridized target molecules remain on the surface of the microarray.

Labels are used to visualize the location of the bound target molecules. By this approach, the colored or fluorescent spots on the surface of the microarray (after the

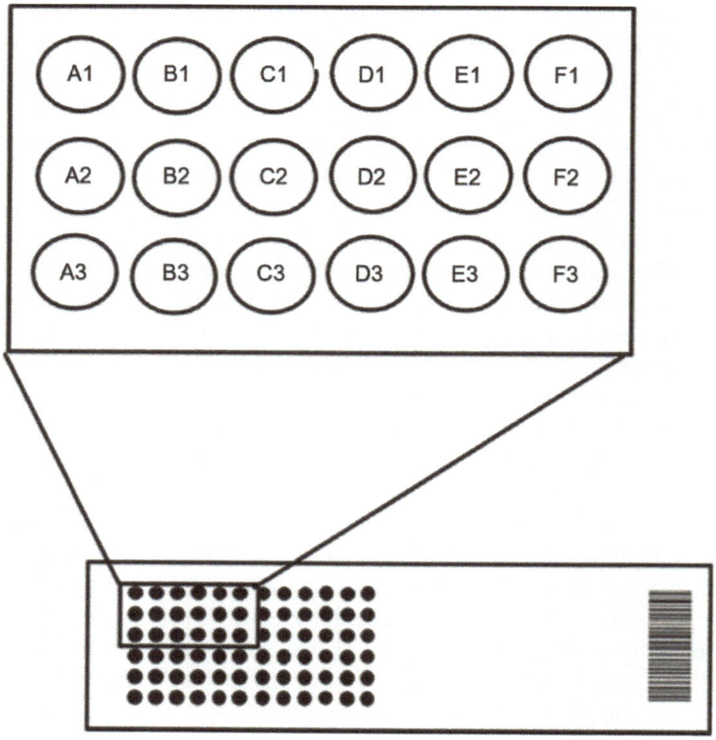

FIG. 4.1

Schematic view of micro spots arrangement in a microarray [1].

Reprinted with permission from Elsevier.

washing steps) indicate the location of the hybridized target molecules. The light signal produced by the labels is then analyzed by scanning photometry methods and each bright spot shows the presence of the target molecule in the sample. Typically, labels are chosen from fluorophores or dyes and the labeling step can be done pre or post hybridization [3–5, 11]. Optimization of microarray protocols includes the patterning of the microarray and the experimental design, immobilization of capture molecules, biorecognition and hybridization of capture and target molecules, scanning, and finally data processing steps [2, 10, 13].

Microarrays can be classified into four general groups depending on their application and their capture probes: (1) DNA microarrays; (2) protein microarrays; (3) cell microarrays; and (4) tissue microarrays.

DNA microarray technology can provide the ability to identify novel compounds and accelerate the discovery of drugs for the treatment of serious diseases like cancer, AIDS, infections, etc. DNA microarrays can analyze genome-wide gene expression patterns and compare gene expression levels in two different samples under or under different conditions. DNA microarrays allow researchers to study the pattern of gene expression in many assays looking at different cellular responses and conditions. Gene expression profiling provides a wealth of data that can be used to develop a more complete understanding of the regulation of gene function in samples from normal and diseased individuals, and in samples from different drug treatment regimens [14–16].

DNA microarrays have different applications in drug discovery and development investigations. For example, identification and validation of antiinfective and anticancer drug targets, mechanisms of drug action and drug metabolism, classification of different types of tumors, identification of protective responses in the host, use of molecular signatures for prediction of disease outcome, and the study of pathogenesis to identify potential new targets for antiinfective drugs [15, 17].

On the other hand, protein microarrays are increasingly being used in drug discovery for a wide range of applications. In recent years many academic research or medical laboratories and industrial biotechnology companies are starting to use antibody arrays in the field of drug discovery. Drug discovery and development includes various aspects like target identification, molecular mechanisms of drug action on the specific target, mechanisms of drug resistance, drug side effects, and applications in clinical trials and in managing patient care. All of these fields can be helped by protein profiling with antibody microarray technology. Antibody arrays have been developed as a novel and helpful approach for drug discovery with a focus on protein activity and behavior in cell biology and disease development. Advanced studies have shown that protein microarrays can give much information about the physiological and pathologic states of organs, tissue, or cells, and can be more accurate and detailed than DNA gene expression microarrays. There are important issues related to proteins and proteomic analysis, which may play a key role in monitoring disease development or progression, and to investigate the drug mechanism of action if the drug affects protein localization, structure, interactions, activities, or function. Proteomic analysis and identification of the expressed proteins could accelerate drug discovery. Protein microarrays can help the progress of drug discovery in different ways such as identification of potential targets, gaining new insight into disease processes, investigation of the molecular mechanisms of drug action, and comparing different drugs to study their effects against the disease, understanding the mechanism of drug resistance, improving drug efficacy during treatment, providing insight into the response to particular drugs or drug combinations, discovering new methods for drug delivery, and advanced study of the pharmacological side effects of drugs [18].

The three main types of microarrays are covered in the next sections.

4.2.1 DNA microarrays

In biology and life sciences, the study of genomics and gene expression in various living organisms has been of great importance. Genomics refers to the entire set of genetic information contained in any organism, and be categorized into structural and functional genomics [2].

There have been many limited and imperfect techniques, but which nevertheless have been used to determine genomic information, e.g., Northern blots. The discovery of microarrays has led to significant advances in genetic sciences, enabling the analysis of gene expression, gene variation, and whole-genome sequencing, that can be carried out simultaneously and also in parallel for thousands of different genes [11]. Additionally, this innovative technology has led to a substantial decline in sequencing costs [4].

In a DNA microarray, the basic principle of detection is the interaction between nucleotide base sequences in DNA strands. Capture probes could be made of sequences of a single strand DNA including 20–1000 bases covalently immobilized on a solid substrate like a glass slide, and acting as elements to hybridize added cDNA or mRNA samples [2, 19].

For sample preparation, the DNA or RNA should be extracted from the desired cells or tissue. The extracted DNA or RNA could be used directly after fragmentation and PCR steps, or in the case of RNA extraction, it could be reverse transcribed to produce cDNA. To detect the occurrence of hybridization between the probes and the target, a labeling step is required. There are two labeling approaches in DNA microarrays: in the first approach, the target nucleic acids are labeled by a linker (e.g., biotin), which can interact with an added fluorescent-labeled moiety (e.g., streptavidin). After the appliance of the sample to the microarray slide and washing, the label is added to interact with the linker attached to the target molecule (DNA fragment, RNA fragment, cDNA fragment). In the second approach, the target is directly attached to the fluorophore and then added to the microarray slide.

In both cases, a washing step is necessary after the hybridization and labeling, to eliminate unhybridized molecules and remove the excess fluorophores.

At the end of the experiment, only the hybridized molecules are detectable by their fluorescent labels. The fluorophores are usually excited by scanning laser a photodetector to measure the intensity of the signals and convert them to quantitative data using image analysis. Fig. 4.2 shows the general steps of an RNA microarray test for gene expression in the biological sample [1, 4, 11].

4.2.1.1 Fabrication methods for DNA microarrays

DNA microarrays use cDNA or DNA fragments or oligonucleotide as capture probes that are immobilized on the surface of the array. There are two general approaches available for manufacturing these biochips. In the first approach, the capture molecules are prepared first and then printed onto the substrate. In the second approach, the capture molecules are synthesized in situ on the surface of the slide. The manufacturing process of DNA microarrays is important due to its influence on the accuracy of the results. If the results obtained from two arrays using the same sample and the same experimental procedure differ from one another, it can be concluded that there must have been an error in the fabrication method [1, 12].

In the 1990s the first microarrays were manufactured using a spotting method. In this technique, the desired nucleotide sequences are first synthesized and then applied on the glass substrate by special spotting probes. The genetic data needed for

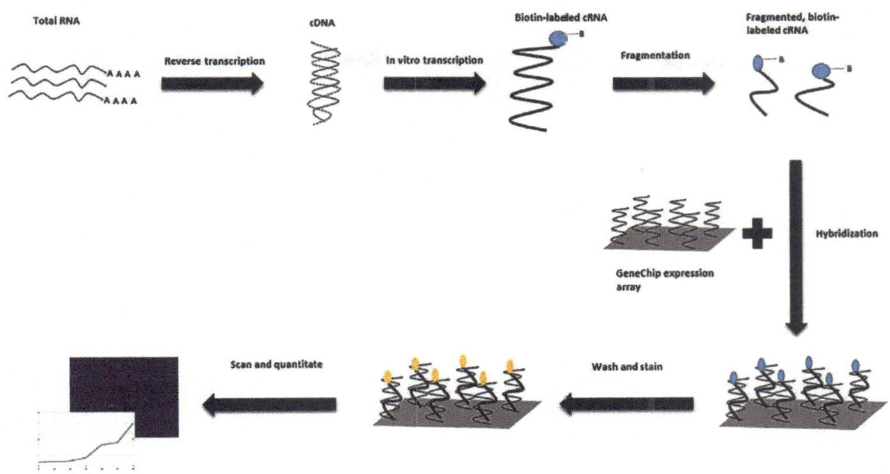

FIG. 4.2

Schematic of the general steps in a microarray device experiment for gene expression by extraction of the RNA from the sample: the experiment starts with reverse transcription of RNA to cDNA. In the next step, the double-stranded cDNA is converted to single strand biotinylated cRNA. Afterward, the biotin-labeled cRNA undergoes a fragmentation step before hybridization with the capture molecules. To eliminate the unhybridized molecules a washing step, and to visualize the binding a labeling step is necessary. Finally, the signals from the fluorophores are detected by scanning the microarray slide [1].

Reprinted with permission from Elsevier.

sequencing the capture probes for diagnosis of a special target is obtained from a gene information database called Genebank.

The glass substrates in this method are similar to glass microscope slides, that have been coated with polylysine for attaching the probes to the surface by the interaction between the functional groups of the surface and the DNA or oligonucleotide probe. There are also other methods for attaching the capture probes, such as aldehyde or acrylamide-based coatings. After spotting the probes a blocking step is required to prevent any interaction between the remaining functional groups on the surface with target molecules.

The capture probe spots are in the range of 50–150 μm printed by an automated spotting device or robot. There are various methods for printing and spotting oligonucleotides or DNAs which are categorized into two main groups: (1) noncontact printing which operates similar to an inkjet printer, including piezoelectric printing or syringe solenoid printing technology; and (2) contact dispensing including the pin printing technique.

Spotted arrays are very sensitive, especially if probes with long nucleotide sequences are used which can lead to a more specific hybridization. On the other hand, this feature causes an increase in the amount of cross-hybridization and reduces the reproducibility rate [2, 3, 11, 20].

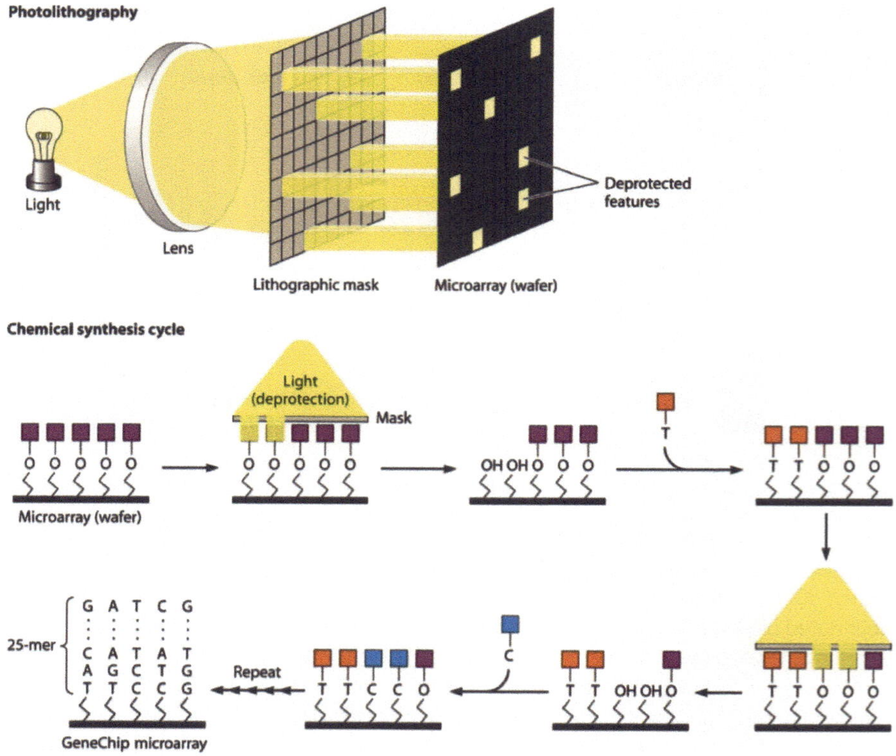

FIG. 4.3

Procedure for the production of Affymetrix oligonucleotide microarrays with the use of photolithography technology [11].

Reprinted with permission from Elsevier.

Because of this issue the Affymetrix company introduced a new method to produce microarrays using photolithography technology, which rapidly became successful in biological and medical applications. In this technique, the capture probes are synthesized on the surface of the microarray in situ.

In this method, the surface of the array is functionalized with molecules, which can interact with nucleotide bases, for example, by modifying the surface with silanes providing hydroxyl groups available for interaction with nucleobases. Next, a protective layer of material such as MeNPOC is reacted with the hydroxyl groups, preventing the interaction between the hydroxyls and the nucleotide bases. This protective layer can be removed by exposure to UV light, thus exposing the hydroxyl group which is activated for bonding to nucleotide bases. As shown in Fig. 4.3 a photolithographic mask covers the locations, which should not bind the nucleotide bases added to the surface. For example, in the first step, the G base will be added to the probes at specific sites. The mask covers other probes for preventing the interaction with the G base, but the probes not covered will lose their protector molecule due to the exposure to UV light, and the G base is attached to the probe site. This procedure can be repeated for up to 70 times to create maximum 25-mer oligonucleotides as capture probes on the array. The advantage of this method is its good reproducibility and the high density of oligonucleotide capture probes. The main downside of this technique is the limitation in the length of the probes which cannot be longer than 25-mers in each sequence [2, 11].

Another method for producing gene microarrays was introduced by Roche NimbleGen and Agilent Technologies, which are both able to produce oligonucleotide probes containing 60–100 base pairs. The Nimblegen method also relies on photolithography technology but instead of a photolithographic mask, a virtual digital mask is created using a digital micromirror device that reflects a pattern of UV light and deprotects the desired oligonucleotides for the addition of the next base. The Agilent technology uses inkjet printing of the bases onto the substrate one by one. In this method, the first row of bases is immobilized on the modified surface by a noncontact inkjet printer, and the succeeding bases are released from the noncontact printing probe to bind at the specific site. The addition of bases continues sequentially until the desired number of base pairs (usually up to 60) in each oligonucleotide is achieved [2, 11].

4.2.2 Protein microarrays

Proteins play a key role in all living systems' manner by mediating cellular reactions and processes. There is, therefore, a great need for studies of the structure and function of proteins, to understand their biological function as catalysts and biomarkers. The term proteomics describes the analysis of proteins for their expression levels, function, structure, and interactions. Proteomics is important for discovering the origin and presence of diseases and also for screening drug delivery systems. Even a small disturbance in the function of various proteins can cause many diseases such as cancer, diabetes, etc.

In recent decades microarray technology has been used for high throughput rapid analysis of thousands of different proteins. The emphasis of this emerging technology is on proteomics encompassing protein expression, biomolecular interactions, drug discovery, diagnosis of disease, and vaccine development. Although this technology still has not advanced as far as DNA microarrays, improvement in proteomics has still had a big impact on life science and medicine.

Radioimmunoassay (RIA) and enzyme-linked immunosorbent assay (ELISA) were the first types of immunoassay technologies, which then led to the emergence of protein microarrays [2, 9, 21–24].

Generally, there are three types of protein microarrays.

4.2.2.1 Analytical protein microarrays

Analytical protein microarrays are the most common type of protein microarrays. Their focus is on protein expression and protein binding affinity, which has a wide application in medical diagnosis. These types of microarrays are suitable for comparison of protein expression profiles in different samples. For instance, to understand the effect of a drug on a special cell type, cell lysates obtained from control cells, and experimental cells can be compared by analytical protein microarrays.

In this technique, a library of probes such as antibodies, aptamers, or affibodies are immobilized on the surface of the microarray substrate. These are designed to bind specifically to their complementary protein targets. To understand the presence and function of proteins as well as their binding affinity within a complex sample, the sample solution and the capture probes are mixed. In other words, the capture molecules are probed by the analyte molecules. To understand interactions between the probe molecules and the target proteins, label-free techniques (such as mass spectrometry or surface plasmon resonance) or chemical labeling techniques can be used. There are two methods available for chemical labeling, direct labeling, and a sandwich assay. These two labeling methods are mainly used in antibody arrays. In the direct labeling or analyte labeled technique, all the proteins in the sample are first labeled with a fluorescent molecule and then applied to the capture antibodies immobilized on the surface of the microarray. If the interaction occurs after the washing steps the fluorophores labeled to the attached analyte molecules, emit light, and generate luminescent spots for data analysis. Some challenges must be overcome in this method, as the lack of specificity in target protein labeling may lead to a decrease in sensitivity. Due to this problem, the sandwich technique has been proposed by researchers to provide higher sensitivity and specificity. In this method, two antibodies are used to interact with the target protein. The first antibody is immobilized on the surface of the microarray and interacts with the target protein. After the washing steps, the second antibody that is labeled by a fluorescent molecule is allowed to interact with a different epitope of the bound target protein. This second labeled antibody is called the reporter or detection antibody and generates the signal for the analysis steps.

4.2.2.2 Functional protein microarrays

In functional protein microarrays, all of the full-length proteins contained in an organism are immobilized on the substrate of the microarray. In this method, the study of biochemical properties of the entire proteome in a single test is possible, due to the use of individually purified proteins. This method permits monitoring of protein interactions and binding activities such as protein-protein, protein-DNA, protein-lipid, protein-drug, protein-peptide, protein-RNA, protein-phospholipid, protein-small molecule, protein-drug, lectin-glycan and lectin-cell interactions, enzyme-substrate relationships, and immune responses.

The principal challenge in this technique is the sensitivity of the proteins. Proteins are widely considered to be very sensitive to their environmental conditions. The portions must retain their native structure during the fabrication process of the protein microarray. If the structure of the protein changes during this process, the interactions will be affected, so the results may not be reliable. One of the solutions to this problem is using affinity tags or linkers to increase the specificity of the interactions, and as a result, obtain a higher signal to noise ratio.

4.2.2.3 Reverse phase microarrays

Reverse phase microarrays are an alternative format of analytical protein microarrays. In this method, cells are isolated from the desired tissue and are then lysed. The lysates or fractionated lysates are then immobilized on a nitrocellulose or glass substrate using a contact pin microarrayer device. This technique aims to recognize a particular target protein on the surface of the cell. For reaching this goal, the lysates are probed by complementary labeled antibodies against the intended target proteins. Additionally, reference peptides could be applied to the surface of the microarray to quantify the results. Reverse phase microarrays are used to determine altered or inefficient proteins or protein pathways. This can help with the diagnosis of diseases, and selecting the proper therapy or drug to affect the desired protein [22–28].

4.2.2.4 Fabrication of protein microarrays

There are some main challenges applicable to the manufacture of a protein microarray:

1. As mentioned before, protein molecules are very sensitive to the environmental conditions and are often denatured in solid-liquid and liquid-air borders.
2. There is no amplification method available for proteins in the same way as PCR functions in DNA microarrays, so all of the proteins must be isolated from the original eukaryotic or prokaryotic organisms, which makes both the sample and the capture probes valuable and difficult to obtain.
3. There is a high probability of cross-reactivity between proteins.
4. The biological activity and functionality of proteins may be lost due to incorrect bonding to the surface of the microarray.

The chemistry of the substrate and the manufacturing process plays a key role in overcoming these obstacles. An ideal substrate for immobilizing the proteins should have several features: maintaining the three dimensional (3D) conformation and functionality of the proteins, preventing the protein denaturation, orienting the protein in the proper direction so that the desired interaction sites are accessible for achieving maximum binding capacity, providing a hydrophilic environment and a long shelf life for proteins, and also allowing a high signal to noise ratio.

Protein chips are prepared on a solid carrier, in the same way as DNA microarrays, including microscope glass slides, silicone, or nitrocellulose slides. The most important factor for arraying the proteins on the solid substrate is the chemistry of the substrate surface. It is vital to consider the orientation of the proteins on the carrier, whether random or uniform? The orientation of the proteins can affect both their affinity and activity. There are three main approaches for providing the proper surface chemistry for immobilizing the proteins.

(a) Covalent immobilization

In covalent immobilization, the hydroxyl groups on the surface of the glass slide are treated with the surface grafted ligands bearing reactive functional groups, such as aldehyde, epoxy, ester, etc. These functional groups can react with the available amine groups in the protein and form a Schiff base linkage. After the attachment of the capture proteins to the surface, the remaining unreacted functional groups are blocked with buffers containing compounds like bovine serum albumin (BSA) or glycine. This technique is suitable for immobilization of a broad range of proteins, but the orientation of the proteins is somewhat random in this method. Additionally, the covalent bond between the capture protein and the surface could affect the chemical reactivity of the protein and consequently cause nonspecific binding to the target molecule.

(b) Noncovalent adsorption

In this method, the surface of the solid substrate is coated with nitrocellulose, gel pads, poly-L-lysine, polyvinylidene fluoride (PVDF), polystyrene, or another substance. The capture proteins are adsorbed physically and passively onto the surface of the microarray. For the coating of these materials to the substrate in a thin layer, physical vapor deposition (PVD) and chemical vapor deposition (CVD) techniques are employed. Although in the noncovalent adsorption technique the proteins are not covalently bonded to the array so their chemical properties and structure will not change, the amount and orientation of the proteins cannot be precisely controlled in this method.

(c) Affinity capture

The affinity capture technique not only minimizes any alteration in the structure and function of the proteins but also overcomes the orientation issue by applying affinity tags for immobilizing the proteins on the surface of the array. The outcome of protein attachment with this method is a uniformly oriented array of capture proteins on the substrate. For instance, the surface can be treated with streptavidin molecules for specific attachment to biotinylated capture proteins. Another popular approach is to coat the glass slide with nickel NTA to bind to HisX6 tagged target proteins.

As mentioned in the production of DNA microarrays, the arraying process is typically done by a contact spotter or a noncontact microarrayer device. This technique employs intricate emerging technologies and robots, such as robotic contact printing, photolithography, inkjet printing, piezoelectric spotting, etc.

The presence of an aqueous environment in all the manufacturing and experimental steps is necessary to avoid protein denaturation. For creating a hydrophilic and aqueous environment, all of the sample buffers should contain a considerable amount of glycerol, and also the immobilization process should be carried out while the humidity environment is regulated carefully [2, 25, 26, 28].

4.2.3 Cell microarrays

One of the important developments in microarray technology is the use of whole live cells as sensing elements and as a source for the target molecules. This technology allows multiplex analysis for understanding cellular responses, behavior, and change in phenotype by analyzing changes in the intended biomolecules. This technology can offer functional analysis as well as analytical analysis as an alternative to conventional nucleic acid and protein microarrays. The term functional analysis means the study of the physiological effect of proteins on the behavior and function of the cells in the body. Initially, these cell-based tests were performed using multiwell plates but miniaturization led to the preparation of cell-based microarrays. To achieve this goal there are two methods available for the immobilization of cells to create a cell-based assay. In the first method, different types of cells are attached to a flat surface (planar arrays or positional arrays), and in the second method, the cells are immobilized on the surface of small particles present in a solution (solution or suspension arrays) [29].

Positional or planar cell microarrays are usually produced by similar methods to protein and DNA microarrays, and then the microspots containing cells are located on the substrate of the array by physical spotting methods or by photolithography. Solution or suspension microarrays contain thousands of microparticles suspended in a liquid. The desired cells are immobilized on the surface of these particles. Suspension microarrays have great flexibility and the capability for multiplexing. In planar or positional arrays the immobilization of different kinds of cells on a single substrate to achieve a multiplexed cell microarray is difficult, due to practical limitations and the complex process. On the other hand, in the case of suspension microarrays, different preparations containing cell-attached microparticles can be mixed to create the final suspension array. To identify the individual microparticles which carry each cell type, the microparticles can be encoded by optical, electrical, or photophysical methods [30–32].

To multiplex these microarrays for high throughput screening and simultaneous assays of different samples, cell microarrays can be combined with microfluidic systems, and also optical or electrical detection systems can be introduced [33].

One of the key points in producing a cell microarray is the physical and chemical properties of the surface of the microarray substrate. The surface of a cell microarray should have proper properties for the attachment, proliferation, and differentiation of living cells. Moreover, the storage conditions and environment of printed living cell microarrays must be considered because of the sensitivity of live cells [2, 34].

4.3 Microfluidic arrays

Microfluidics can provide many advantages in combination with other scientific technologies. By merging microfluidics with microarrays, the new field of microfluidic arrays was introduced. Microfluidic arrays simultaneously take advantage of the more efficient sample handling of fluidic systems, as well as the rapid and accurate diagnosis of microarray technology. To provide an efficient microfluidic array system, a collaboration of scientific fields, including physics, chemistry, biochemistry, and engineering is required. Microfluidic arrays are typically made up of microscale constructions making this device a valuable solution for clinical diagnosis and measurement of biomolecules [6–8].

4.3.1 Advantages of microfluidic array technology

Conventional microarrays suffer from a series of pitfalls. One of these limitations is the lengthy incubation times needed for the hybridization of target molecules with the capture probes immobilized on the surface of the microarray. In conventional microarrays, the target molecule (which is generally in solution) must diffuse to the surface of the array to interact with its complementary capture probe. Moreover, the target molecules must move a large distance across the array to encounter their proper capture probe. Due to the slow mass transfer, the incubation and processing time in conventional arrays can increase to several hours. Another downside of the conventional microarray method, is the high consumption of samples, due to the need for complete coverage of the array surface and all of the capture probes by the sample solution. The diagnostic samples used in these experiments are obtained from the human body by a complex, expensive, and time-consuming procedure, which makes them very valuable. The addition of microfluidics to microarray systems leads to many beneficial consequences, which could overcome the mentioned obstacles. Firstly, the hybridization time is decreased due to the presence of microscale flow through the channels and pumps, which enhances the mass transfer by forced flow, and also the diffusional distance is reduced by the use of shallow microchannels. As a result, the incubation time for the interaction of capture probes and target molecules is significantly reduced to less than 1 min.

Pappaert et al. reported that in a microarray analysis that took 24 h, the binding efficiency was lower than 0.2%, and 6-day analysis time was required to raise the binding efficiency to 2% [8, 35, 36]. Another benefit of microfluidic arrays is the reduction of the sample volume and reagent consumption, due to the lower surface area needed to be covered by the sample. Using this method, the required sample volume could be reduced to 1 pL. Furthermore, microfluidic arrays provide the ability to analyze multiple samples simultaneously. Generally speaking, the direct comparison of samples on a single chip is very effective due to the small differences in a single assay, but larger differences from batch to batch. This is achieved by the integration of multiple fluidic channels and separate fluidic processors.

Nowadays, the early diagnosis of diseases is not as widespread as might be expected, because of the high price of the technology needed for these analyses. Using microfluidic arrays, a dramatic drop in the cost of assays could be expected due to mass production.

One of the most important points in protein microarray experiments is the maintenance of sufficient humidity, which is needed to prevent the denaturation of proteins during sample preparation and the microarray experimental steps. Microfluidic arrays can offer a suitable environment for proteins during the experiment due to closed architectures and special packaging systems. This closed system structure also eliminates the entrance of contaminants into the test environment. These contaminants can cause a remarkable increase in noise and false-positive signals [7, 8].

4.3.2 Disadvantages of microfluidic array technology

Although several advantages have been suggested for microfluidic arrays, there are also some disadvantages to this technology. By merging microfluidics and microarrays, the fabrication of the device becomes more complicated due to, material specification, fabrication method, and production costs. One point that should be considered is the large surface area covered by the small scale fluidic channels. The large surface area to volume ratio can cause surface effects, e.g., the adsorption of sample molecules to the surface. A high level of nonspecific adsorption in the sample can lead to false-positive results. To avoid this unwanted adsorption, some precautions should be taken. For example by selecting a substrate, which avoids nonspecific adsorption, or by using special dynamic or covalently-bonded coatings to eliminate this problem. On the other hand, the substrate itself should show no optical features to allow the reporter molecules to provide a sensitive readout. Polymers are generally attractive materials for making microfluidic systems owing to their low cost, versatility, and easy handling, but many polymers are not suitable to be used in a microarray system, especially when the fluorescent labeling readout is in the visible or near IR spectral region. Additionally, because of the comparatively small volumes of sample and reagents, and consequently the small number of target molecules, the microarray, and the signal transducer should be highly sensitive, and could be designed with the ability to analyze the sample even at the single-molecule level. Another important process in microfluidic arrays is the appliance of the sample and the reagents. Macrodevices such as conventional pipets are sometimes used for sample loading. As a result, for the proper analysis using microfluidic array systems, this source of error should be considered for increasing the accuracy of the obtained results [7].

4.3.3 Fabrication of microfluidic arrays

The design and fabrication techniques for microarrays was described in previous sections, but an important point in the manufacturing of a microfluidic array is the design and fabrication of the fluidic channels. The manufacturing of a microfluidic array system can use various materials and different methods. In a microfluidic system, the sample and reagents should flow through a series of microscale thin channels to reach the capture probes in the microarray area. Although the very small volume of the sample used increases the sensitivity of the system, it is still necessary that the sample and reagents transfer paths be as thin as possible to minimize the transfer time. When the channels and chambers are fabricated at the microscale, the surface area increases which may lead to an increase in nonspecific sample adsorption and also increased flow resistance, and as a result, the flow rate may not increase past a specific limit. To obtain the desired flow rate in the microchannels, several approaches are available such as electrokinetic control, centrifugal force, vacuum suction, and syringe pumping. The vacuum suction and syringe pumping techniques work with the help of pressure and are mostly used due to their compatibility with different media. The centrifugal force technique is mostly used in the case of parallel hybridization. In this method, the sample and reagents are driven by the force of a rotating disc and are directed by hydrophobic barriers.

In microfluidic systems, it is important to consider that the buffer solutions and reagents used in a microarray experiment often contain a large number of salts, which may lead to the corrosion of metallic components [7, 8, 37].

The most common materials used for the fabrication of microfluidic systems are, silicon, glass, or polymers. Glass and quartz substrates have good compatibility with the microfluidic arrays due to their suitable optical properties (transparency) and also their well-defined surface. The optical properties of the glass substrate have a great impact on the signal readout of the array when using fluorescent labeling techniques. The microfabrication techniques for producing microfluidic arrays using glass or quartz substrates include plasma etching, reactive ion etching, and lithography. Although these materials are suitable for microfluidic arrays, the fabrication techniques can be highly time-consuming, labor-intensive, and expensive.

Polymers have also been used to create microfluidic devices, as an alternative to glass and quartz substrates. The advantage of polymer materials is their capacity to be optimized according to the properties needed for the desired application. Additionally, they are appropriate for the microfabrication of structures in a microfluidic device, as well as having low cost. The techniques used for producing polymeric microfluidic channels and networks in a microfluidic array system include lithography, UV laser ablation, hot embossing, injection molding, or direct micromilling. In the hot embossing and injection molding method, there is a mold master is employed, which can stamp the desired microfluidic structures onto the substrate. The patterns can be created on the mold masters by micromachining or by a lithography-based method. The LIGA technique is one lithography-based method, which is used for the patterning of the mold masters and creating high aspect ratio microstructures. Liga is the German abbreviation for Lithographie Galvanoformun Abformun (Lithography Electroplating Molding). The processing steps required to prepare a microstructured mold master are X-ray LIGA and molding. The advantage of this technique is that although the process for making the mold master is time consuming, complex, and expensive, nevertheless this procedure needs to be undertaken only once, and after that many microfluidic devices could be mass-produced using this mold master by injection molding or hot embossing. In hot embossing, the polymeric substrate is placed between two metal plates, where one of them is the mold master containing the required micropattern on its surface. Then the system is heated till the temperature is above the glass transition temperature of the polymer, and after that, the metal plates compress the polymer substrate. This causes the micropattern to appear on the surface of the mold master plate stamp polymer substrate. This procedure can be completed in less than 5 min and also this technique is relatively inexpensive for mass production [7, 37].

Polydimethylsiloxane (PDMS) is a suitable material for the fabrication of microflow channels because of its high inertness in contact with biomolecules. PDMS is an elastomeric polymer that is useful to produce three-dimensional structures. The fabrication technique for producing microfluidic structures using PDMS is called soft lithography. In this method, a microstructured mold is filled with the prepolymer of PDMS and a curing agent. After curing and cross-linking are completed the PDMS has conformed to the shape of the relief and is removed. These steps result in a PDMS substrate containing microscale networks. Finally, the PDMS microfluidic structure is plasma oxidized to increase the hydrophilicity and is sealed by a pressing step.

Typically, after the microfluidic network is formed, a sealing step is needed to avoid leakage and entry of contaminants. This sealing could be by using a cover plate of the same material as the microfluidic substrate, or by the use of low temperature or high pressure.

Other methods for enclosing and sealing the microfluidic arrays include the use of adhesives or pressed flexible polymers. Adhesives are applied to single-use microfluidic arrays, but flexible polymers allow changing the microarray substrate. In the case of the polymers which need a pressing step for sealing the system, such as silicone and polytetrafluoroethylene (PTFE), the amount of applied pressure is important because if the pressure passes a certain limit, it may damage the flow cell [7, 37].

4.3.4 Automated microfluidic arrays (lab-on-a-chip systems)

The development of automated microfluidic arrays has become increasingly important for the potential to integrate various experimental steps in a single device. Microarray experiments typically include multiple sample preparation and fluid handling steps. In the conventional microarrays, all of these steps are carried out manually by the operator. This procedure is not only very time-consuming but also can increase the number of variables and errors. Automated platforms provide the integration of several manual steps including, sample preparation, delivery of sample and reagents, washing steps, hybridization, and detection into one automated system.

For gene expression assays an automated microfluidic device can provide a direct solution for DNA analysis including, sample and reagent delivery, electrophoresis, cell capture, preconcentration, purification, PCR, hybridization, washing steps, and detection. Automation in the hybridization and post hybridization processes is important in clinical diagnostics because of being user-friendly and also reproducible in operation. Additionally, this approach minimizes the run-to-run and operator-to-operator variation, such as temperature, the stringency of the hybridization, and washing buffer conditions [36, 38].

In an automated flow-through microarray, a robot pipetting system or an autosampler is used to apply the sample and reagents. Other robotic work-stations including valves, pumps, detection systems, and electronics carry out the analysis procedure automatically. Autosamplers can also apply the proper volumes of many solutions when the array is used to analyze several samples [8, 37].

These bench-top instruments for the processing and readout of the microarray data are generally expensive and large. As a result, these devices are generally only used in clinical laboratories. Moreover, they are neither reconfigurable nor scalable after manufacture. Therefore, there is a need for the design and fabrication of low-cost and portable automated microarrays.

Microfluidic systems have solved the abovementioned problems and also made a revolution in rapid biological diagnosis. They have evolved from simple setups to lab-on-a-chip devices over the years [38]. The lab-on-a-chip also called a microfluidic biochip can perform multiple steps and a wide range of tasks including, sample preparation, analysis, separation, DNA amplification, clean up, and detection by replacing cumbersome equipment with the help of miniaturized assemblies such as valves, pressure systems, metering systems, reaction chambers, and detection systems. This emerging technology has advantages in comparison with more passive conventional microarrays. The lab-on-a-chip device is compact, miniaturized, cost-effective, automated, and it can handle small amounts of solution at microliter or nanoliter scales. The main idea of this invention is to offer a single device, which integrates all essential functions needed for a biochemical analysis by the combination of electronics, chemistry, and biology using microfluidics technology [8, 36, 39, 40].

There are two different approaches available for liquid handling in microfluidic biochips.

(1) Continuous flow biochips

In this method, a continuous liquid flow is manipulated in microstructured flow channels. The actuation force for the creation of liquid flow in this system can be applied by permanently etched micropumps, microvalves, and microchannels, which can work by one or a mixture of approaches such as, external pressure sources, integrated mechanical micropumps, microfluidic large scale integration (mLSI), electrokinetic mechanisms, and by combination with capillary forces. Electroosmosis is a frequently used electrokinetic method for microfluidic arrays. In this method, the flow of an ionic liquid is caused by the application of an electrical field. The continuous flow technique has a great application in the well-defined biological analysis as a result of its simplicity and lower sensitivity to protein fouling problems. On the other hand, this method is not suitable for complicated tasks, which need complex manipulation of the array solutions. Additionally, it is very hard to scale up this fluidic system because the parameters which control and affect the liquid flow, such as pressure fluid resistance and electrical field may vary from region to region within the fluidic system. Another problem with this technique is the possibility of contaminant entry and the creation of dead volumes because of the shear flow and diffusion within the microchannels [40–42].

(2) Droplet-based biochips

Droplet-based biochips are an alternative to continuous flow chips, which may solve many of the shortcomings of the continuous flow method. In this technique, there are two kinds of fluid employed, which are immiscible with each other. This forms a two-phase system including a continuous phase and a dispersed phase. The continuous phase is the medium in which the droplets are generated and moved through the dispersed phase containing the intended sample or reagent in the shape of microliter or nanoliter droplets. These droplets could be actuated by external electrical or magnetic fields. This system is more scalable in comparison to the automated microfluidic arrays operating with a continuous flow system [43–45].

The solution droplets can be created in active or passive mode. In the active mode, the droplets are formed and manipulated by the help of external devices such as valves, centrifuge, and magnetic or electric fields. In the passive mode, there is no external energy needed, and the droplets are formed continuously using pressure-driven flow and a different geometry of the channels. The three different methods available for creating droplets in passive mode, include T-junction, flow focusing, and a co-flow setup. In these three techniques, an inert oil shears the aqueous phase, which could contain the sample or the reagent solution. The specific design of the microchannels helps the production of the droplets [46, 47].

4.3.5 Examples of microfluidic arrays

Microfluidic arrays can be used to study a variety of samples, and conventional microarrays require only small volumes of sample and reagents. Microfluidic arrays can study enzymatic reactions (e.g., glucose and lactate assays), DNA analysis for gene expression and genotyping, polymerase chain reaction (PCR) and nucleic acid sequencing, proteomics and immunoassays, drug discovery and toxicity screening. These devices have a wide application in clinical laboratories because of their real-time biomolecular detection ability [40]. Here we review some of the microfluidic arrays which have been designed for special purposes.

Liu et al. designed a DNA microarray silicon chip with 12,000 separate features for screening the gene expression of the human leukemia cell line (K562). This microarray was merged with a microfluidic system for automation of the sample and reagent handling. This microfluidic system was fully automated and completely self-contained including washing and labeling steps. The device showed comparable results to a similar test using a conventional microarray [48].

In another research, Kadimisetty et al. fabricated a novel automated microfluidic array for the detection of multiple proteins in trace amounts with the help of three-dimensional (3D) printing. The detection was done by using an electro-chemiluminescent (ECL) detection technique and a CCD camera. A paper-thin pyrolytic graphite microwell preparation was merged with a microfluidic system to complete the sandwich immunoassay where the sample and reagents were delivered to the chip automatically. The total cost of this fully automated microfluidic array was reported to be 0.65$ [49].

For early detection of leukemia and tumor heterogeneity, the rapid isolation and analysis of single leukemia cells is a desirable goal. There are two methods at present for isolation and identification of leukemia cells from white blood cells (WBCs) because of their size overlap: immunolabeling or cytogenetic assays. Hyun Lee and coworkers proposed a novel method for the rapid and label-free identification of single leukemia cells directly from blood cells. In this study, a high-density microfluidic trapping array was used for the separation of hemocytes. This high-density microfluidic trapping array, which was made from 1600 densely packed single-cell traps was able to filter and trap both red and white blood cells [50].

4.4 Conclusion

Microfluidic systems are produced by the merging of microarray technology and microfluidic systems and can take advantage of efficient sample handling by the fluidic system and rapid and accurate diagnosis of microarray technology within a single device.

Microfluidic arrays have an interesting and unique set of features including the ability to analyze small sample volumes on the scale of picoliters, nanoliters, or microliters. In the microarray system, the samples are obtained directly from the human body and as a result, they are precious. This method minimizes the amount of required sample for analysis, as well as reducing its hybridization time and providing the possibility for mass production of diagnostic devices at a low cost.

The automated microfluidic systems have revolutionized biochemical diagnosis by offering a system that could analyze multiple samples simultaneously because of its separate fluidic pathways. Automated microfluidic arrays (lab-on-a-chip device) can considerably reduce the reagent costs and time consumption. On the other hand, this technology minimizes the variables and eliminates errors caused by the operator-dependent manual steps.

Although there are lots of promising advantages for microfluidic array technology, there are still some shortcomings and challenges such as complexity in the materials, fabrication methods, and high production costs. As a result, further research and work still need to be carried out to improve this useful technology [7].

References

[1] R. Gonzalo, A. Sánchez, Introduction to microarrays technology and data analysis, in: Data analysis for omic sciences: methods and applications, vol. 82, Elsevier, 2018, p. 37.
[2] P.N. Prasad, Introduction to biophotonics, Wiley-Interscience, 2003.
[3] M. Dufva, DNA microarrays for biomedical research, Springer, 2009.
[4] F.D. Park, R. Sasik, T. Reya, Microarrays: an introduction and guide to their use, in: Basic science methods for clinical researchers, Elsevier, 2017, pp. 57–76.
[5] H. Shi, et al., A review: fabrications, detections and applications of peptide nucleic acids (PNAs) microarray, Biosens Bioelectron 66 (2015) 481–489.
[6] H. Zhang, et al., Detection of single-base mutations using 1-D microfluidic beads array, Electrophoresis 28 (24) (2007) 4668–4678.
[7] C. Situma, M. Hashimoto, S.A. Soper, Merging microfluidics with microarray-based bioassays, Biomol Eng 23 (5) (2006) 213–231.
[8] L. Wang, P.C. Li, Microfluidic DNA microarray analysis: a review, Anal Chim Acta 687 (1) (2011) 12–27.
[9] H. Sun, G.Y. Chen, S.Q. Yao, Recent advances in microarray technologies for proteomics, Chem Biol 20 (5) (2013) 685–699.
[10] S. Nimse, et al., Immobilization techniques for microarray: challenges and applications, Sensors 14 (12) (2014) 22208–22229.
[11] A. Sánchez-Pla, DNA microarrays technology: overview and current status, in: Comprehensive analytical chemistry, Elsevier, 2014, pp. 1–23.
[12] I. Barbulovic-Nad, et al., Bio-microarray fabrication techniques—a review, Crit Rev Biotechnol 26 (4) (2006) 237–259.
[13] F.S. Ligler, C.R. Taitt, Optical biosensors: today and tomorrow, Elsevier, 2011.
[14] S. Khan, et al., DNA microarray technology and drug development, Chron Young Sci 1 (1) (2010) 1.

[15] K.D. Kumble, S. Kumble, Microarrays in drug discovery and development, in: Pharmaceutical sciences encyclopedia: drug discovery, development, and manufacturing, 2010, pp. 1–28.
[16] D. Castel, et al., Cell microarrays in drug discovery, Drug Discov Today 11 (13-14) (2006) 616–622.
[17] S. Wang, Q. Cheng, Microarray analysis in drug discovery and clinical applications, in: Bioinformatics and drug discovery, Springer, 2006, pp. 49–65.
[18] W. Huang, et al., Integration of antibody array technology into drug discovery and development, Assay Drug Dev Technol 16 (2) (2018) 74–95.
[19] M. Dehmer, F. Emmert-Streib, Analysis of microarray data: a network-based approach, John Wiley & Sons, 2008.
[20] D. Rose, Microfluidic technologies and instrumentation for printing DNA microarrays, in: Microarray biochip technology, 2000, pp. 19–38.
[21] W.C. Cho, Proteomics technologies and challenges, Genomics Proteomics Bioinformatics 5 (2) (2007) 77–85.
[22] B. Aslam, et al., Proteomics: technologies and their applications, J Chromatogr Sci 55 (2) (2017) 182–196.
[23] G. MacBeath, Protein microarrays and proteomics, Nat Genet 32 (4s) (2002) 526.
[24] K. Pratsch, R. Wellhausen, H. Seitz, Advances in the quantification of protein microarrays, Curr Opin Chem Biol 18 (2014) 16–20.
[25] F.R. Sutandy, et al., Overview of protein microarrays, Curr Protoc Protein Sci 72 (1) (2013) 27.1.1–27.1.16.
[26] D.A. Hall, J. Ptacek, M. Snyder, Protein microarray technology, Mech Ageing Dev 128 (1) (2007) 161–167.
[27] J.M. Blackburn, A. Shoko, N. Beeton-Kempen, Miniaturized, microarray-based assays for chemical proteomic studies of protein function, in: Chemical genomics and proteomics, Springer, 2012, pp. 133–162.
[28] H. Zhu, J. Qian, Applications of functional protein microarrays in basic and clinical research, in: Advances in genetics, Elsevier, 2012, pp. 123–155.
[29] M.L. Yarmush, K.R. King, Living-cell microarrays, Annu Rev Biomed Eng 11 (2009) 235–257.
[30] H. Hong, W. Koom, W.-G. Koh, Cell microarray technologies for high-throughput cell-based biosensors, Sensors 17 (6) (2017) 1293.
[31] A. Vafajoo, et al., Multiplexed microarrays based on optically encoded microbeads, Biomed Microdevices 20 (3) (2018) 66.
[32] S.F. Parsa, et al., Early diagnosis of disease using microbead array technology: a review, Anal Chim Acta 1032 (2018) 1–17.
[33] O.I. Berthuy, et al., Multiplex cell microarrays for high-throughput screening, Lab Chip 16 (22) (2016) 4248–4262.
[34] R. Jonczyk, et al., Living cell microarrays: an overview of concepts, Microarrays 5 (2) (2016) 11.
[35] W. Qiao, Biomedical applications for microfluidic devices, UC San Diego, 2013.
[36] K. Pappaert, et al., Enhancement of DNA micro-array analysis using a shear-driven micro-channel flow system, J Chromatogr A 1014 (1-2) (2003) 1–9.
[37] M. Seidel, R. Niessner, Automated analytical microarrays: a critical review, Anal Bioanal Chem 391 (5) (2008) 1521.
[38] R.H. Liu, et al., Integrated microfluidic biochips for DNA microarray analysis, Expert Rev Mol Diagn 6 (2) (2006) 253–261.

[39] D. Figeys, D. Pinto, Lab-on-a-chip: a revolution in biological and medical sciences, ACS Publications, 2000.
[40] F. Su, K. Chakrabarty, R.B. Fair, Microfluidics-based biochips: technology issues, implementation platforms, and design-automation challenges, IEEE Trans Comput Aided Des Integr Circuits Syst 25 (2) (2006) 211–223.
[41] H. Chang, L. Yeo, Electrokinetically driven microfluidics and nanofluidics, Cambridge University Press, 2010.
[42] T.-M. Tseng, et al., Columba 2.0: a co-layout synthesis tool for continuous-flow microfluidic biochips, IEEE Trans Comput Aided Des Integr Circuits Syst 37 (8) (2017) 1588–1601.
[43] W.L. Hwang, F. Su, K. Chakrabarty, Automated design of pin-constrained digital microfluidic arrays for lab-on-a-chip applications, in: 2006 43rd ACM/IEEE design automation conference, IEEE, 2006.
[44] M. Sesen, T. Alan, A. Neild, Droplet control technologies for microfluidic high throughput screening (μHTS), Lab Chip 17 (14) (2017) 2372–2394.
[45] P. Zhu, L. Wang, Passive and active droplet generation with microfluidics: a review, Lab Chip 17 (1) (2017) 34–75.
[46] M. Tenje, et al., Particle manipulation methods in droplet microfluidics, ACS Publications, 2017.
[47] N. Shembekar, et al., Droplet-based microfluidics in drug discovery, transcriptomics and high-throughput molecular genetics, Lab Chip 16 (8) (2016) 1314–1331.
[48] R.H. Liu, et al., Fully integrated miniature device for automated gene expression DNA microarray processing, Anal Chem 78 (6) (2006) 1980–1986.
[49] K. Kadimisetty, et al., Automated 3D-printed microfluidic array for rapid nanomaterial-enhanced detection of multiple proteins, Anal Chem 90 (12) (2018) 7569–7577.
[50] D.-H. Lee, et al., Rapid and label-free identification of single leukemia cells from blood in a high-density microfluidic trapping array by fluorescence lifetime imaging microscopy, Lab Chip 18 (9) (2018) 1349–1358.

CHAPTER

Microfluidics: Organ-on-a-chip 5

Shahin Aghamiri[a,b], Navid Rabiee[c,*], Sepideh Ahmadi[a,b], Mohammad Rabiee[d], Mojtaba Bagherzadeh[c], and Mahdi Karimi[e,f,g,h]

[a]Student Research Committee, Department of Medical Biotechnology, School of Advanced Technologies in Medicine, Shahid Beheshti University of Medical Sciences, Tehran, Iran
[b]Cellular and Molecular Biology Research Center, Shahid Beheshti University of Medical Sciences, Tehran, Iran
[c]Department of Chemistry, Sharif University of Technology, Tehran, Iran
[d]Biomaterials Group, Department of Biomedical Engineering, Amirkabir University of Technology, Tehran, Iran
[e]Cellular and Molecular Research Center, Iran University of Medical Sciences, Tehran, Iran
[f]Department of Medical Nanotechnology, Faculty of Advanced Technologies in Medicine, Iran University of Medical Sciences, Tehran, Iran
[g]Oncopathology Research Center, Iran University of Medical Sciences, Tehran, Iran
[h]Research Center for Science and Technology in Medicine, Tehran University of Medical Sciences, Tehran, Iran
**Corresponding author. E-mail: nrabiee94@gmail.com*

The conventional platforms for cell characterization and drug delivery do not fully satisfy the demands of researchers. Because of numerous advantages like miniaturization, low cost, flexibility, and precision, microfluidic systems have become robust research tools heralding a new era in molecular medicine and drug delivery [1]. A special type of microfluidic system, called "organ-on-a-chip," is a combination of cell biology techniques and microfluidic technology [2].

Organ-on-a-chip systems create a tunable tissue culture microenvironment for various types of cells to mimic their micrometer-scale structure and function. In other words, these systems duplicate the biomechanical, biochemical, and biochemical properties of the extracellular matrix (ECM) and the cellular microenvironment [3]. In the past few years, the feasibility and simplicity of organ-on-a-chip systems for biological cell characterization and the development of disease models for drug delivery and discovery have been established by several groups. To date, the creation of many "suborgans," which can emulate the microstructure and partial function of tissue units, has been reported [4]. In this chapter, we will discuss the cutting-edge advances in the organ-on-a-chip field, like heart-on-a-chip, vessel-on-a-chip,

Biomedical Applications of Microfluidic Devices. https://doi.org/10.1016/B978-0-12-818791-3.00001-2

liver-on-a-chip, neuron-on-a-chip, and kidney-on-a-chip. Furthermore, the most important drawbacks and principles of microfabrication of the current devices will be described.

5.1 Traditional systems drawbacks

In this part, the drawbacks of traditional drug screening and drug delivery devices will be discussed. A normal drug development effort consists of three phases, (1) preclinical phase, (2) clinical phase, and (3) postmarketing phase. The two most central steps of the preclinical phase are drug-delivery testing, in vitro drug screening, and laboratory tests that are largely animal tests [5].

To check the efficacy and safety of new drugs, some novel platforms, which can emulate the in vivo environment, have recently emerged. All drug-delivery agents, such as nanoparticles, liposomes, implanted depots, and free naked drugs can be studied using in vitro models [6]. At the first stage, two-dimensional (2D)-based cell culture methods are the most often employed in vitro platforms. In this platform, as the first step, a monolayer of cells must be cultured. Then, at the second step, drug candidates for screening are added into the culture flask. After the desired time, the responses of the cells to the tested drugs are documented. At last, the biological and chemical signals produced by cells are evaluated. Drug-cell interaction screening can be provided by 2D in vitro platforms [7–9]. However, it has been realized that a 2D cell monolayer culture cannot properly imitate the three-dimensional (3D) cellular microenvironment of the human body, partly due to the oversimplification of the extracellular matrix (ECM). The remarkable difference between the ECM properties of in vivo and in vitro models has been established [10].

To address the aforementioned limitation, numerous 3D culture platforms, including spheroids, cell sheets, and cell aggregates have been designed [11, 12]. The 3D ECM microenvironment in vitro can be generated as a result of cell accumulation and specific 3D structure formation, like multicellular layers and aggregates. In these structures, cells easily can interact with each other in a 3D environment. All these platforms have been used successfully to generate a 3D ECM microenvironment in vitro. But serious problems still remain because the cellular microenvironment also consists of mechanical and electrical interactions, which 3D cell structures cannot easily provide. To investigate in vivo cell response to drugs, electrical and mechanical changes in cells must be considered in the same way as chemical changes [13].

The toxicological and metabolic effects of drugs are two important factors, which should be evaluated for drug discovery testing. As already mentioned, drug-delivery testing is one of the most important preclinical trial stages for the prediction of drug performance [14, 15]. Animal models are central elements in conventional drug discovery testing because the microenvironment of cells in living animals in vivo is the closest to humans. But there are several challenges like the difficulty in obtaining reproducible results as a consequence of poorly controllable and different characteristics of individual animals. Moreover, in many studies, the effect of the drug is evaluated just by monitoring the changes in the concentrations of chemical compounds, which does not allow a deeper understanding of toxicity and interaction mechanisms [16, 17].

To solve the above-mentioned limitations, the organ-on-a-chip platform was created as a new cutting-edge approach. The organ-on-a-chip platform can simplify many types of studies such as drug screening and delivery tests and analysis, cell-ECM, cell-cell, and cell-tubular flow interactions studies, and moreover, investigations for characterization of cell physical properties. High controllability, low cost, and imitation of different organ functions are the most important advantages of this revolutionary platform [18, 19].

5.2 Microfabrication principles

The process of fabrication of organ-on-a-chip platforms has great importance for more accurate imitation of in vivo microenvironments. For advanced organ-on-a-chip platforms, microfabrication techniques have received much attention because the tissue environment can be constructed at the microscale [20]. Several techniques like soft lithography, microcontact printing, and replica molding have been used to fabricate organ-on-a-chip platforms.

Polydimethylsiloxane (PDMS) is one of the most important materials in organ-on-a-chip platform fabrication, due to its flexibility and biodegradability. Because of its optically clear properties, high-quality microscopic images of cultured cells can be captured [21]. The PDMS stamp can be fabricated using the replica molding method. In this method, a uniform photoresist layer is used to coat the silicon wafer. By using ultraviolet (UV) light, the photoresist layer can be cross-linked to the silicon wafer layer. The use of a photomask allows just the desired parts of the photoresist to be irradiated. Afterward, the pattern is transferred to the silicon wafer substrate that then becomes a mold. The patterned mold is filled with the PDMS and then the product is polymerized by oven-baking. After this step, the PDMS is peeled off from the substrate. The substrate can be used again and again for successive fabrications; therefore, the procedure is called replica molding. Replica molding is derived from the soft lithography technology. Soft lithography also can be applied to create PDMS channels for flowing fluids. The creation stages are very similar to the replica molding technique, with just one difference: the strength of bonds between the PDMS device and the substrate is higher [21–23].

Porous membranes, fluidic channels, and microwells are some of the most commonly used components for organ-on-a-chip platforms constructed to investigate cell behavior, cell-cell interactions, and cell responses to mechanical and chemical stimulation [21]. Microfabrication is a cutting-edge technology, which can make possible the generation of organ-on-a-chip platforms to investigate in vivo microenvironmental effects.

5.3 Significant organ-on-a-chip platforms

In this section, we discuss some significant organ-on-a-chip platforms like heart-on-a-chip, liver-on-a-chip, lung-on-a-chip, vessel-on-a-chip, neuron-on-a-chip, kidney-on-a-chip, tumor-on-a-chip, and multiorgans-on-a-chip to demonstrate the high potential of these platforms for future clinical applications.

5.3.1 Lung-on-a-chip

Because of several serious lung-related diseases like cancer, emphysema, chronic bronchitis, and asthma, research into lung biology has a great significance. Moreover, the lung epithelial barrier is a critical challenge for the treatment of lung-related diseases [24, 25]. Fortunately, microfluidic systems can be a great help for studying cell-matrix interactions, cell-cell interactions, cell-gas flow, and cell-blood flow, all of which are vital for lung physiology and research into drug discovery and delivery [26].

The last decade has witnessed a rapid growth in lung-on-a-chip platforms for studies on lung diseases like pulmonary edema [5]. In 2010, a microfluidic device was used by Huh et al. [27] to design a biomimetic microsystem that could imitate the alveolar-capillary interface of the living human lung. They showed that this microchip system could be a low-cost alternative to clinical and animal research for toxicology and drug screening tests.

In another interesting study, the simulation of alveoli was reported by Douville et al. [13] who studied the combined effects of fluid and solid mechanical stresses on the behavior of a microfluidic lung model.

Despite many advances in the modeling of the capillary-alveolar interface, several lung diseases require a more complex 3D model to imitate the vascular system and nutrient-oxygen transport to the tissue. In order to address this problem and provide a more complex model, Kniazeva and colleagues [28] synthesized a microfluidic-based capillary channel device for blood delivery with a large-area membrane for oxygen exchange. By combining this architecture with the lung-on-a-chip platform, an efficient 3D lung model could be generated.

5.3.2 Intestine-on-a-chip

Since 2004, there has been a rapid rise in the use of intestine-on-a-chip platforms, due to the interest into gastrointestinal (GI) chronic diseases such as celiac disease, Crohn's disease, and gastroenteritis, and also for modeling the uptake of orally administered drugs by absorption in the small intestine [29–31]. These models should have the correct structural features including villi and mucus, special cell types (goblet cells, enterocytes, and vascular endothelial cells (ECs)), and dynamic properties (peristalsis) [32, 33]. Kimura and colleagues [34] provided some of these features. They produced a novel intestinal-on-a-chip device with detection functionality. Their microfluidic architecture consisted of two channels, with a semipermeable membrane separating them from each other. They demonstrated that the cultured cells could survive for more than two weeks, and also rhodamine 123 transport through a cell monolayer could be monitored. As previously mentioned, villi are a critical feature of an intestinal model. Kim et al. [35] designed an intestine-on-a-chip system which can allow villi formation. Their device could imitate the intestinal peristaltic motion that is critical for cell proliferation and villi generation. In another study conducted by Sung et al. [36], the GI scaffold produced villi by several different mechanisms. In the most important one, a perforated membrane was combined with the cell layer and another microfluidic channel emulated the tissue, which lies behind the endothelial walls. The effects of consumption of dairy products on the immune system function in the GI tract were studied using the NutriChip, a microfluidic intestine-on-a-chip, designed by Ramadan and colleagues [37].

Within the next few years, intestine-on-a-chip and gut-on-a-chip are set to become important tools for studying nutrikinetics, drug development, and drug delivery studies.

5.3.3 Blood vessel-on-a-chip

The network of blood vessels has an important role in the circulatory system of vertebrates and connects tissues and organs to each other [38]. There are three different types of blood vessels. Capillaries are responsible for oxygen, carbon dioxide, water, and chemical exchange between the tissue and blood. Arteries carry blood away from the heart to the various organs and tissues of the body. Veins carry blood from different organs and tissues back to the heart [39]. Generally, blood vessels are composed of three different layers, which are generally known as tunica. The tunica externa, also called tunica adventitia, is the outermost and thickest layer in veins. The middle layer in vessels and also the thickest part in the arteries is called tunica media. The tunica intima is the innermost layer of a vein or artery [40], as shown in Fig. 5.3. ECs are responsible for the selective permeability barrier between blood and tissue. Recently, because of the importance of ECs in numerous physiological functions like inflammation, barriers, angiogenesis, clotting, tumor metastasis, and vasoconstriction or vasodilation, there have been many reports about vessel-on-a-chip devices. A perfusable 3D microvascular network on a chip was designed by Kim et al. [38]. They showed that the microvasculature allowed the delivery of chemical compounds, biomolecules, cell suspensions, and nutrients. This system could be used in many types of vascular physiology research and may be a great model for drug development and delivery for human diseases.

5.3.4 Heart-on-a-chip

Among the deadliest diseases in the world, is cardiovascular disease (CVD) [41, 42]. The mammalian heart has several critical functions like autorhythmicity (beating) for pumping blood [43]. Therefore, studies on drug development and delivery, drug adverse effects, and drug interactions for cardiac applications have increased. A heart-on-a-chip platform could be a time-saving and cost-efficient approach for assays and screening in preparation for clinical trials [44, 45]. In one the most important studies, a functional cardiac tissue construct on a flexible substrate was generated by Parker and colleagues [46]. They cultured heart muscle cells in the form of tiny tissue strips. A contractile response was observed and also the cardiotoxic effects of some drugs could be quantified. In another study by Aubin et al. [47] the 3D structure of functional cardiac tissue was investigated using microscale hydrogels. They encapsulated cardiomyocytes inside hydrogels with various micropatterns. Fiber-like structures were efficiently generated. This study demonstrated that microscale scaffolds could be designed to emulate the shape and size of in vivo cardiac fibers. Human embryonic stem cells (hESCs) were used to make a microstructural cardiac bioreactor, an attractive model for drug testing. The effects of nitric oxide on the beating of cardiac biowires was investigated, showing the spontaneous beating could be retarded [48].

5.3.5 Liver-on-a-chip

The liver is the largest glandular organ in the body on the right of the abdomen, with two large sections, the left and right lobes [49]. There are two practical units in the liver, lobules, and acini. They are very important for life and can carry out more than 500 tasks, such as removal of toxins (detoxification), blood glucose regulation, and storage of fat-soluble vitamins (A, D, E, and K). Other functions of the liver are to purify the blood, by trapping and neutralizing toxins and pathogens. Because of these functions, the liver is a vulnerable and sensitive organ. An overdose of different drugs can cause severe damage to liver tissue. For this purpose, the liver is considered a drug-induced toxicity target and hepatotoxicity must be avoided. Unfortunately, the prediction of liver response to drugs challenging and it is difficult to fully mimic the liver in vitro.

Microfluidic systems can offer valuable information on the response of the human liver to drug administration. For research on drug development and screening, primary hepatocytes can be cultured in microfluidic devices. Lee et al. established the possible application of PDMS- microfluidic channels for emulating the liver anatomy (Fig. 5.1) [50]. For the microfabrication procedure, an epoxy-based negative photoresist (SU-8) was used for silicone replicate molding and used to make cell-loaded channels. The functional unit in this microsystem consisted of a hepatic cell culture chamber with surrounding nutrient flow channels isolated by microbarrier structures (2 μm in width) that could mimic the highly permeable endothelial barrier between hepatocytes and liver sinusoidal cells. The most important features of this microfluidic device included the constant exchange of nutrients between cells, imitating the natural endothelial barrier layer, and cultured liver cells that could survive for more than 7 days.

Numerous researches have also been performed to prepare other types of liver-on-chip microdevices to study the potential side effects of drugs and treatment strategies. Bhushan and coworkers developed a 3D microfluidic devices to imitate the acinus of human liver tissue, which consists of four various cell types: ECs, hepatocytes, stellate cells, and Kupffer cells, as shown in Fig. 5.2 [51]. This chip provided metabolic

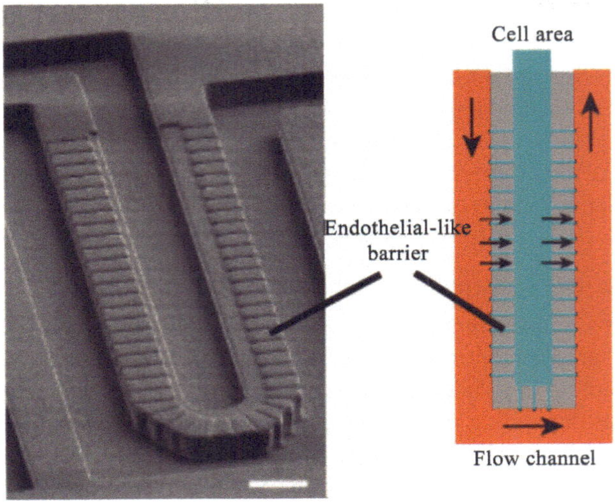

FIG. 5.1

SEM micrograph of in vitro microfluidic liver sinusoidal layer.

Reprinted with permission from Lee PJ, Hung PJ, Lee LP. An artificial liver sinusoid with a microfluidic endothelial-like barrier for primary hepatocyte culture. Biotechnol Bioeng 2007;97(5):1340–6, Copyright (2007) Wiley.

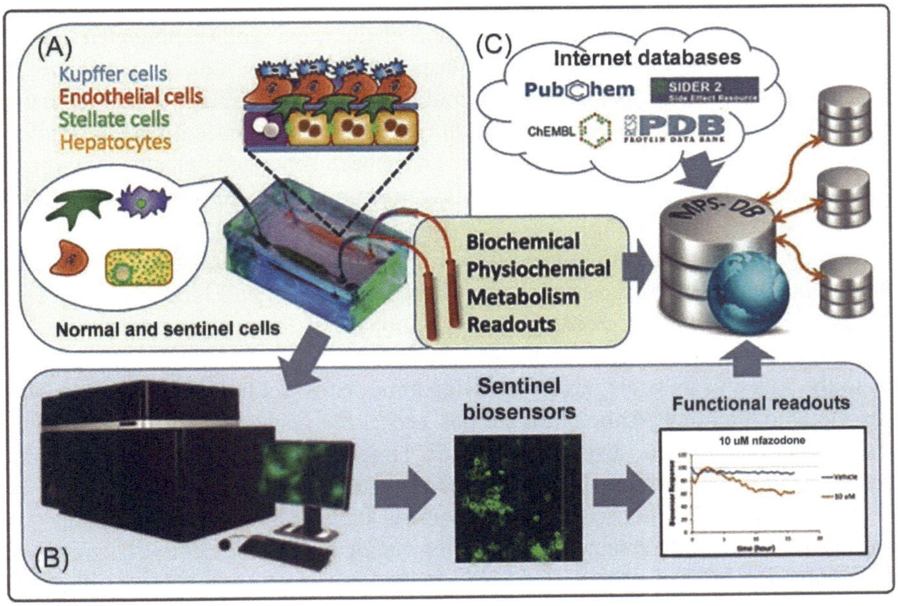

FIG. 5.2

Schematic illustration of liver-on-a-chip to mimic the liver acinus: (A) four types of liver cells in the acinus microchip model; (B) examination of the microchip function by sentinel biosensors; (C) providing external resources by analyzing graphs in a database.

Reprinted with permission from Bhushan A, Senutovitch N, Bale SS, McCarty WJ, Hegde M, Jindal R, et al. Towards a three-dimensional microfluidic liver platform for predicting drug efficacy and toxicity in humans. Stem Cell Res Ther 2013;4(1):S16, Copyright (2020) Elsevier.

and biochemical information by allowing cell co-culture with enzymatic and biosynthetic activity. The bio-chip contained fluorescent markers allowing changes in cell function to be observed when a toxic drug was added, which could possibly lead to the generation of free radicals and liver failure.

Liver-on-a-chip systems are able to provide databases that make possible real-time monitoring of cell death, cell damage after drug exposure, as well as the ability to create predictive models of human hepatotoxicity (Fig. 5.2) [51].

5.3.6 Tumor-on-a-chip

The tumor-on-a-chip is another area of interest in organ-on-a chip studies. This technique has great potential for discovering novel anticancer therapies to target cancer cells more specifically. The tumor-on-a-chip can be categorized into three major subtypes depending on the purpose; (a) monitoring antiangiogenesis, vascularization, migration of cancer cells; (b) screening and evaluating the effects of drugs or nanodrugs on tumor cells, and (c) detection of blood-borne cancer markers [52].

Microfluidic devices have many applications in cancer, including the creation of size-tunable 3D tumor spheroids, sorting of tumor cells, and balancing of cell density in co-culture. Recently, new 3D platforms have been generated to explore the cross-talk between normal cells and cancer cells. Microfluidics also has great importance for developing new targeted drug delivery systems [53].

Tumor marker detection devices are one of the most well-documented tumor-on-a-chip platforms. Generally, these devices can be used for collecting and detecting circulating tumor cells (CTCs) that could improve cancer diagnosis in the early stages. To imitate the microenvironment of tumor cells and adjacent vessels, numerous nanoparticle-based screening platforms have been generated, which can improve drug delivery and drug screening [54]. A tumor-on-a-chip device emulating a breast tumor is shown in Fig. 5.3 [5].

The endothelium was mimicked by a single layer of vascular ECs on a porous membrane, and the lymph vessel was emulated by the red and blue channels. This strategy can simplify the screening of both nanoparticle transport and cross-talk between nanoparticles and tumor cells [5].

In the past 8 years strategies for studying tumor neovascularization have received considerable attention. Although there has been little research on the microfluidic generation of capillaries, several microfluidic strategies have been designed in order to explore the relationship between tumor cells and blood vessels [56].

This method is composed of three channels including the central channel (for seeding ECs) and side channels (for seeding tumor cells). The central channel and side channels were linked to each other by filled gelatin pathways. The tumor cells could be seeded on the tumor-vessel co-culture devices. After that, the tumor cells accumulate in the adjacent pathway to the vessels, allowing the investigation of transport and invasion mechanism [56]. This tumor-on-a-chip platform could be an outstanding tool to investigate how tumor cells grow in tissues.

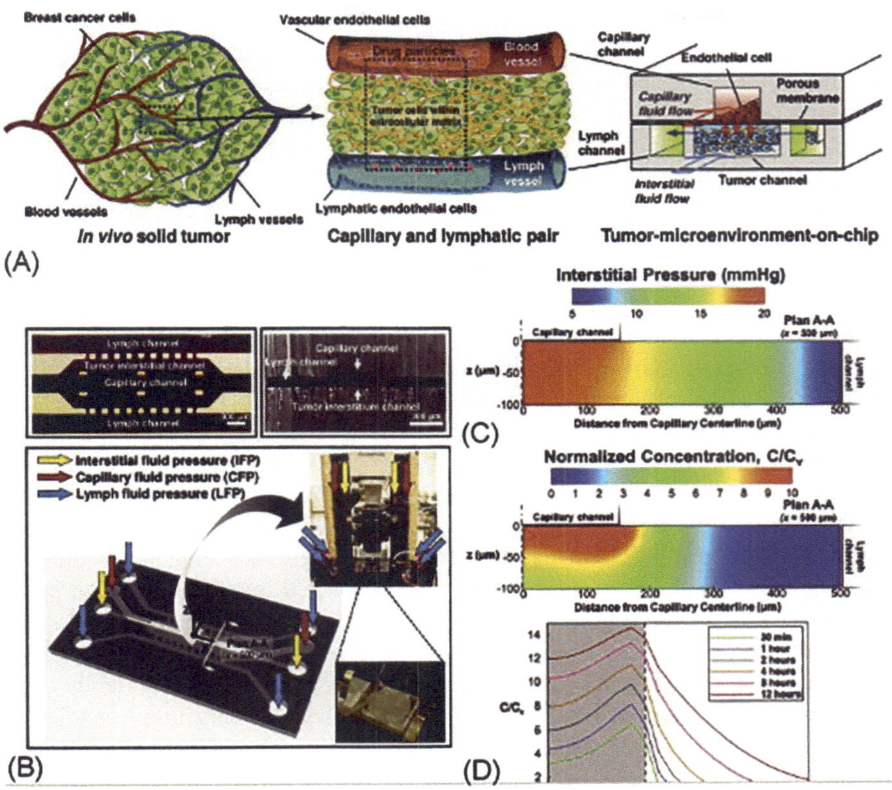

FIG. 5.3

Tumor-on-a-chip device [55]. (A) In vivo tumor microenvironment including lymphatic endothelial, and tumor cells. (B) The tumor-microenvironment-on-chip. Computational model of (C) IFP and (D) concentration of nanoparticles in the tumor-microenvironment-on-chip [5].

Tumor-on-a-chip platforms have been used for many tumor types, like lung, bone marrow, brain, urinary system, intestine, liver, and breast.

5.3.7 Bone marrow-tumor-on-a-chip

In one study, Bruce and his coworkers [57] investigated the microenvironment of acute lymphoblastic leukemia (ALL) in 2D and 3D static microenvironments, as well as a 3D dynamic microenvironment. Leukemia cancer begins in the bone marrow and then spreads throughout the body. Various types of cancer cells along with primary bone marrow stromal cells and osteoblasts can be cultured in the model. The microchannels can be manufactured by PDMS soft lithography methods and bonded onto a glass plate. Numerous rows and columns have been developed to close the inlet and outlet valves to keep the cells within the microchannels at the center of the microchip. Ethanol (70%) and UV exposure have been applied for the sterilization of the microchip. Following loading of the cells suspended in culture medium into the microchannels, the collagen was gelatinized, and then in the 3D dynamic model, the culture medium was pumped continuously into the microchannels using a syringe pump. They investigated cancer drug resistance to Ara-C, which is used as a chemotherapy drug for the therapy of hematologic neoplasms, employing the 2D and 3D static and 3D dynamic platforms. The cancer cells were exposed to diluted concentrations of Ara-C for 48 h. Immunofluorescence and flow cytometry image analysis was used to study the viability of the cells. In the tri-culture platform treated with Ara-C, the survival rate of leukemic cells was higher than the monoculture system. The microenvironmental protection in the 3D dynamic platform was higher than the 3D static platform, which in turn was higher than the 2D static platform. They ascribed the difference between 2D and 3D platforms to differences in cell-matrix interactions, causing cell-cell signal transduction and integrin activation. The collagen matrix can also restrict drug delivery in this model [58].

Young et al. [59] studied the effects of two drugs, bortezomib and tumor necrosis factor (TNF)-α on multiple myeloma (MM) cells. Their microfluidic system consisted of a central chamber and side chamber connected by radial diffusion ports. HS-5 cells were cultured in the central chamber and RPMI 8226 cells in the side chambers. The advantage of this system was that it maintains cells in the microchannels without any cell traps and aids their growth. After 16 h, 99% of cell viability was maintained. Bortezomib is an inhibitor of NF-κB activation. This drug was injected into the microchamber and then a fluorescence-based cell viability assay was used to study the chemoresistance of the cells. The results showed that by increasing drug concentration, the cell viability was reduced. They also developed a microfluidic single-cell nuclear translocation (μSCeNT) ECM-cell interaction assay to study the activation of transcription factors such as STAT3 and NF-κB, which have an important role in the regulation of cellular processes in cancer. They studied NF-κB activation and inhibition after drug and cytokine delivery, and also the activation of STAT3 in MM cells in the co-culture model with bone marrow stromal cells (BMSCs).

Pak and his colleagues [60] studied the chemoresistance of MM cells to bortezomib when cultured in the microfluidic system used in their previous work. A microfluidic-cis-coculture (MicroC3) system was prepared by co-culturing patient-derived $CD138^+$ MM cells with the patient's own $CD138^-$ tumor-associated mononuclear cells. This platform showed a very good correlation between the MicroC3 readout and patient clinical responses and could be used as a predictive method for MM treatment by bortezomib.

5.3.8 Brain-tumor-on-a-chip

Glioblastoma multiforme (GBM) is the most lethal type of brain cancer and has an average survival time of only 12–15 months. Various microdevices have been fabricated to culture GBM cancer cells. Conventional 2D cell culture is well-accepted because of its simplicity; however, it cannot emulate the physiological behavior of living tissue [61, 62]. As a consequence, cell spheroids and organoid technologies have been studied to better mimic the in vivo tumor microenvironment. Nevertheless, none of these 3D cell culture devices have the ability to completely recapitulate the complexity of living organs.

Screening of anticancer agents is one of the most important applications of microfluidic systems for the treatment of GBM. In order to culture the C6 cell line, a four-chamber microfluidic system was developed using PDMS soft lithography [63]. C6 glioblastoma cells were cultured in a continuous flow of Dulbecco's improved Eagle's medium (DMEM) plus fetal bovine serum (FBS) and at low hydrostatic pressure. After 48 h, the cellular response to various concentrations of colchicine (0.05–10 μg/mL) was investigated. The viability of C6 cells was investigated by fluorescent imaging after staining with propidium iodide (PI). By increasing the concentration of colchicine or the time of treatment, the rate of cell death was increased.

Chang et al. [64] used GBM8 cells to assess the anti-GBM effect of TMZ. In this work, tumor tissue was used instead of cancer cells. After GBM8 cell injection into the brain of mice, GBM xenograft sections with 400 μm thickness were obtained. A microdevice has been developed using multilayer PDMS soft lithography. A poly-tetrafluoroethylene (PTFE) porous membrane was used to culture tissue fragments. A 96-well plate was placed underneath the PTFE porous membrane. The two components of the microfluidic device were connected to each other through several microchannels [64]. To study drug the delivery mechanism to tissue fragments, COMSOL Multiphysics™ was applied. Fluorescent cell probes were used for experimental visualization. In this method, the drug channels were divided by buffer channels to allow delivery of different drug doses. The profile of dose-dependent chemosensitivity was obtained using fluorescent staurosporine (STS) labeled cells. Quantified readouts were obtained from fluorescence images of tissue after various doses of drug exposure. This method could be valuable in anticancer drug screening and rapid treatment of cancer in the early stage.

It has been suggested that the lack of oxygen leads to glioma progression. GMB pseudopalisades can occur by the migration of cancer cells to areas that are high in nutrients and oxygen. Ayuso et al. [65] investigated the generation of pseudopalisades in glioblastoma by a microfluidic device. U-251-MG cells were cultured within a SU-8 based microchip [66] with tuned flow via lateral microchannels that recapitulated the nutrient starvation situation. In the initial phase when nutrients were sufficient, U-251-MG cells showed a nonaggressive behavior. But following the reduction of nutrients, the tumor cells started to migrate toward areas with high nutrients and oxygen, resulting in the generation of pseudopalisades.

The gold standard diagnostic technique for solid tumors is immunohistochemistry (IHC). Unfortunately, the IHC technique has disadvantages such as experimental variability and difficult data analysis. This is not the case for flow cytometry, but the sample and reagent consumption is high. Therefore, investigators have developed a miniaturized model for more economic and sensitive diagnostic methods. For instance, Sun and his colleagues [67] developed a microfluidic imaging flow cytometer (MIC) for single-cell proteomic analysis using cultured U87 cells. They evaluated four important signaling proteins (PTEN, EGFR, phosphorylated-S6, and phosphorylated-Akt) simultaneously using a PDMS microdevice consisting of 24 cell culture chambers. Their measurements were validated by clinical IHC experiments. In addition, a comparison of multiparameter MIC data sets was performed using bioinformatics techniques, such as self-organizing maps.

Haung et al. [68] used PDMS microdevices to investigate the migration behavior of GBM cancer stem cells. These contained three sections: a seeding chamber, a receiving chamber, and bridging microchannels. In this device, the migration of brain tumor stem cells (BTSC) passes through different parts of the microfluidic system to simulate the migration and proliferation of cancer cells through the intercellular space. Recently, it was shown that a microfluidic electrophoresis device could play an important role in the verification of brain cancer cell lines. In the study, another Qian et al. [69] studied the stability of DNA profiling of various cell lines by applying a microfluidic-electrophoresis model. They assessed the consistency of DNA profiling on various subcultures. This technique was suggested to be easier and more efficient for fragment length analysis (FLA) compared to capillary electrophoresis. Moreover, this method could be used to size and quantify RNA, DNA, cells, and proteins.

5.4 Conclusion and future perspectives

Although various organ-on-a-chip devices have been reported to mimic many different organs and tissues, much work remains to be done to produce more efficient organ-on-a-chip devices. Generally, the idea of an organ-on-a-chip system is to employ cells and tissues that can be used as a substitute for animal testing. To attain this goal, the reliability and controllability of organ-on-a-chip devices must be improved, to make them comprehensive platforms for metabolic testing of drugs. The present models mainly focus on cell behaviors, such as cell fusion, cell-cell and ECM-cell interactions.

In terms of feasibility, the optimization of the design, and the use of physical models with high precision have yet to be explored. Even though computational fluid dynamics (CFD) has been established for many years, and there are various CFD-based simulation models available, the study of cell flow in complex media conditions remains challenging. Furthermore, the mathematical analysis of cell properties is another related problem. Current platforms focus on cell behavior, including ECM-cell and cell-cell interactions. Those platforms require further refinement to better simulate in vivo cell activities. Machine learning technology could be applied to study complex platforms of human-on-a-chip systems. Such algorithms could optimize the design of human organs-on-a-chip. Researchers need to be able to analyze the different properties of organs by mathematical equations. These expressions could be modeled using computers with numerical computation methods (FEM, Monte Carlo) in order to improve and expedite a more precise design process.

The long-term reliability of the organ-on-a-chip devices must be proven. Also, these systems should be able to maintain their structural integrity after prolonged exposure to different chemicals. In fact, in order to provide greater resistance to chemicals and high compatibility with lithography techniques, etc., the extensively used PDMS materials need to be enhanced or replaced to achieve higher resistance to chemicals.

In the near future, microchip devices could be more than a new type of drug testing tool. This method also has the potential to be applied as a high-speed, and noninvasive platform to address patient-to-patient differences in drug responses. Besides clinical applications, organ-on-a-chip devices also have important roles in biochemical and biological mechanistic studies. Combined with other technologies, an organ-on-a-chip platform could be synthesized as a comprehensive platform for cell-tissue and organ-level characterization. Using this model, biologists could better understand the mystery of the cellular organization of humans, animals, or plants.

In conclusion, microdevices are laboratory-generated systems recapitulating several functions of natural living organs. These models may be useful tools for discovering drugs and probing cellular functions at the microscale in various biology research fields.

References

[1] A. Polini, L. Prodanov, N.S. Bhise, V. Manoharan, M.R. Dokmeci, A. Khademhosseini, Organs-on-a-chip: a new tool for drug discovery, Expert Opin Drug Discovery 9 (4) (2014) 335–352.

[2] E.W. Esch, A. Bahinski, D. Huh, Organs-on-chips at the frontiers of drug discovery, Nat Rev Drug Discov 14 (4) (2015) 248–260.

[3] P. Neužil, S. Giselbrecht, K. Länge, T.J. Huang, A. Manz, Revisiting lab-on-a-chip technology for drug discovery, Nat Rev Drug Discov 11 (8) (2012) 620–632.

[4] A. Skardal, T. Shupe, A. Atala, Organoid-on-a-chip and body-on-a-chip systems for drug screening and disease modeling, Drug Discov Today 21 (9) (2016) 1399–1411.

[5] D.Z. Wang, S. Roya, K.-I. Koo, K. Kim, Organ-on-a-chip platforms for drug delivery and cell characterization: a review, Sens Mater 27 (2015).

[6] G. Du, Q. Fang, J.M.J. den Toonder, Microfluidics for cell-based high throughput screening platforms—a review, Anal Chim Acta 903 (2016) 36–50.

[7] B.J. Papenburg, J. Liu, G.A. Higuera, A.M.C. Barradas, J. de Boer, C.A. van Blitterswijk, et al., Development and analysis of multi-layer scaffolds for tissue engineering, Biomaterials 30 (31) (2009) 6228–6239.

[8] Y.-C. Tung, A.Y. Hsiao, S.G. Allen, Y.-S. Torisawa, M. Ho, S. Takayama, High-throughput 3D spheroid culture and drug testing using a 384 hanging drop array, Analyst 136 (3) (2011) 473–478.

[9] B. Duan, State-of-the-art review of 3D bioprinting for cardiovascular tissue engineering, Ann Biomed Eng 45 (1) (2017) 195–209.

[10] J.M. Karp, J. Yeh, G. Eng, J. Fukuda, J. Blumling, K.-Y. Suh, et al., Controlling size, shape and homogeneity of embryoid bodies using poly(ethylene glycol) microwells, Lab Chip 7 (6) (2007) 786–794.

[11] V. van Duinen, S.J. Trietsch, J. Joore, P. Vulto, T. Hankemeier, Microfluidic 3D cell culture: from tools to tissue models, Curr Opin Biotechnol 35 (2015) 118–126.
[12] E. Fennema, N. Rivron, J. Rouwkema, C. van Blitterswijk, J. de Boer, Spheroid culture as a tool for creating 3D complex tissues, Trends Biotechnol 31 (2) (2013) 108–115.
[13] N.J. Douville, P. Zamankhan, Y.-C. Tung, R. Li, B.L. Vaughan, C.-F. Tai, et al., Combination of fluid and solid mechanical stresses contribute to cell death and detachment in a microfluidic alveolar model, Lab Chip 11 (4) (2011) 609–619.
[14] L. Kang, B.G. Chung, R. Langer, A. Khademhosseini, Microfluidics for drug discovery and development: from target selection to product lifecycle management, Drug Discov Today 13 (1) (2008) 1–13.
[15] D.L. Stirland, J.W. Nichols, S. Miura, Y.H. Bae, Mind the gap: a survey of how cancer drug carriers are susceptible to the gap between research and practice, J Control Release 172 (3) (2013) 1045–1064.
[16] T. Lammers, F. Kiessling, W.E. Hennink, G. Storm, Drug targeting to tumors: principles, pitfalls and (pre-) clinical progress, J Control Release 161 (2) (2012) 175–187.
[17] T.S. Fröde, Y.S. Medeiros, Animal models to test drugs with potential antidiabetic activity, J Ethnopharmacol 115 (2) (2008) 173–183.
[18] D. Huh, G.A. Hamilton, D.E. Ingber, From 3D cell culture to organs-on-chips, Trends Cell Biol 21 (12) (2011) 745–754.
[19] K.-J. Jang, A.P. Mehr, G.A. Hamilton, L.A. McPartlin, S. Chung, K.-Y. Suh, et al., Human kidney proximal tubule-on-a-chip for drug transport and nephrotoxicity assessment, Integr Biol 5 (9) (2013) 1119–1129.
[20] X. Mu, W. Zheng, J. Sun, W. Zhang, X. Jiang, Microfluidics for manipulating cells, Small 9 (1) (2013) 9–21.
[21] S.N. Bhatia, D.E. Ingber, Microfluidic organs-on-chips, Nat Biotechnol 32 (2014) 760.
[22] A. Bernard, J.P. Renault, B. Michel, H.R. Bosshard, E. Delamarche, Microcontact printing of proteins, Adv Mater 12 (14) (2000) 1067–1070.
[23] H.V. Prentice-Mott, C.-H. Chang, L. Mahadevan, T.J. Mitchison, D. Irimia, J.V. Shah, Biased migration of confined neutrophil-like cells in asymmetric hydraulic environments, Proc Natl Acad Sci U S A 110 (52) (2013) 21006.
[24] J.A. Barta, C.A. Powell, J.P. Wisnivesky, Global epidemiology of lung cancer, Ann Glob Health 85 (1) (2019) 8.
[25] L. Zhao, Z. Wang, S. Fan, Q. Meng, B. Li, S. Shao, et al., Chemotherapy resistance research of lung cancer based on micro-fluidic chip system with flow medium, Biomed Microdevices 12 (2) (2010) 325–332.
[26] D.D. Nalayanda, C. Puleo, W.B. Fulton, L.M. Sharpe, T.-H. Wang, F. Abdullah, An open-access microfluidic model for lung-specific functional studies at an air-liquid interface, Biomed Microdevices 11 (5) (2009) 1081.
[27] D. Huh, B.D. Matthews, A. Mammoto, M. Montoya-Zavala, H.Y. Hsin, D.E. Ingber, Reconstituting organ-level lung functions on a chip, Science 328 (5986) (2010) 1662.
[28] T. Kniazeva, J.C. Hsiao, J.L. Charest, J.T. Borenstein, A microfluidic respiratory assist device with high gas permeance for artificial lung applications, Biomed Microdevices 13 (2) (2011) 315–323.
[29] M.K. Chen, E.A. Beierle, Animal models for intestinal tissue engineering, Biomaterials 25 (9) (2004) 1675–1681.
[30] F.G. Rocha, E.E. Whang, Intestinal tissue engineering: from regenerative medicine to model systems, J Surg Res 120 (2) (2004) 320–325.

[31] J.P. Vacanti, Tissue and organ engineering: can we build intestine and vital organs? J Gastrointest Surg 7 (7) (2003) 831–835.
[32] A.J. Macpherson, E. Slack, M.B. Geuking, M.C. KD (Eds.), The mucosal firewalls against commensal intestinal microbes, in: Seminars in immunopathology, Springer, 2009.
[33] A.M. Ghaemmaghami, M.J. Hancock, H. Harrington, H. Kaji, A. Khademhosseini, Biomimetic tissues on a chip for drug discovery, Drug Discov Today 17 (3) (2012) 173–181.
[34] H. Kimura, T. Yamamoto, H. Sakai, Y. Sakai, T. Fujii, An integrated microfluidic system for long-term perfusion culture and on-line monitoring of intestinal tissue models, Lab Chip 8 (5) (2008) 741–746.
[35] H.J. Kim, D. Huh, G. Hamilton, D.E. Ingber, Human gut-on-a-chip inhabited by microbial flora that experiences intestinal peristalsis-like motions and flow, Lab Chip 12 (12) (2012) 2165–2174.
[36] J.H. Sung, J. Yu, D. Luo, M.L. Shuler, J.C. March, Microscale 3-D hydrogel scaffold for biomimetic gastrointestinal (GI) tract model, Lab Chip 11 (3) (2011) 389–392.
[37] Q. Ramadan, H. Jafarpoorchekab, C. Huang, P. Silacci, S. Carrara, G. Koklü, et al., NutriChip: nutrition analysis meets microfluidics, Lab Chip 13 (2) (2013) 196–203.
[38] S. Kim, H. Lee, M. Chung, N.L. Jeon, Engineering of functional, perfusable 3D microvascular networks on a chip, Lab Chip 13 (8) (2013) 1489–1500.
[39] C. Porth, Essentials of pathophysiology: concepts of altered health states, Lippincott Williams & Wilkins, 2011.
[40] W. Karwowski, B. Naumnik, M. Szczepański, M. Myśliwiec, The mechanism of vascular calcification—a systematic review, Med Sci Monit 18 (1) (2012) RA1–RA11.
[41] F. An, Y. Qu, X. Liu, R. Zhong, Y. Luo, Organ-on-a-chip: new platform for biological analysis, Anal Chem Insights 10 (2015). ACI.S28905.
[42] D. Mozaffarian, J. Benjamin Emelia, S. Go Alan, K. Arnett Donna, J. Blaha Michael, M. Cushman, et al., Executive summary: heart disease and stroke statistics—2016 update, Circulation 133 (4) (2016) 447–454.
[43] M. Reinecke, Neurotensin: immunohistochemical localization in central and peripheral nervous system and in endocrine cells and its functional role as neurotransmitter and endocrine hormone, Prog Histochem Cytochem 16 (1) (1985) III-172.
[44] M.P. van den Berg, K.Y. van Spaendonck-Zwarts, D.J. van Veldhuisen, J.A. Gietema, A. Postma, J.P. van Tintelen, Familial dilated cardiomyopathy: another risk factor for anthracycline-induced cardiotoxicity? Eur J Heart Fail 12 (12) (2010) 1297–1299.
[45] L. Gianni, E.H. Herman, S.E. Lipshultz, G. Minotti, N. Sarvazyan, D.B. Sawyer, Anthracycline cardiotoxicity: from bench to bedside, J Clin Oncol 26 (22) (2008) 3777–3784.
[46] A. Grosberg, P.W. Alford, M.L. McCain, K.K. Parker, Ensembles of engineered cardiac tissues for physiological and pharmacological study: heart on a chip, Lab Chip 11 (24) (2011) 4165–4173.
[47] H. Aubin, J.W. Nichol, C.B. Hutson, H. Bae, A.L. Sieminski, D.M. Cropek, et al., Directed 3D cell alignment and elongation in microengineered hydrogels, Biomaterials 31 (27) (2010) 6941–6951.
[48] Y. Xiao, B. Zhang, H. Liu, J.W. Miklas, M. Gagliardi, A. Pahnke, et al., Microfabricated perfusable cardiac biowire: a platform that mimics native cardiac bundle, Lab Chip 14 (5) (2014) 869–882.

[49] Encyclopædia Britannica, Liver in encyclopædia britannica, Encyclopædia Britannica, London, UK, 2019.
[50] P.J. Lee, P.J. Hung, L.P. Lee, An artificial liver sinusoid with a microfluidic endothelial-like barrier for primary hepatocyte culture, Biotechnol Bioeng 97 (5) (2007) 1340–1346.
[51] A. Bhushan, N. Senutovitch, S.S. Bale, W.J. McCarty, M. Hegde, R. Jindal, et al., Towards a three-dimensional microfluidic liver platform for predicting drug efficacy and toxicity in humans, Stem Cell Res Ther 4 (1) (2013) S16.
[52] M.L. Shuler, Advances in organ-, body-, and disease-on-a-chip systems, Lab Chip 19 (1) (2019) 9–10.
[53] N. Kashaninejad, M.R. Nikmaneshi, H. Moghadas, A. Kiyoumarsi Oskouei, M. Rismanian, M. Barisam, et al., Organ-tumor-on-a-chip for chemosensitivity assay: a critical review, Micromachines 7 (8) (2016).
[54] Y. Chen, P. Li, P.-H. Huang, Y. Xie, J.D. Mai, L. Wang, et al., Rare cell isolation and analysis in microfluidics, Lab Chip 14 (4) (2014) 626–645.
[55] B. Kwak, A. Ozcelikkale, C.S. Shin, K. Park, B. Han, Simulation of complex transport of nanoparticles around a tumor using tumor-microenvironment-on-chip, J Control Release 194 (2014) 157–167.
[56] I.K. Zervantonakis, C.R. Kothapalli, S. Chung, R. Sudo, R.D. Kamm, Microfluidic devices for studying heterotypic cell-cell interactions and tissue specimen cultures under controlled microenvironments, Biomicrofluidics 5 (1) (2011), 013406.
[57] A. Bruce, R. Evans, R. Mezan, L. Shi, B.S. Moses, K.H. Martin, et al., Three-dimensional microfluidic tri-culture model of the bone marrow microenvironment for study of acute lymphoblastic leukemia, PLoS One 10 (10) (2015), e0140506.
[58] J. Ruppen, F.D. Wildhaber, C. Strub, S.R. Hall, R.A. Schmid, T. Geiser, et al., Towards personalized medicine: chemosensitivity assays of patient lung cancer cell spheroids in a perfused microfluidic platform, Lab Chip 15 (14) (2015) 3076–3085.
[59] E.W. Young, C. Pak, B.S. Kahl, D.T. Yang, N.S. Callander, S. Miyamoto, et al., Microscale functional cytomics for studying hematologic cancers, Blood 119 (10) (2012) e76–e85.
[60] C. Pak, N.S. Callander, E.W.K. Young, B. Titz, K. Kim, S. Saha, et al., MicroC3: an ex vivo microfluidic cis-coculture assay to test chemosensitivity and resistance of patient multiple myeloma cells, Integr Biol 7 (6) (2015) 643–654.
[61] F. Hanif, K. Muzaffar, K. Perveen, S.M. Malhi, S.U. Simjee, Glioblastoma multiforme: a review of its epidemiology and pathogenesis through clinical presentation and treatment, Asian Pac J Cancer Prev 18 (1) (2017) 3–9.
[62] D.W. Parsons, S. Jones, X. Zhang, J.C.-H. Lin, R.J. Leary, P. Angenendt, et al., An integrated genomic analysis of human glioblastoma multiforme, Science 321 (5897) (2008) 1807.
[63] W. Liu, P. Sun, L. Yang, J. Wang, L. Li, J. Wang, Assay of glioma cell responses to an anticancer drug in a cell-based microfluidic device, Microfluid Nanofluid 9 (4) (2010) 717–725.
[64] T.C. Chang, A.M. Mikheev, W. Huynh, R.J. Monnat, R.C. Rostomily, A. Folch, Parallel microfluidic chemosensitivity testing on individual slice cultures, Lab Chip 14 (23) (2014) 4540–4551.
[65] J.M. Ayuso, R. Monge, A. Martínez-González, G.A. Llamazares, J. Berganzo, A. Hernández-Laín, et al., Abstract B04: an in vitro model for glioblastoma using microfluidics: Generating pseudopalisades on a chip, Cancer Res 75(23 Suppl.) (2015) B04.

[66] J.M. Ayuso, R. Monge, G.A. Llamazares, M. Moreno, M. Agirregabiria, J. Berganzo, et al., SU-8 based microdevices to study self-induced chemotaxis in 3D microenvironments, Front Mater 2 (37) (2015).
[67] J. Sun, M.D. Masterman-Smith, N.A. Graham, J. Jiao, J. Mottahedeh, D.R. Laks, et al., A microfluidic platform for systems pathology: multiparameter single-cell signaling measurements of clinical brain tumor specimens, Cancer Res 70 (15) (2010) 6128.
[68] Y. Huang, B. Agrawal, P.A. Clark, J.C. Williams, J.S. Kuo, Evaluation of cancer stem cell migration using compartmentalizing microfluidic devices and live cell imaging, JoVE 58 (2011), e3297.
[69] Q. An, H.L. Fillmore, M. Vouri, G.J. Pilkington, Brain tumor cell line authentication, an efficient alternative to capillary electrophoresis by using a microfluidics-based system, Neuro Oncol 16 (2) (2013) 265–273.

CHAPTER

Microfluidic devices for pathogen detection

6

Sepideh Ahmadi[a,b,*], Navid Rabiee[c], Mojtaba Bagherzadeh[c], and Mahdi Karimi[d,e,f,g]

[a]*Student Research Committee, Department of Medical Biotechnology, School of Advanced Technologies in Medicine, Shahid Beheshti University of Medical Sciences, Tehran, Iran*
[b]*Cellular and Molecular Biology Research Center, Shahid Beheshti University of Medical Sciences, Tehran, Iran*
[c]*Department of Chemistry, Sharif University of Technology, Tehran, Iran*
[d]*Cellular and Molecular Research Center, Iran University of Medical Sciences, Tehran, Iran*
[e]*Department of Medical Nanotechnology, Faculty of Advanced Technologies in Medicine, Iran University of Medical Sciences, Tehran, Iran*
[f]*Oncopathology Research Center, Iran University of Medical Sciences, Tehran, Iran*
[g]*Research Center for Science and Technology in Medicine, Tehran University of Medical Sciences, Tehran, Iran*
**Corresponding author. E-mail: speahmadi@yahoo.com*

6.1 Introduction

The microorganisms that are capable of causing disease in animals and humans, including bacteria, viruses, protozoa, and fungi are called pathogenic microorganisms [1]. Generally, in the developing world, up to 95% of mortality due to infections may be related to the lack of effective pathogen detection, and pathogen detection is accepted as a basic requirement for the prevention of infectious diseases. Despite recent advances in diagnosis, infectious diseases are still regarded as an important factor in mortality all around the world, such as lung infections, malaria, acquired immunodeficiency syndrome (AIDS), and COVID-19, etc. [2]. Additionally, in order to monitor the patients' response to treatment and disease progression, diagnostic tests that can measure (for instance the rate of viral load) are required to be repeated periodically.

The rapid, sensitive, and specific diagnosis of pathogens is very important to identify the source of infection, to improve the care of the patient by selecting the appropriate treatment, and to control the spread of diseases [3, 4]. The complexity and wide variety of pathogens as well as the different incubation periods before the onset of clinical symptoms (ranging from a few minutes to years after the initial infection) have made the detection of infectious pathogens a challenging problem.

Biomedical Applications of Microfluidic Devices. https://doi.org/10.1016/B978-0-12-818791-3.00006-1

When foods are contaminated, foodborne illnesses can be caused by pathogens, such as *Salmonella* [5], *Listeria monocytogenes* [6], *Vibrio parahaemolyticus* [7], *Escherichia coli* O157:H7, and *Shigella* [8], leading to a public health problem in food safety. Individuals infected with foodborne illnesses often have symptoms of diarrhea that can even lead to death, which is an important health problem worldwide. The World Health Organization (WHO) estimates that about 420,000 deaths in 2010 are due to infections caused by foodborne pathogens [9]. The portability and simplicity of a diagnostic microdevice could provide a platform for point-of-care (POC) diagnostics for foodborne pathogens, where rapid validation of food quality is needed.

In recent years, different techniques have been developed to diagnose microbial infections, which have both advantages and disadvantages, but many require culturing the bacteria and take 18–24h. The common methods that are available cannot completely eliminate the problems. For example, culture methods are the gold standard for the detection of bacteria but are time-consuming and limited by their inability to distinguish bacteria at the strain and species level [10]. In recent years, new molecular and immunological diagnostic methods have been established for pathogen identification. Molecular techniques such as nucleic acid-based-methods, e.g., polymerase chain reaction (PCR) [10–12], NASBA [13], loop-mediated isothermal amplification (LAMP) [14] and immunological-based methods, e.g., enzyme-linked immunosorbent assay (ELISA) [15], enzyme-linked fluorescent assay (ELFA) [16], lateral flow assays (LFAs) [17], and other methods such as next-generation sequencing (NGS) [18, 19]. Immunological-based such as ELISA [20], enzyme-linked fluorescent immunoassay (ELFA) [16], and molecular-based PCR [21] or mass spectroscopy methods [22], are used for rapid identification of pathogens. Although these techniques have high sensitivity, specificity, and reproducibility, they require labor-intensive sample preparation. Delay in the diagnosis of bacterial infections can be dangerous in emergencies like pandemics and epidemics. In addition, precision analysis and complex instruments are needed to diagnose pathogen infections, and some of the chemicals used in these diagnostic methods have a very limited shelf-life which limits their use. This limitation is more pronounced, especially in developing countries and rural areas where infectious microbial infections are more common and are likely to cause major health problems [23]. Table 6.1 describes the current techniques used for detection of various pathogens.

Much effort has been made to develop novel strategies based on microfluidic principles, for high-throughput and rapid pathogen detection to gain accurate evidence from samples containing different and unknown pathogens [34]. Microfluidics is the science of using and controlling very small amounts of fluids with volumes in the range of picoliters to microliters based on the regulation of layered fluid flow in small microchannels. These microchannels with desired shape and dimensions (10–100μm) are often constructed from a polydimethylsiloxane (PDMS) polymer and provide the possibility of establishing fluid flow with adjustable pressure [35]. Microfluidic chips can reduce the time gap between diagnosis and treatment, allow the consumption of only a small volume of fluid, control the process better, and provide a high accuracy due to the quick response of the system. These advantages could be necessary for the patients' survival [36, 37].

Table 6.1 The benefits and disadvantages of current methods used for detection of various pathogens.

	Advantages	Limitations	Refs.
Culture-based	Bacterial isolation for subsequent analysis (virulence determinants and antimicrobial susceptibility testing). Appropriate for slower-growing pathogens Qualitative and quantitative information	Risk of contamination High skill level is necessary for optimal results. Time-consuming (generally needs 2–3 days) False-positive results	[24, 25]
Biochemical test	Short analysis times, and the capability for simultaneous detection of more microorganisms than culture based	Requires a long time, low sensitivity and specificity, no direct detection from clinical samples, labor intensive, only possible on solid media, not possible for a specific microorganism	[25–28]
Immunoassay-based (i.e., ELISA)	High sensitivity, efficiency, and specificity, based on antigen-antibody reaction	Expensive to prepare antibody, instability, false positive/negative results, laborious assay	[29, 30]
Molecular-based (i.e., PCR)	High specificity, high sensitivity, automated, faster than culture methods, rapidly identify pathogens directly from clinical samples	False positive and false negative results, requires complex DNA extraction procedure	[12, 31]
Whole-genome sequencing (WGS)	Increased accuracy, diagnosis time is a few hours	Short sequence reading, restricted in identifying types of mutations	[32, 33]

Lab-on-a-chip (LOC) describes the use of microfluidics in chemical and biological studies and in analyte identification. The main purpose of LOC devices is to integrate several laboratory features on a single microfluidic chip [38]. LOC devices provide benefits for pathogen diagnosis such as a small sample volume, miniaturization, and a short diagnosis time [39].

Appropriate detection methods must be coupled to microfluidic devices in order to analyze the samples in an accurate and sensitive manner. This chapter discusses the preparation of microfluidic devices and different classes of LOC devices based on the detection technique involved, such as optical, electrochemical, mass spectrometry, or PCR-based methods. The main purpose of having the detection system incorporated into the microfluidic chip is to integrate it as an inseparable part of a transportable device with a rapid response and high sensitivity.

6.2 Sample preparation for microfluidics devices

Sample preparation plays an important role in increasing the diagnostic sensitivity, speed, and accuracy of microfluidic chips. Therefore, sample preparation is a key part of the analysis [40]. To carry out PCR-based techniques, we need to extract the DNA or RNA, which may be very time-consuming and problematic [41]. Moreover, it is required to increase the concentration of the extracted DNA, if the original concentration is not adequate. Other detection methods, such as optical analysis, fluorescence detection, or electrochemical analysis may reduce the required preprocessing of the sample, and enable automatic, easy, and rapid detection of bacterial infections [42–44]. Biological samples can be either simple or complex. In simple samples, even if the sample purification or preparation procedure has not been carried out extensively, the diagnosis procedure may still work well. Nevertheless, in complex samples, like foodborne pathogens, soil pathogens, or for some viruses, there may be difficulties. Very few individual pathogen entities may be contained in food, so that enrichment of the cells or analytes may be of great importance for efficient diagnosis [45, 46].

Microfluidic devices are able to rapidly and efficiently obtain results from small volumes of complex samples, and can also be used to concentrate pathogens into a smaller volume. This can increase the efficiency of the detection of pathogens. In 2005, researchers were able to collect dengue virus RNA using superparamagnetic beads inside a microfluidic system. Microbeads such as magnetic iron oxide nanoparticles (IONPs), are often used in microfluidic devices to increase the efficiency of pathogen identification. One of the strategies to prepare samples is to use ligand-functionalized beads (for instance antibodies) to extract the pathogens from contaminated samples. Pathogens attach to the beads, that can be enriched and collected by using an external magnetic field, called immunomagnetic separation (IMS). Molecules such as quantum dots or fluorescent dyes can be used to label the bacteria and separate unlabeled bacteria from labeled ones. First, magnetic beads are modified with antibodies to bind the pathogens, then a magnetic field is used to separate the labeled targets.

Kim et al. reported the concentration of *Salmonella typhimurium* bacteria using anti-Salmonella polyclonal antibody-conjugated QDs that bound to antibody-conjugated magnetic beads that isolated bacteria present at 10^3 CFU/mL in a food extract. After isolating the bacteria at ambient temperature, enrichment, and washing, two solutions of Ab-conjugated QDs and the captured cells were injected into the microfluidic device, and by using an external magnetic field, the labeled cells were visualized in the detection zone [47].

Kim et al. [48] used a three-dimensional (3D)-printed microfluidic platform (3DpμFD) and magnetic silica beads (MSBs) to purify the genomic DNA (gDNA) from *Staphylococcus aureus* and *E. coli* O157:H7. After the bacteria bound to the MSBs, the next step involved extracting the genomic RNA from the lysis buffer and then removing the buffer and bacteria. Finally, the ribonucleic acid (RNA) product could be eluted from the beads. With this system, *E. coli* was successfully detected from only a single colony-forming unit.

Although magnetic beads can help to enrich pathogens using a microdevice to rapidly and robustly identify pathogens in contaminated food, this procedure has several limitations, such as its high cost [49, 50].

Continuous flow separation microfluidic approaches have been used for rapid and low cost sample separation. Separation and concentration of foodborne bacteria from a large volume of sample (10 mL) using a nickel nanowire (NiNW) bridge was able to isolate 74% of the target bacteria in 3 h. The NiNW were first attached to bacteria-specific Abs, then, were injected into the microchannels to create bridges. Then, a large volume of bacterial suspension was injected into the microchannels using continuous flow, and the target bacteria bound to the Abs. The process is illustrated in Fig. 6.1 [51].

In continuous-flow separation, forces such as magnetophoretic, mechanical, dielectrophoretic, etc. can be used. One of the most widely used forces is acoustophoresis. Acoustophoresis is a technique that allows the label-free separation of micrometer-sized particles or bacteria based on their density and size. Ngamsom et al. employed an acoustophoretic method to collect bacteria on a chip. This system consisted of three inlets, a central channel, and three outlets all assembled on the chip. In side inlets, samples were injected, and the buffer was loaded through the central inlet. Upon ultrasound actuation, pathogenic cells remained adjacent to the channel walls, while large debris particles were separated into the center of the flow channel. This system was successfully validated with *Salmonella typhimurium* contaminated samples from chicken meat with 10(3) CFU/mL and a pathogen recovery of 60%–90% [52] (Fig. 6.2).

6.3 Microfluidic devices integrated with different technologies for the detection of pathogens

6.3.1 Biosensor-based microfluidics

The healthcare system is moving from physician-centered care toward patient-centered care, and diagnostic systems are no exception. Diagnostic systems are used to choose an individual treatment plan by rapid analysis of patient samples [53]. The development of the necessary systems to satisfy this demand must detect pathogenic bacteria related to health problems and food safety issues. Laws and regulations are applied in the food industry to avoid adverse consequences caused by microbial contamination. Although, achieving results in the shortest possible time is essential, nevertheless results often take 7 to 8 days using traditional and standard methods for pathogen detection [54]. So, many researchers have focused their efforts on more rapid techniques. The development of novel technologies, such as biosensors, has attracted much attention.

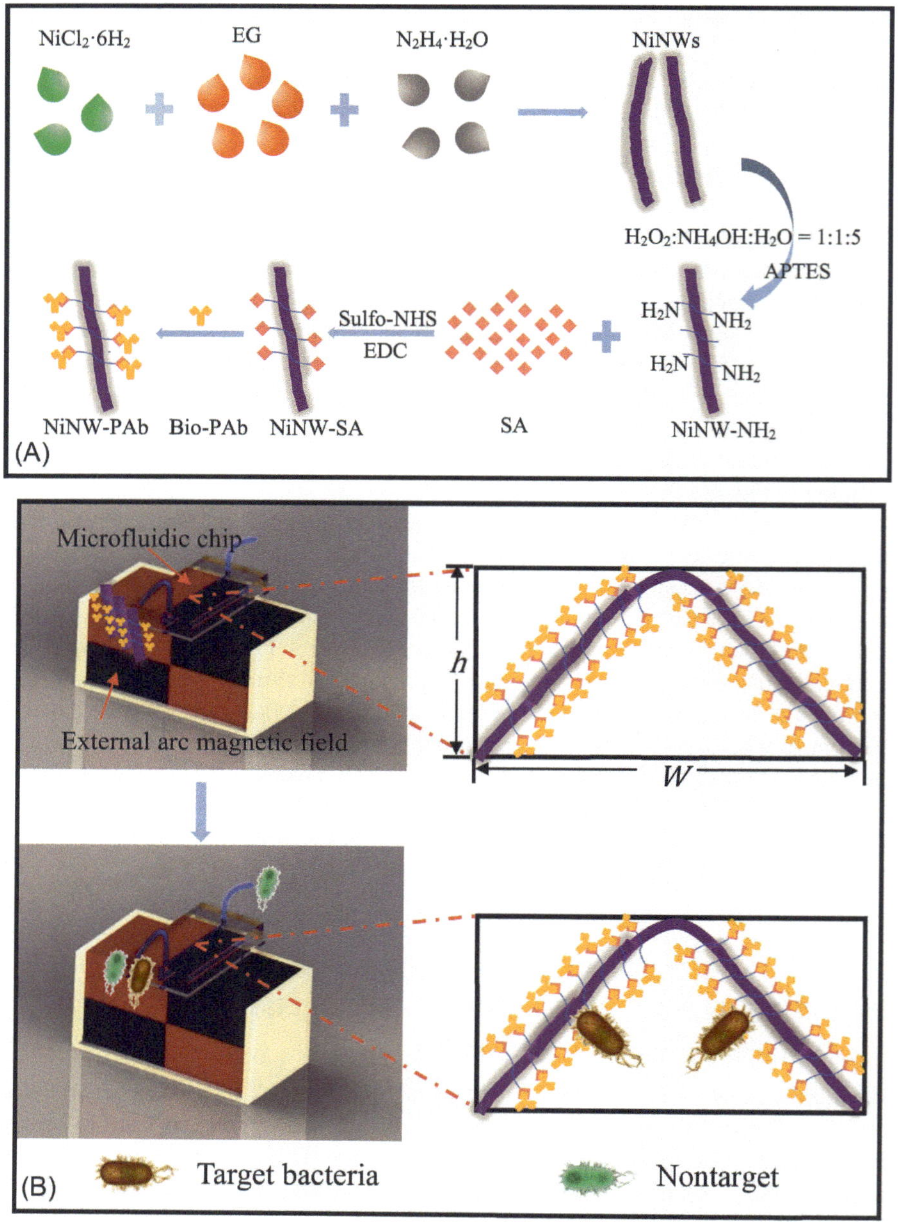

FIG. 6.1

Schematic illustration synthesis of immune nickel nanowires (NiNWs) (A) and continuous-flow separation of the large volumes of targeted bacteria using NiNWs (B) [51].

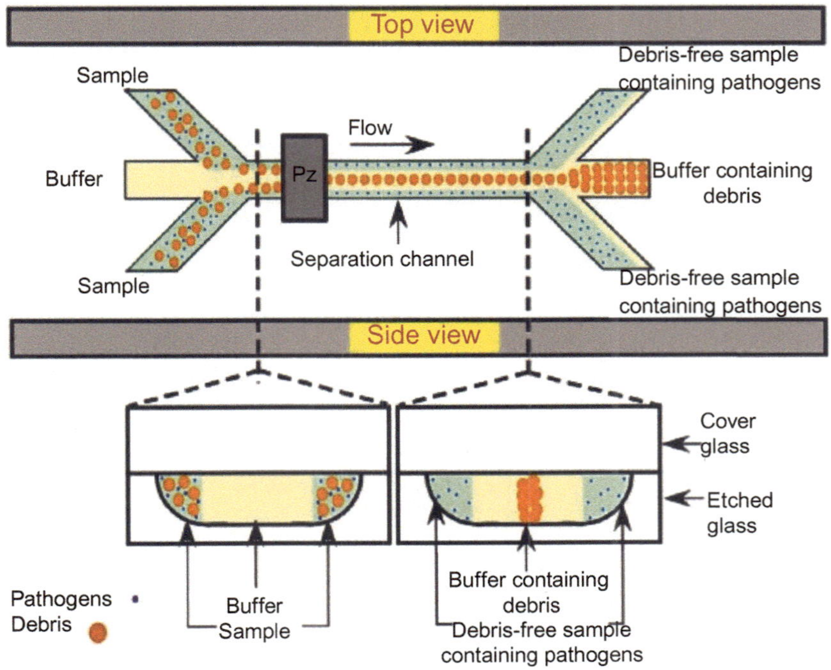

FIG. 6.2

An acoustophoresis microfluidic system for separation of *Salmonella typhimurium* [52].

Reprinted with permission from Elsevier.

The first biosensor was a glucose detection system invented by Professor Clark in 1962. Recently the integration of biosensors with microfluidic devices has allowed the combination of biological and chemical components into a single platform for pathogen detection and analysis of various analytes. Furthermore, biosensor-based microfluidics can increase the sensitivity and specificity, and also decrease the time and cost compared to conventional detection assays. Biosensors consist of two main components: (1) a biological element (such as aptamers, enzyme-based biosensor, or antibody-based biosensor) and (2) a signal transducer element.

Problems that are encountered in the conventional detection of pathogens include difficulties in DNA or RNA extraction, and inadequate amounts of sample. Microfluidics systems using optical or electrochemical readouts can directly detect very small numbers of bacterial cells. Biosensors can be categorized into several types depending on the type of transducer, such as optical fluorescence, chemiluminescence (CL), surface plasmon resonance (SPR), surface-enhanced Raman spectroscopy (SERS), electrochemical (amperometric, impedance, and potentiometric), or mass spectrometry (MS).

Advanced biosensors are very accurate, but require training to operate satisfactorily. Such devices are not very practical in resource-limited settings, because laboratories are rare, and the end-users may not know how to use them. Therefore, an autonomous microfluidic chip system that uses a smartphone for analysis is desirable. Novel methods, such as optical, acoustic, and electrochemical techniques, are included in the "noncell culture" diagnostic category. The most rapid and accurate techniques among the noncell culture procedures rely on optical techniques [55].

6.3.2 Optical-based microfluidics

The development of optical diagnostic methods in medicine has become an active area of photonics research. The reason is that some therapeutic bioanalytes have special optical spectral properties, such as fluorescence and absorption. These analytes include cholesterol, glucose, uric acid, therapeutic drugs, lactate, toxins, etc. [56]. The spectroscopic properties of these analytes are attributed to the presence of specific chromophores in these biomolecules. Optical biosensors have a broad application in the field of drug discovery and food safety. Optical biosensors are one of the most common types of diagnostic biosensor, that combine a biorecognition element and a signal recognition device to provide a rapid, sensitive and durable detection ability.

Examples of a microfluidic device for pathogen detection have been based on optical fibers [57], CL [58], fluorescence [59], or surface plasmon resonance (SPR) [60]. Optical-based microfluidics in general are composed of light sources and detectors.

Light sources can include commercial light-emitting diodes (LEDs) or diode lasers that are often used in microfluidics due to their availability and low price. Organic LEDs are newer alternatives and older dye lasers could also be used. Light sources should be fully integrated into the microfluidic and for maximum versatility [61]. Different detectors can be used for optical detection, the most common of which are charge-coupled device (CCD) sensors and photomultiplier tubes (PMTs), organic-OPDs, as well as CMOS sensors (complementary metal-oxide semiconductor). CCDs make possible multiplexed assays and the use of CMOS sensors and OPDs allow lens-free imaging [62, 63].

Optical biosensors for the identification of microorganisms can be characterized into sensor-based and substrate-based approaches. In the substrate-based approach, a glass slide or silicon wafer [64], polymer or paper films [65], have been used as platforms. The most common substrate for the recognition of microbes is glass slides that are often used for the detection of *Pseudomonas aeruginosa* [64, 66].

Despite recent advances in the use of electrochemical or mechanical biosensors in diagnosis, there are still challenges facing their application in microfluidics. The application of optical sensors is an interesting solution, which has received much attention given the ubiquity of laboratory optical methods and the desire for cost-effective devices for point of care (POC) applications [67]. However, there are still concerns about the application of optical sensors in LOC systems, including their cost-effectiveness and miniaturization ability. Over recent years, methods have been developed that can help solve these problems. Fluorescence and luminescence are among the common optical biosensors, which have been integrated into microfluidic chips and used to detect pathogens [68].

6.3.3 Fluorescence-based microfluidics

Optofluidic systems can employ surface-enhanced Raman scattering, light-scattering, or fluorescence-based methods for readouts. Fluorescence intensity measurement is a common technique in LOC devices, and combining fluorescent sensors with microfluidic chips, leads to increased sensitivity and efficiency [68, 69]. The use of fluorescence requires the sample to be conjugated to specific dyes that emit fluorescence when excited by a suitable light source [70, 71]. The fluorescence detection procedure depends on the parameters of excitation, excited-state lifetime, and fluorescence emission. The sensing process uses filters that can separate the emitted photons from excitation photons so that the emission can be quantified [72].

Fronczek et al. [73], prepared a rapid, sensitive paper-based microfluidic chip made from cellulose and nitrocellulose equipped with a smartphone-based fluorescence imaging system using a LED lamp for detection of *Salmonella typhimurium* with a LOD of 10^3 CFU/mL within 5 min.

In another study, a microdevice employed fluorescence labeling, immunomagnetic separation and smartphone video for the sensitive and rapid detection of *Salmonella typhimurium*. First, MNPs were modified by mAbs for separation of *Salmonella* from biological samples and a bacteria-mAb complex was formed. These bound to fluorescent microspheres (FMSs) attached to polyclonal antibodies (PAbs) and the final MNP-bacteria-FMS complex was formed. After the magnetic separation of fluorescent bacteria, this complex was injected into the microfluidic chip (PDMS microchannel and glass plate) and imaged with a smartphone-based fluorescent microscopy system (Fig. 6.3). This consisted of three parts: the smartphone App for real-time video processing, the light source for fluorescent excitation, and the fluorescent microscope as an optical amplifier. The results allowed quantitative bacterial analysis with a LOD of 58 CFU/mL within 2 h [74].

6.3.4 Chemiluminescence-based microfluidics

CL refers to light emission from the excited state product of a chemical reaction when it returns to its ground state [75]. In fact, when an electron reaches a lower energy level from the excited or higher energy level and emits its energy in the form of light, it is called a luminescence reaction. Several types of luminescence phenomena have been recognized (fluorescence, phosphorescence, and CL). CL phenomenon differs from other luminescence phenomena. In this phenomenon, the chemical or electrochemical reaction leads to electronic excitation, but the result is similar to fluorescence and light is emitted when the electron returns to the base energy level [76].

The types of CL are electrochemiluminescence (ECL), bioluminescence (BL), and thermochemiluminescence (TCL) [77]. The main advantages of using CL are high-quality measurement, good detection in low sample volumes and short times,

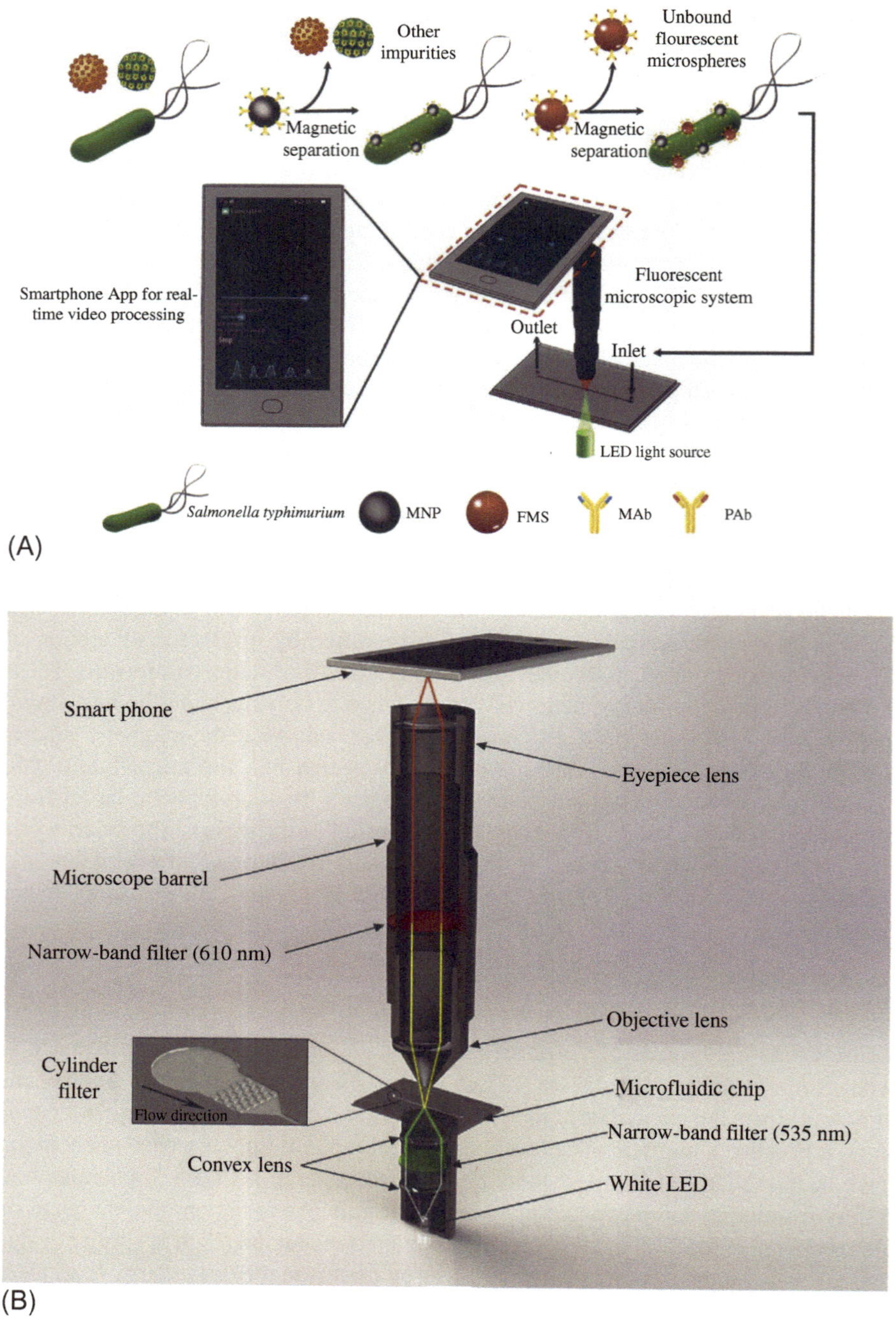

FIG. 6.3

(A) Schematic illustration of microdevice for sensitive and rapid dignosis of *Salmonella typhimurium*, (B) The structure of the smartphone based-fluorescent microscopic device [74].

Reprinted with permission from Elsevier.

integration with imaging systems, and simple equipment required for its measurement (no filters or light source) [77]. Light is produced by the oxidation of a chemoluminescent reagent, the most common of which are *p*-iodophenol (PIP) and luminol [78].

Chemoluminescence signals can be identified by a CCD camera, or a CMOS and a smartphone via an optical fiber [79, 80]. Zangheri et al. developed a new system based on the integration of a disposable portable microfluidic cartridge with a thin-film of a-Si:H photosensor for quantitative and multiplex detection of viral DNA (parvovirus B19 genotypes). One side of the glass slide consisted of three specific oligonucleotide probes coupled to the PDMS layer and the other side contained a thin film of a photosensor. Target probes were labeled with biotin and avidin-horseradish peroxidase (HRP) conjugate, binding was identified using CL, and signal measurement was performed by a CCD camera. This procedure offered advantages such as high specificity, high detectability in low volume samples (50-μL) during 1 h [58] (Fig. 6.4).

6.3.5 Plasmonic-based microfluidics

One of the outstanding developments in sensors has been plasmonic sensors for pathogen recognition. Two main plasmonic sensors apply local SPR, SERS, and localized SPR (LSPR) [81]. In the following section, we will discuss these types of plasmonic sensors and their application in microfluidics for the detection of pathogens.

SPR describes the excitation of electrons at the interface of a thin metal film such as gold and a surrounding dielectric medium. The coupling of a light wave with the metal film excites surface plasmons [81]. SPR technologies can involve metal NPs (silver, gold, magnetic) or thin gold films to identify pathogens [82, 83], nucleic acids [84], drugs [85], or proteins [86].

In the sensor, the target receptors are located on the metal surface and electromagnetic radiation of a certain wavelength interacts with the electron cloud of the thin metal and produces a strong resonance when pathogens have been bound to the metal surface, leading to wavelength changes. High-sensitivity and real-time detection are the advantages of SPR biosensors [87]. SPR sensors have low sensitivity, due to the limited penetration depth of SPR into a metal surface (< 300 nm) [88]. LSPR is an indirect assay to increase the SPR sensitivity, and allow real-time, cost-effective, and label-free pathogen detection. The use of a modified LSPR-based sensing platform allowed the identification of whole-cell bacteria *Pseudomonas aeruginosa* strain PAO1 with a LOD 10–10^3 CFU/mL in ~3 h using a single sensor [89].

An LSPR sensor using Au trigonal nanoprisms modified with a mixture of Bt-PEG thiols was prepared for the ultrasensitive identification of whole-cell *Acinetobacter baumannii* with a LOD of 80 bacterial cells. The sensitivity of LSPR sensors can be increased by improving the stability of the Bt-siderophore and optimizing the conditions [90].

However, SPR biosensors have some limitations: (1) Sensitivity to the environment, (2) Sample volume required, and (3) Refractive index of the target [91].

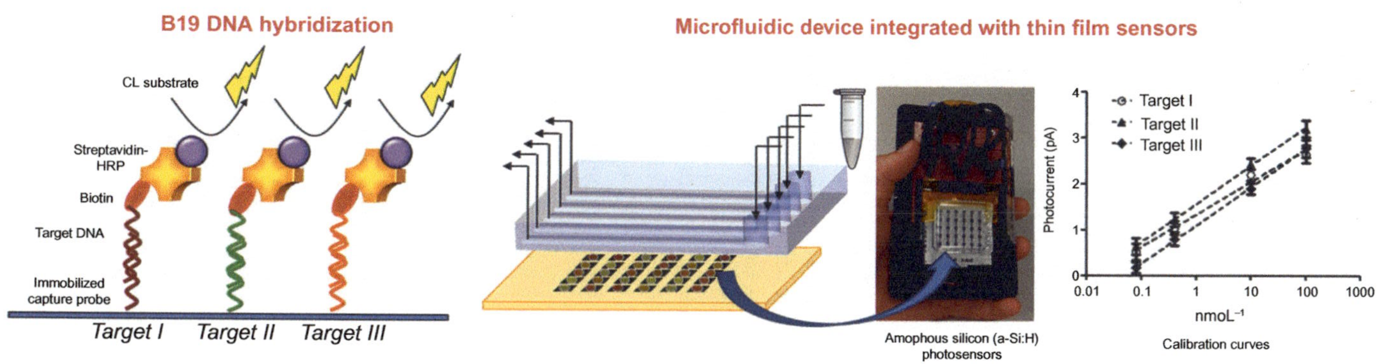

FIG. 6.4

Schematic illustration of microfluidic cartridge with thin-film of a-Si:H photosensor for quantitative and multiplex detection of parvovirus B19 genotypes [58].

Reprinted with permission from Elsevier.

Microfluidics chips allow the easy detection of very small amounts of samples using SPR or LSPR when integrated onto chips [92]. Coupling SPR sensors to chips is achieved by a metal grating, prism, or waveguide. In the prism coupling mode, a layer of gold is placed onto the walls of the microfluidic channels and used to detect the analyte binding after it flows over the film [93].

Tokel et al. [94] developed a cheap, label-free, portable microfluidic-based SPR system for the identification of *E. coli* and *Staphylococcus aureus* in PD and PBS fluid with LOD of 10^5 and 3.2×10^7 CFU/mL (Fig. 6.5). The gold-coated glass substrate was placed on the rectangular prism, modified with *N*-(3-dimethylaminopropyl)-*N′*-ethyl carbodiimide hydrochloride (EDC), 11-mercaptoundecanoic acid (MUA), *N*-hydroxysuccinimide (NHS), and antibodies that recognized *E. coli* lipopolysaccharide (anti-LPS) and lipoteichoic acid of *Staphylococcus aureus* (anti-LAT). The bacteria were captured by the antibodies on the gold-coated surface, leading to alterations in the local refractive index. This alteration creates a signature in the reflected light, which was transmitted to the computer for analysis. SPR is also a promising technique to detect other pathogens such as AIDS, influenza, and hepatitis viruses.

Zordan et al. [95] developed an SRP-microdevice for multiplexed diagnosis of *E. coli* O157:H7. The antibody was placed on the surface of the chip to specifically bind to *E. coli* O157:H7, and not bind to negative controls. The bacteria were fluorescently labeled and then added to the chip surface. Therefore, when the bacterial cells were captured by the antibody, the SPRi images allowed differentiation of fluorescent living pathogenic cells from dead cells and negative control cells simultaneously.

SPR-based microfluidic systems can be small devices that are portable and allow rapid pathogen detection. However, there is a need for improvement due to the low concentration of food pathogens, the complexity of the samples, to need to optimize and adapt the SPR sensors, and to improve cost-effectiveness. The limits on temperature difference and the high cost of the chips are considered as other disadvantages of SPR systems, which would need to be considered for point-of-care (POC) diagnostics.

SERS is a surface method to increase the sensitivity of Raman scattering signals from molecules adsorbed on the metal surface (an optical characteristic of specific materials) [96]. The enhancement coefficient can be as high as 10^{10} and it can detect single molecules as well [97]. SERS refers to the study of samples that have been adsorbed and interact with metals surfaces in geometries. In fact, SERS is a surface effect obtained by the application of a metal substrate, and the target molecule or molecule is adsorbed onto the metal, and the Raman scattering signal is significantly enhanced, compared to normal Raman spectroscopy [98]. Fleischmann [99] introduced this technique for the first time and showed a Raman scattering signal from pyridine on a silver electrode.

SERS methods are becoming progressively more widespread and are now available for specific and accurate, real-time detection of pathogens. However, the reproducibility of SERS-based methods is a challenge due to the complex signals. This problem can be overcome by integrating the SERS techniques into a microdevice, which can provide a continuous flow condition for SERS measurement. SERS based

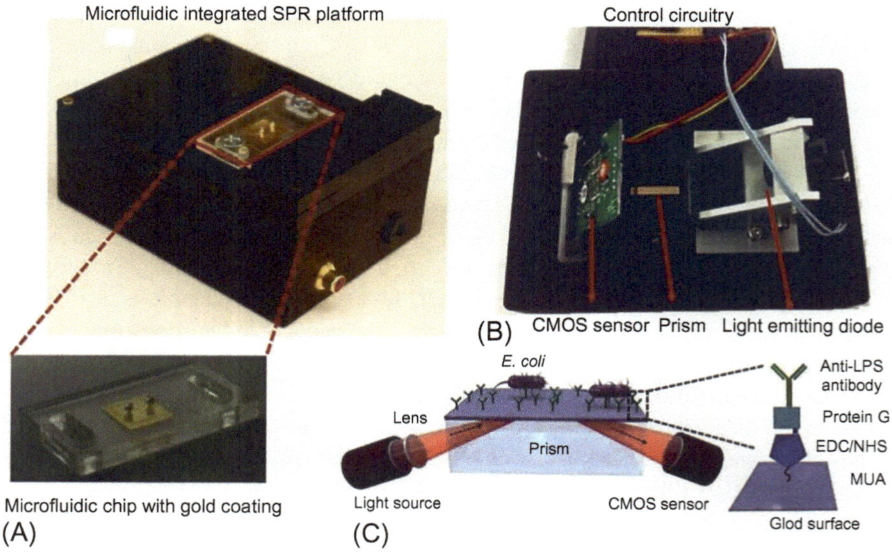

FIG. 6.5

Plasmonic chip for multiplex and inexpensive diagnosis of *E. coli* and *Staphylococcus aureus*. (A) Microfluidic chip with gold coating, (B) The electronic setup of the device, and (C) Schematics illustration of the microfluidic integrated SPR platform [94].

microfluidic devices or lab-on-a-chip SERS (LoC-SERS) can perform elaborate sample processing for accurate analysis of pathogens. Microfluidic chips combined with SERS and dielectric electrophoretic (DEP) enrichment methods were constructed which could allow the enrichment and detection of *Staphylococcus aureus* in 15 s.

A microfluidic device was constructed by combining a nano-DEP enrichment strategy and integrating it with SERS reporters, in a self-referencing platform with the capacity to identify 10 CFU/mL of *E. coli* O157:H7 with 95% accuracy [100]. In this study, to increase the LOD for an on-site recognition system, a bacterial concentration mechanism based on Nano-DEP enrichment was applied to increase the SERS signal.

6.3.6 Colorimetric-based microfluidics

Colorimetric biosensors are label-free optical sensors that allow the operator to directly observe (using the naked eye) the detection of pathogenic agents in samples producing a color change. There is no need for complex optical devices, and this method is qualitative or semiquantitative. Colorimetric sensor arrays have been used for the detection of 15 cultured bacterial pathogens, with high specificity (99.4%) and sensitivity (91%) over 2 h [101]. Colorimetric sensors can be divided into two different types: (1) solution based [102, 103], and (2) substrate based [104]. Solution-based colorimetric biosensors using nanomaterials can be used for sensitive and rapid detection, but need large volumes of samples for the assay. In solution-based biosensors, AuNPs are commonly employed and the color change can be observed through the aggregation of the Au-NPs [12]. In the substrate-based assays, materials include glass, polymers, nanomaterials (nanoparticles, nanotubes, nanoplate), silicon, and paper and need only a small volume of sample. The substrate can be made more sensitive using optical conductive layers, such as gold layers, or magnetic beads to capture pathogens such as *E. coli* cells.

In one study, Zheng et al. [105] developed a colorimetric based on-chip bioreactor microfluidic chip using a glass substrate to rapidly identify *E. coli* by aggregation of AuNPs and a smartphone imaging system. This microfluidic device consisted of two serpentine mixing channels, a separation chamber, and a detection chamber. Catalase was mixed with the bacterial sample in the first mixing channel, after addition of AuNPs and a cross-linking agent, the MNPs-*E. coli*-PS complex moved to the separation chamber. Then after injection of H_2O_2 the MNPs-*E. coli*-PS reacted with the bound catalase in the second mixing channel. If a sample was present, a color change from blue to red was observed. The LOD was 50 CFU/mL within 1 h and this method had high sensitivity and specificity. But this method could not attain the LOD of 1 CFU/mL needed for foodborne pathogen detection. This microfluidic device enabled mixing between the nanoparticles and liquid samples and had the ability to use a small microscale fluid volume.

A paper chip offers an analytical platform for POC experiments for bacterial identification and detection of contamination in water [106, 107]. For the first time in 2007, the Whitesides team reported the construction of microfluidic paper-based analytical devices (μPAD) [108].

A μPAD used hydrophilic paper and permits hydrophobic regions to be made with different polymers for colorimetric detection [109]. Colorimetry is commonly regarded as the most appropriate detection method to be integrated with μPADs, due to its compatibility with low-cost reporting systems, including scanners and smartphones [110, 111].

Kim and Yeo [112] described a wax-printed microfluidic μPAD for in situ detection of *E. coli* in environmental samples. This sensor relies on a combination of catalysts and Fenton chemistry for colorimetric detection. First, a suspension containing *E. coli* is mixed with hydrogen peroxide and then the residual hydrogen peroxide reacts with a compound of iron (II) in the paper-based LOC chambers, and the color changes from pale yellow to brown. Therefore, the color intensity increases as the microorganism number increases.

Lately, a μPAD was employed for colorimetric detection of human papillomavirus (HPV16) DNA from cervical samples in less than an hour [113]. The system was fabricated from pressure-sensitive adhesive sheets and paper to extract, amplify, and detect nucleic acids, and was developed for rapid detection of cervical cancer, human immunodeficiency virus-1 (HIV-1), *E. coli*, and *Staphylococcus aureus* pathogens [114].

They first modified the AuNPs with specific identification elements and then transferred the modified AuNP solution to a cellulose paper strip. If the samples are recognized, the NPs accumulate and change color. The color change of the AuNPs was detectable by the naked eye. A mobile camera was also used to capture the spot image of the NPs, and LOD was reported as 8 CFU/mL.

μPADs have been prepared using numerous techniques, photolithography or chemical vapor deposition (CVD) [115]. CVD and photolithography offer good accuracy, but they are costly and complex procedures [116, 117]. Cheaper printing methods include screen, inkjet, and wax printing [118, 119]. Wax printers and inkjet printers need to be modified to construct μPAD. A laser printed microfluidic paper-based analytical device (LP-μPAD) was constructed with benefits such as simplicity, low cost, rapidity, and user-friendly operation. It used a microwell spot assay and lateral flow for the rapid diagnosis of *E. coli* and nitrate. The microwell spot assay for the diagnosis of living *E. coli* worked after the functionalization of LP-μPAD with APETS, and the β-galactosidase enzyme from lysed *E. coli* was immobilized on the surface of the LP-μPAD. By the addition of a chlorophenyl red β-galactopyranoside (CPRG) substrate, the detection of the lowest concentration of *E. coli* (10^4 CFU/mL) was achieved by a color change from yellow to red-violet in a short time [117].

6.3.7 Electrochemical-based microfluidics

Electrochemical recognition is another option for miniaturized analytical approaches. Due to its numerous benefits such as simplicity, the possibility of miniaturization, portability, low cost, using a small sample size, and high sensitivity, electrochemical biosensors have received considerable attention [120, 121]. Therefore, electrochemical biosensors have a high potential to become POC sensors for sensitive diagnosis of diseases [122]. The application of electrochemical biosensors for pathogen detection is favorable due to the above-mentioned advantages [123, 124]. Electrochemical biosensor systems can be integrated within a microfluidic system, with advantages such as ease of sample preparation, high adaptability, and sensitivity [125].

In electrochemical sensors, the electrode is used as a transducer to convert biological information to an electronic signal, and the electrical signals (potentials) produced by the electrochemical reaction are measured at the electrode surface [126]. This enables the quantitative analysis of analytes. The electrochemical biosensor is able to combine the analytical ability of electrochemical techniques with the specific recognition function of the biological element. The receptor is immobilized on an appropriate electrode and the interaction of the analyte (measured substance) with the bioreceptor leads to the generation of the electrical signal (potentiometric, amperometric response, etc.), which is proportional to the analyte concentration [127].

Potentiometric, impedimetric, and amperometric/voltammetric, are the electrochemical sensor approaches that can be integrated into microdevices [128]. In potentiometric sensors, changes in the voltage signal are detected [129], in amperometric sensors, changes in current are detected [130]. The impedance signal is produced by the obstruction of the electron-transfer with the electrode surface, subsequent to the specific binding of element and analyte. Compared to other electrochemical sensors, these sensors are label-free and are also a good choice for small molecule toxins, while sometimes multipart arrays and high-density electrodes have to be combined to increase the LOD [128]. Compared to optical methods, this type of electrochemical sensor can analyze turbid samples and has low costs, although they are not significantly different in terms of sensitivity and selectivity. In both voltammetric and amperometric sensors, the transducer is an electrode made of materials such as gold (Au), carbon or platinum (Pt) [131, 132].

Altintas et al. developed an automated microfluidic-based electrochemical biosensor for real-time amperometric measurement of the waterborne pathogen *E. coli*. The microfluidic device was integrated with a HRP-conjugated biosensor and eight Au electrodes. Bacterial cells could be bound on the surface of the Au electrodes. HRP-labeled antibodies were used to form a sandwich structure with the captured bacterial cells for electrochemical measurement of the reaction between HRP and 3,3′,5,5′-tetramethylbenzidine (TMB). This system identified *E. coli* with a LOD as low as 50 CFU/mL [133]. The advantage of this sensor was that its surface had the ability to be regenerated multiple times, which could significantly reduce the cost of the system. It could also be useful in identifying other pathogens in addition to *E. coli* [134].

The impedimetric method is based on material conductivity measurement. It was first used to quantitatively determine the biomass or biological mass within a sample. The advantage of this method over the two others is that it does not need markers and has ease of integration [135–137]. The disadvantages of the impedimetric method are its low sensitivity, low reproducibility, and time consumption [138]. The microfluidic device can increase the sensitivity of an impedance biosensor by integrating the electrode into a small microfluidic channel. In addition, the microdevice can improve reproducibility by reducing the chance of electrode fouling, which is an important problem in microelectrode based impedance detection. Lastly, the microdevice enables better control and management of small volumes of liquid samples for impedance detection [135]. The rapid response of the impedance biosensors makes them appropriate for diagnostic applications. Rapid diagnosis of *Salmonella typhimurium* by integrating microfluidics with a vertical electrode led to a 10-fold increase in sensitivity compared to nonmicrofluidic methods. Anti-Salmonella monoclonal Abs were coated on a high-density electrode inside a microfluidic chip which used an impedance analyzer for selective detection [139].

The application of integrated DEP technology on microfluidic chips enriches the bacteria and increases diagnostic sensitivity. The DEP performance in increasing the detection sensitivity is limited. Improving the performance and sensitivity of DEP with the use of metal NPs such as silver, gold, could be advantageous.

Wang et al. [140] designed a multifunctional microfluidic chip with a Tesla mixing zone, interdigital microelectrodes and a detection zone in order to increase the sensitivity of impedimetric detection of *E. coli* using silver NPs to improve the impedance signals, and reached a LOD of 500 CFU/mL. In this study, bacteria were coated with PDDA, and after adding AuNPs into the mixing zone in the microfluidic device, it formed an *E. coli*/PDDA/AuNP complex. By adding silver NPs, the complex was enriched at the edge of microelectrode within the detection zone.

In another study, Ghosh Dastider et al. [134] successfully prepared a microfluidic MEMS biosensor for the specific and sensitive detection of *E. coli* O157:H7 using antibody-antigen recognition and impedance spectroscopy in order to detect bacteria at concentrations of 39 CFU/mL in 2 h.

The microfluidic MEMS biosensor contained two focusing and sensing areas. The sensing area contained three sets of interdigitated microelectrode arrays (IDEAs) resulting in the detection of very low numbers of bacteria with very high sensitivity, and a focusing electrode pair was located within the microfluidic channel. The anti-*E. coli* antibody was bound to the sensing IDEAs, the impedance change occurred after antigen binding, and changes were measured in the 100 Hz–10 MHz frequency range. Moreover, in this system, the sensing area electrodes used a positive dielectrophoretic force (*p*-DEP) resulting in the concentration of the bacteria within the central channel.

An electrode array interdigitated (IDE array) could be used to simultaneously detect two different serotypes of *Salmonella* with a concentration of 300 CFU/mL. This system had a structure such that two sets of IDE arrays in two channels (antibody and antigen channels) could be used for the simultaneous identification of two *Salmonella* species without any cross-contamination. In this system, the bacterial sample flowed through the sample inlet into the area of sensing IDE and after the area was filled, the flow was stopped in a few minutes to further increase the association between the antigen and the antibody. Just like techniques such as PCR, this technique does not require extraction or amplification and in case of the increased concentration of bacteria, impedance flow rate increases, too [141].

Potentiometric assay or potentiometry is less common than other types of biosensors and employs a membrane with selective permeability to ions or other bioactive substances such as enzymes. During the reaction which is catalyzed by an enzyme, the materials are consumed or produced which are then detected by the electrode. Using this sensor, very small changes in concentration can also be detected. Guilbault and Montalvo in 1969 reported the first potentiometric biosensor to detect urea [142]. However, despite the significant benefits of electrochemical based microfluidic devices, they still have limitations, such as their difficult production.

6.3.8 PCR-based microfluidic systems

In nucleic acid-based diagnostics, DNA or RNA is used for the diagnosis. In order to identify pathogens such as *Streptococci*, *E. coli*, *Helicobacter pylori* or fungi, an adequate volume of genetic material and sample size are required [143, 144]. Nucleic acid-based microfluidic pathogen detection has been expanded to cover a wide range of bacteria, viruses, and fungi. By improving integration, tuning, amplification, and signal detection, LOC technology can reduce the time required for assays as well as sample consumption and cost reduction [145].

The first microfluidic-PCR device was reported by Kopp et al. [146]. After transferring the 10-μL sample through the microfluidic channel and passing it repeatedly through three controlled temperature zones, they observed that 20 PCR cycles could be accomplished in approximately 2 min. Henceforth, numerous researchers have been endeavoring to develop improved PCR-based microfluidic devices to increase sensitivity and reduce production costs.

There are plentiful examples of rapid microfluidic diagnosis of pathogenic genomic material, but they still have problems. These concerns include low concentrations of targets as well as a rather complex biological sample matrix. Accordingly, there is a balance between the minimum sample size, the rapid assessment, and the sensitivity of the detection, that should be optimized in manufacturing the final device. PCR and real-time PCR are widely used for amplification in most of these systems. PCR is one of the most commonly used techniques in DNA technology. Integrating PCR with microfluidic systems makes it possible to control the small volume consumption of samples, a higher surface to volume ratio, as well as the rapid transfer of mass and heat. There is a need for a well-controlled temperature-time cycle in microfluidic PCR systems, as well as a requirement for rapid heat transfer and temperature uniformity within the system [147]. Therefore, there is a need for preparation steps of the sample, including lysis of the cells, and purification to remove contaminants as well as nucleic acid purification in microfluidic PCR systems [66].

Microfluidic PCR has a lower thermal mass than conventional PCR systems, as well as high surface-to-volume ratio of microfluidic PCR systems that leads to rapid heat transfer [148]. As a result, the time required to achieve the equilibrium temperature during the denaturing and annealing steps can be significantly reduced. In this system, the consumption of expensive materials is also significantly reduced [147]. In addition, the integration of pre- and post-PCR steps involves identification, sample handling, mixing, and isolation in a single chip, which may be advantageous for system integration and system automation [149, 150].

The synthesis of PCR-based microchannels or microchambers employs silicon, glass, polycarbonate [151], PMMA [152] or polydimethylsiloxane (PDMS) [153]. Although new materials like cyclic olefin copolymer (COC), SU-8 [154], or $LiNbO_3$ [155] have also been tested in PCR microfluidic devices. The identification of PCR products is performed using fluorescence microscopy or real-time fluorescence detection [156, 157].

Three main types of microfluidic PCR devices include shunting PCR, chamber-based stationary, and continuous flow. Northrup et al. [158] developed the first PCR chip based on a stationary chamber. In this PCR device, the PCR solution was kept stationary and the temperature of the reaction chamber was cycled between the different temperatures.

However, a chamber-based stationary PCR microfluidic setup has limitations such as a lack of flexibility to change the PCR speed and is more time-consuming [159].

Continuous-flow PCR can overcome the limitations of chamber-based stationary PCR chips, with faster cooling and heating times and a decrease in the total time of the PCR reaction. Continuous-flow PCR can be classified into two types, single-phase microfluidic PCR, and droplet microfluidic PCR. In continuous-flow PCR microfluidics, the following features were found to be critical: heater spacings, chip material choice, number of cycles, and length ratio of the channels [160]. In the single-phase system, the chamber or channel is filled with a single aqueous phase containing the PCR components. This system has some challenges, such as causing contamination between samples, and low sensitivity [161, 162].

Combining nested PCR with single-phase systems can partially solve their challenges and increase diagnostic sensitivity. Nested PCR uses two sets of primers (outer and inner). The first-round target sequence is amplified by PCR using the outer primers. In the second round, the first-round product acts as a template for the inner primers. This can increase the level of microfluidic-PCR sensitivity by increasing the concentration of the analyte and reducing the probability of producing nonspecific products and nonspecific binding to the target [163]. For example, the identification and genotyping of 11 human RNA viruses present in feces, oysters samples, or sewage, using microfluidic nested PCR on an array chip and MiSeq sequencing, enabling more than 20,000 reads in low virus samples (LOD = 10^0 to 10^3 copies/mL in cDNA sample, 10^1–10^4 copies/mL in sewage, and 10^5–10^8 copies/g in human feces or oysters) [164].

High sensitivity detection of *Listeria monocytogenes* at 0.2 copies/μL by single-phase continuous-flow nested PCR (SP-CF-NPCR) was achieved (Fig. 6.6A). In the three isothermal regions of the cylindrical cavity channel, the reaction mixture flowed continuously thus completing the first and second PCR. The role of the disposable polytetrafluorethylene (PTFE) tube reactor was to not only provide the correct sample, but it could also be replaced with new tubing to avoid cross-contamination of the samples (Fig. 6.6) [165].

Due to the disadvantages of single-phase systems, recent research has concentrated on droplet systems and digital microfluidics. In droplet microfluidic systems using two immiscible fluids forming droplets in microchannels using the mixing flow of immiscible fluids. These systems decrease analysis times, increase sensitivity, and allow high-throughput screening [166, 167]. In any single droplet, PCR can be well controlled, efficient, and repeatable. It also produces less cross-contamination. Digital microfluidics are widely used in applications with low consumption of samples. Splitting and merging droplets into digital microfluidics allows better sample performance. Droplet-based microfluidics and digital microfluidics now play important roles in advanced nucleic acid (NA) amplification assays [66, 168].

Bian et al. designed a droplet digital PCR (ddPCR) device for the simultaneous detection of *E. coli* and *Listeria monocytogenes* in water samples. This system consists of a polyethylene siloxane saturated mineral oil (OSP) chip that could prevent the evaporation of water droplets. The system integrated droplet production, on-chip amplification, and end-point fluorescence readout in other to detect *Listeria monocytogenes* and *E. coli* with a LOD of 10 CFU/mL in 2 h [169].

The loop-mediated isothermal amplification technique (LAMP) carries out NA amplification and has received much attention due to its advantageous properties. LAMP operates without a thermal cycler and is more tolerant of inhibitory

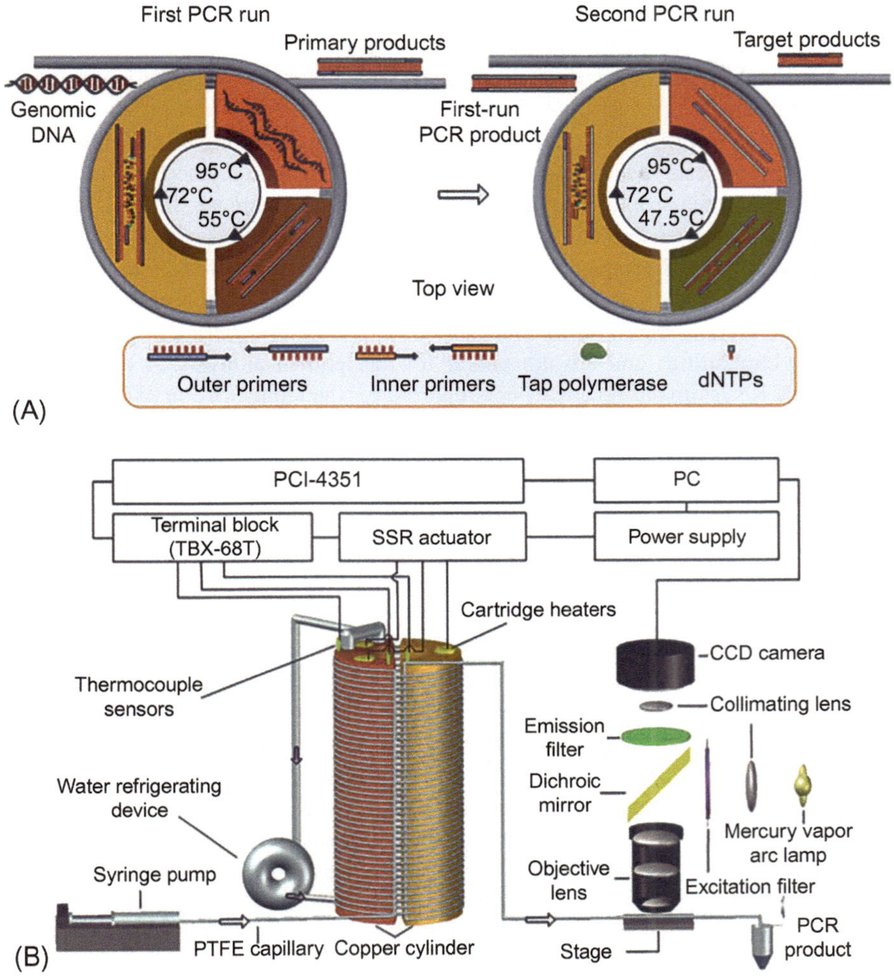

FIG. 6.6

Schematic illustration of the SP-CF-NPCR (A) and cylindrical helical-channel continuous-flow nested PCR microfluidics device (B) [165].

compounds than PCR, therefore has been effectively employed for the identification of pathogens. It also produces 50 times more signal than PCR [170]. The specific stem-loop design of primers (4–6 primers), strand displacement specificity of Bst DNA polymerase enzyme, and the use of DNA-reactive dyes have made this method independent from thermocycling and electrophoresis equipment. The use of the LAMP method in microdevices for the rapid detection of pathogens has become a new trend. This technology has advantages such as short reaction time and constant temperature amplification. It has great potential in POC testing as a combination of LAMP and droplet microfluidics.

The combination of the LAMP with microfluidic droplets provided an accurate and sensitive biosensor for the detection of RNA extracted from *Salmonella typhimurium*. Millions of water-in-oil droplets were combined with the LAMP reaction cocktail using a microfluidic flow-focusing system. After incubating the droplets at 68°C for 30 min, the droplets were then photographed using a ZOE fluorescent cell imager, and positive and negative droplets could be distinguished. In this experiment, the greater the droplet size (20 μm), the greater the diagnostic limit (10^5 X) and 40 μm droplets showed ≥ 10(5) X [171].

Occasionally, PCR products may be extracted and subsequent analysis performed for diagnostic purposes, such as real-time PCR with gel electrophoresis. However, microfluidic systems based on chamber-based stationary and continuous flow setups, lack these capabilities and are not useful for subsequent analysis. A microfluidic shunting PCR system has recently been reported for the identification of 0.7 ng/μL of *E. coli* [172]. This system consisted of a polycarbonate chip, a shunting thermal cycler, and a fluorescence detector with advantages such as faster heating and cooling times as well as the ability to extract the PCR product. The use of a shunting thermal cycler can provide rapid temperature cycles. It also reduces the amplification time and reduces temperature overshooting. This system is capable of carrying out PCR with different annealing temperatures ranging from 54°C to 68°C and amplifying three different PCR products with sizes of 250, 552, and 1500 bp.

Nowadays, various commercial microfluidic PCR devices are able to detect a variety of pathogens. In fact, they make it possible to use low volume samples in clinical trials. Also, they allow the performance of medical tests in the doctors' office and with no need for further testing. One example is the use of a commercial microfluidic-based PCR system such as, the BioMark. 48.48 Dynamic Array which is manufactured by Fluidigm (San Francisco, California). In fact, this system is able to perform 2304 reactions per chip, despite the fact that fewer liquid loading steps are required. This chip has the ability to perform several reactions that could be used to detect different types of bacteria involved in lignocellulose decomposition [173].

Current commercial digital PCR (dPCR) systems include the QX100 and QX200 instruments (Bio-Rad), 3D instruments and QuantStudio 12 K Flex (Thermo Fisher, Waltham, Massachusetts), RainDrop (RainDance, Billerica, Massachusetts) that have been developed for the detection of pathogens. For example, a low copy number of HIV DNA can be measured by QX100 (Bio-Rad) or Quantstudio 3D (Life Technologies). In QX100 and Bio-Rad, droplets are produced in the microfluidic system, and these droplets are used in the thermal cycler for performing amplification [174].

However, there are still barriers to further use of commercial microfluidic systems, including lack of FDA-approved tests, and high costs of these systems preventing their use in developing countries.

6.3.9 Mass spectrometry-based microfluidics

Mass spectrometry (MS) can allow highly selective detection of the mass of ions using magnetic and electrical fields [175]. In recent years, the coupling of microfluidic chips with several MS systems, particularly liquid chromatography-mass spectrometry (LC-MS) or LC-ESI-MS system, electrospray ionization (ESI), matrix-assisted laser desorption/ionization (MALDI), has allowed the detection of pathogens, especially bacteria and fungi. Chip-MS has been used for medical diagnosis, treatment of diseases, microbial metabolism studies, and single-cell analysis. However, MS-microfluidic systems have not been developed as much as other methods such as optical and electrochemical detection methods. One of the most difficult problems is the coupling of the detection performed in the microfluidic system with off-chip MS analysis. However, the results of this system may worth the trouble in the future [176].

In one study, Bian et al. constructed a PDMS LC-MS microfluidic system for collection (using a microfluidic trapping device) and detection (LC-MS) of three different bacterial samples in an aerosol, *E. coli*, *Vibrio parahemolyticus*, and *Listeria monocytogenes*. The air sampler consisted of a double spiral microchannel as well as a pump in the inlet area. The pump transmitted airflow containing various types of bacteria into the spiral channel and trapped them. Compared to current methods, this system could collect and enrich samples with very high efficiency (100%). Overall, this system showed lower cost and greater efficacy than conventional approaches, with promise in future diagnostic applications [177].

Table 6.2 shows a list of microfluidic devices that have been integrated with different technologies for the detection of pathogens.

6.4 Conclusions

Rapid and effective detection of disease-causing and foodborne pathogens is important for the treatment of diseases and preventative clinical applications. Microfluidic technology can replace conventional methods such as culture and biochemical tests, increasing the sensitivity and diagnostic specificity. One of the problems is the process of identifying, preparing, and condensing complex samples. However, efficient multipathogen capture from complex food samples for high-throughput analysis is possible but still challenging. This is mostly due to the absence of generally applicable bacterial adsorbents, with a high affinity for pathogens. In recent years, aptamers and antibodies have been widely used to identify pathogens in food samples in integrated microfluidic devices. Other molecules, include phages, lectins, etc. have been investigated. All these recognition systems can be developed in microfluidic devices to improve sample preparation and preconcentration steps. The combination of microfluidic systems with other biosensors, such as optical, electrochemical, as well as, nucleic acid amplification using LAMP and PCR, can be used for rapid identification of pathogens. While optical methods are usually more sensitive to electrochemical detection, most of these systems are expensive and complex. Electrochemical-based microfluids also need to be improved with regards to performance and reproducibility. To reduce diagnostic costs, microfluidic systems are changing to paper or polymer-based systems that can still function effectively. For example, replacing

Table 6.2 Pathogen detection based on microfluidic systems made of different materials.

	Methods	Pathogens	Materials used	Limit of detection (LOD)	Refs.
Optical-based microfluidic					
	SERS-based optofluidics	*Listeria monocytogenes* and *Listeria innocua*	PDMS	–	[178]
	SERS-based microfluidic	*Staphylococcus aureus, Escherichia coli, Pseudomonas aeruginosa*	PDMS	5×10^3 CFU/mL	[179]
	Microfluidic chip, NanoGene assay	*E. coli* O157:H7	PMMA	49×10^{15} mol/L	[180]
	Hybrid microfluidic SPR	*E. coli* O157:H7	Microfluidic chip assembly of SF10 glass chip, SU-8 and PDMS chip	–	[95]
	Immunofluorescence microfluidic	*Aspergillus niger*	SU-82025, PDMS	20 spores	[181]
	SEB LOC system	Staphylococcal enterotoxin B (SEB)	PMMA	0.1 ng/mL	[182]
	Impedance microfluidic	*E. coli* O157:H7 and *Staphylococcus aureus*	PDMS	10^2 CFU/mL	[183]
	Centrifugal microfluidic automatic wireless endpoint detection system integrated with loop-mediated isothermal amplification (LAMP)	*E. coli*, *Salmonella* spp., and *Vibrio cholerae*	PMMA	3×10^{-5} ng μL^{-1}	[184]

Electrochemical based microfluidic					
	Graphene oxide-based impedance electrochemical immunosensor	Influenza viruses	PDMS chips	1 to 10^4 PFU mL^{-1}	[185]
	Microfluidic multiplex electrochemical LAMP (μME-LAMP) device	*Mycobacterium tuberculosis* (MTB), *Haemophilus influenza* (HIN), and *Klebsiella pneumonia* (KPN)	PDMS chips	28, 17, and 16 copies μL^{-1} for MTB, HIN, and KPN	[186]
	Electrochemical microfluidic paper-based immunosensor array (E-μPIA)	HIV/HCV	–	LODs of 300 pg/mL and 750 pg/mL for HIV and HCV	[187]
PCR-based microfluidic					
	POC RTPCR platform	Zika virus or chikungunya virus	–	10 RNA copies per microliter	[188]
	qRT-PCR	Influenza viruses	–	less than 10 RNA copies per reaction	[189]
	On-chip mixed-dye-based LAMP (CMD-LAMP)	*Vibrio parahemolyticus*	PDMS, silicon	1×10^3 CFU/mL	[190]
	Continuous flow high-throughput PCR microfluidic	Airborne pathogens	PDMS	18 Cells per reaction were achieved for *E. coli*	[191]
	Digital PCR chip	Antibiotic resistance bacteria (*E. coli*)	Glass	5 pg genomic DNA, equivalent to 900 blaCTX-M-15 copies	[192]
	LAMP-droplet microfluidic	*Salmonella typhimurium*	PDMS, Glass	5000 CFU/mL in the sample, or 25 RNA template	[171]

silicon systems with polymer or polycarbonate chips can overcome the limitations. In general, laboratory diagnostic methods are moving forward today, and many tests are being designed based on microfluidic systems, which can be very effective in early diagnosis and medical and diagnostic sciences.

References

[1] A. Godfree, 17—Health constraints on the agricultural recycling of wastewater sludges, in: D. Mara, N. Horan (Eds.), Handbook of water and wastewater microbiology, Academic Press, London, 2003, pp. 281–298.

[2] M.T. Caballero, et al., Mortality associated with acute respiratory infections among children at home, J Infect Dis 219 (3) (2019) 358–364.

[3] A.M. Caliendo, et al., Better tests, better care: improved diagnostics for infectious diseases, Clin Infect Dis 57 (Suppl. 3) (2013) S139–S170.

[4] T. Briese, et al., Diagnostic system for rapid and sensitive differential detection of pathogens, Emerg Infect Dis 11 (2) (2005) 310–313.

[5] I.R. Lake, Food-borne disease and climate change in the United Kingdom, Environ Health 16 (Suppl. 1) (2017) 117.

[6] A. Chlebicz, K. Śliżewska, Campylobacteriosis, salmonellosis, yersiniosis, and listeriosis as zoonotic foodborne diseases: a review, Int J Environ Res Public Health 15 (5) (2018) 863.

[7] S.-W. Jung, A foodborne outbreak of gastroenteritis caused by Vibrio parahaemolyticus associated with cross-contamination from squid in Korea, Epidemiol Health 40 (2018) e2018056-0.

[8] J. Tataryn, et al., Outbreak of E. coli O157:H7 associated with lettuce served at fast food chains in the Maritimes and Ontario, Canada, Dec 2012, Can Commun Dis Rep 40 (Suppl. 1) (2014) 2–9.

[9] A.H. Havelaar, et al., World Health Organization global estimates and regional comparisons of the burden of foodborne disease in 2010, PLoS Med 12 (12) (2015) e1001923.

[10] J. Zhang, et al., Development of Candida-specific real-time PCR assays for the detection and identification of eight medically important Candida species, Microbiol Insights 9 (2016) 21–28.

[11] Y. Yamamoto, PCR in diagnosis of infection: detection of bacteria in cerebrospinal fluids, Clin Diagn Lab Immunol 9 (3) (2002) 508–514.

[12] S. Ahmadi, et al., Thiol-capped gold nanoparticle biosensors for rapid and sensitive visual colorimetric detection of Klebsiella pneumoniae, J Fluoresc 28 (4) (2018) 987–998.

[13] N. Cook, The use of NASBA for the detection of microbial pathogens in food and environmental samples, J Microbiol Methods 53 (2) (2003) 165–174.

[14] Y. Li, et al., Loop-mediated isothermal amplification (LAMP): a novel rapid detection platform for pathogens, Microb Pathog 107 (2017) 54–61.

[15] J. Wang, et al., Enzyme-liked immunosorbent assay for the detection of pathogenic spiroplasma in commercially exploited crustaceans from China, Aquaculture 292 (3) (2009) 166–171.

[16] K. Rohonczy, et al., Comparison of an automated ELFA and two different real-time PCR techniques for Salmonella detection in poultry samples, Acta Microbiol Immunol Hung 61 (3) (2014) 261–272.

[17] Z. Li, H. Chen, P. Wang, Lateral flow assay ruler for quantitative and rapid point-of-care testing, Analyst 144 (10) (2019) 3314–3322.

[18] E. Anis, et al., Evaluation of targeted next-generation sequencing for detection of bovine pathogens in clinical samples, J Clin Microbiol 56 (7) (2018) e00399-18.

[19] M. Gwinn, D. MacCannell, G.L. Armstrong, Next-generation sequencing of infectious pathogensnext-generation sequencing of infectious pathogensnext-generation sequencing of infectious pathogens, JAMA 321 (9) (2019) 893–894.

[20] M. Feng, et al., Development of a monoclonal antibody-based ELISA to detect Escherichia coli O157:H7, Food Agric Immunol 24 (4) (2013) 481–487.

[21] M.F. Anjum, E. Zankari, H. Hasman, Molecular methods for detection of antimicrobial resistance, Microbiol Spectr 5 (6) (2017) 0011-2017.

[22] L. Krásný, R. Hynek, I. Hochel, Identification of bacteria using mass spectrometry techniques, Int J Mass Spectrom 353 (2013) 67–79.

[23] H. Kim, D.-R. Chung, M. Kang, A new point-of-care test for the diagnosis of infectious diseases based on multiplex lateral flow immunoassays, Analyst 144 (8) (2019) 2460–2466.

[24] R.A. Deshmukh, et al., Recent developments in detection and enumeration of waterborne bacteria: a retrospective minireview, Microbiologyopen 5 (6) (2016) 901–922.

[25] L. Váradi, et al., Methods for the detection and identification of pathogenic bacteria: past, present, and future, Chem Soc Rev 46 (16) (2017) 4818–4832.

[26] B.A. Pinsky, et al., Comparison of real-time PCR and conventional biochemical methods for identification of Staphylococcus lugdunensis, J Clin Microbiol 47 (11) (2009) 3472–3477.

[27] R. Franco-Duarte, et al., Advances in chemical and biological methods to identify microorganisms-from past to present, Microorganisms 7 (5) (2019) 130.

[28] C.M. O'Hara, Manual and automated instrumentation for identification of Enterobacteriaceae and other aerobic gram-negative bacilli, Clin Microbiol Rev 18 (1) (2005) 147–162.

[29] S. Sakamoto, et al., Enzyme-linked immunosorbent assay for the quantitative/qualitative analysis of plant secondary metabolites, J Nat Med 72 (1) (2018) 32–42.

[30] S. Hosseini, et al., Advantages, disadvantages and modifications of conventional ELISA, in: S. Hosseini, et al. (Eds.), Enzyme-linked immunosorbent assay (ELISA): from A to Z, Springer Singapore, Singapore, 2018, pp. 67–115.

[31] A.-K. Järvinen, et al., Rapid identification of bacterial pathogens using a PCR- and microarray-based assay, BMC Microbiol 9 (2009) 161.

[32] S.E. Hasnain, et al., Whole genome sequencing: a new paradigm in the surveillance and control of human tuberculosis, Tuberculosis 95 (2) (2015) 91–94.

[33] S. Quainoo, et al., Whole-genome sequencing of bacterial pathogens: the future of nosocomial outbreak analysis, Clin Microbiol Rev 30 (4) (2017) 1015.

[34] A.M. Foudeh, et al., Microfluidic designs and techniques using lab-on-a-chip devices for pathogen detection for point-of-care diagnostics, Lab Chip 12 (18) (2012) 3249–3266.

[35] T.A. Duncombe, A.M. Tentori, A.E. Herr, Microfluidics: reframing biological enquiry, Nat Rev Mol Cell Biol 16 (9) (2015) 554–567.

[36] D. Zhang, et al., Detection of pathogenic microorganisms by microfluidics based analytical methods, Anal Chem 90 (9) (2018) 5512–5520.

[37] K. Kaarj, P. Akarapipad, J.-Y. Yoon, Simpler, faster, and sensitive zika virus assay using smartphone detection of loop-mediated isothermal amplification on paper microfluidic chips, Sci Rep 8 (1) (2018) 12438.

[38] H. Jayamohan, H.J. Sant, B.K. Gale, Applications of microfluidics for molecular diagnostics, Methods Mol Biol 949 (2013) 305–334.
[39] S.L. Karsten, et al., Point-of-care (POC) devices by means of advanced MEMS, Talanta 145 (2015) 55–59.
[40] J. Yin, et al., Integrated microfluidic systems with sample preparation and nucleic acid amplification, Lab Chip 19 (17) (2019) 2769–2785.
[41] A. Mäki, et al., Sample preservation, DNA or RNA extraction and data analysis for high-throughput phytoplankton community sequencing, Front Microbiol 8 (2017) 1848.
[42] X. Zhao, M. Li, Y. Liu, Microfluidic-based approaches for foodborne pathogen detection, Microorganisms 7 (10) (2019) 381.
[43] H.E. Giana, et al., Rapid identification of bacterial species by fluorescence spectroscopy and classification through principal components analysis, J Fluoresc 13 (6) (2003) 489–493.
[44] Y. Huang, et al., Disease-related detection with electrochemical biosensors: a review, Sensors 17 (10) (2017) 2375.
[45] Y. Zhao, et al., Rapid multiplex detection of 10 foodborne pathogens with an up-converting phosphor technology-based 10-channel lateral flow assay, Sci Rep 6 (1) (2016) 21342.
[46] K.A. Stevens, L.A. Jaykus, Bacterial separation and concentration from complex sample matrices: a review, Crit Rev Microbiol 30 (1) (2004) 7–24.
[47] G. Kim, et al., A microfluidic nano-biosensor for the detection of pathogenic Salmonella, Biosens Bioelectron 67 (2015) 243–247.
[48] Y. Kim, J. Lee, S. Park, A 3D-printed millifluidic platform enabling bacterial preconcentration and dna purification for molecular detection of pathogens in blood, Micromachines 9 (9) (2018) 472.
[49] G. Jenikova, J. Pazlarova, K. Demnerova, Detection of Salmonella in food samples by the combination of immunomagnetic separation and PCR assay, Int Microbiol 3 (4) (2000) 225–229.
[50] X. Li, et al., Rapid sample processing for detection of food-borne pathogens via crossflow microfiltration, Appl Environ Microbiol 79 (22) (2013) 7048–7054.
[51] X. Huo, et al., Continuous-flow separation and efficient concentration of foodborne bacteria from large volume using nickel nanowire bridge in microfluidic chip, Micromachines 10 (10) (2019) 644.
[52] B. Ngamsom, et al., On-chip acoustophoretic isolation of microflora including S. typhimurium from raw chicken, beef and blood samples, J Microbiol Methods 123 (2016) 79–86.
[53] M. van der Eijk, et al., Moving from physician-centered care towards patient-centered care for Parkinson's disease patients, Parkinsonism Relat Disord 19 (11) (2013) 923–927.
[54] O. Lazcka, F.J. Del Campo, F.X. Munoz, Pathogen detection: a perspective of traditional methods and biosensors, Biosens Bioelectron 22 (7) (2007) 1205–1217.
[55] G. Luka, et al., Microfluidics integrated biosensors: a leading technology towards lab-on-a-chip and sensing applications, Sensors 15 (12) (2015) 30011–30031.
[56] S.K. Krishnan, et al., A review on graphene-based nanocomposites for electrochemical and fluorescent biosensors, RSC Adv 9 (16) (2019) 8778–8881.
[57] C.L. Lin, et al., A microfluidic system integrated with buried optical fibers for detection of Phalaenopsis orchid pathogens, Biosens Bioelectron 63 (2015) 572–579.

[58] M. Zangheri, et al., Microfluidic cartridge with integrated array of amorphous silicon photosensors for chemiluminescence detection of viral DNA, Sens Biosens Res 7 (2016) 127–132.

[59] W. Zhang, et al., Microfluidics using a thiol–acrylate resin for fluorescence-based pathogen detection assays, Lab Chip 15 (21) (2015) 4227–4231.

[60] C. Liu, D. Cui, H. Li, A hard–soft microfluidic-based biosensor flow cell for SPR imaging application, Biosens Bioelectron 26 (1) (2010) 255–261.

[61] P.K. Dasgupta, et al., Light emitting diode-based detectors: absorbance, fluorescence and spectroelectrochemical measurements in a planar flow-through cell, Anal Chim Acta 500 (1) (2003) 337–364.

[62] S. Rezaei-Mazinani, et al., Monitoring fluorescent calcium signals in neural cells with organic photodetectors, J Mater Chem C 7 (29) (2019) 9049–9056.

[63] G. Williams, C. Backhouse, H. Aziz, Integration of organic light emitting diodes and organic photodetectors for lab-on-a-chip bio-detection systems, Electronics 3 (1) (2014) 43–75.

[64] L. Preiss, S. Neethirajan, Single cells of Pseudomonas aeruginosa exhibit electrotaxis and durotaxis behaviours, bioRxiv (2015) 020511.

[65] C.-C. Lin, et al., Microfluidic immunoassays, J Assoc Lab Autom 15 (3) (2010) 253–274.

[66] L. Gorgannezhad, H. Stratton, N.-T. Nguyen, Microfluidic-based nucleic acid amplification systems in microbiology, Micromachines 10 (6) (2019) 408.

[67] N.M.M. Pires, et al., Recent developments in optical detection technologies in lab-on-a-chip devices for biosensing applications, Sensors 14 (8) (2014) 15458–15479.

[68] B. Srinivasan, S. Tung, Development and applications of portable biosensors, J Lab Autom 20 (4) (2015) 365–389.

[69] Z. Shu, et al., Highly sensitive on-chip fluorescence sensor with integrated fully solution processed organic light sources and detectors, RSC Adv 7 (42) (2017) 26384–26391.

[70] D. Musumeci, et al., Fluorescence sensing using DNA aptamers in cancer research and clinical diagnostics, Cancer 9 (12) (2017) 174.

[71] Á. Szabó, et al., The effect of fluorophore conjugation on antibody affinity and the photophysical properties of dyes, Biophys J 114 (3) (2018) 688–700.

[72] M.Y. Berezin, S. Achilefu, Fluorescence lifetime measurements and biological imaging, Chem Rev 110 (5) (2010) 2641–2684.

[73] C.F. Fronczek, et al., Paper microfluidic extraction and direct smartphone-based identification of pathogenic nucleic acids from field and clinical samples, RSC Adv 4 (22) (2014) 11103–11110.

[74] S. Wang, et al., A microfluidic biosensor for online and sensitive detection of Salmonella typhimurium using fluorescence labeling and smartphone video processing, Biosens Bioelectron 140 (2019) 111333.

[75] D. Christodouleas, et al., Flow-based methods with chemiluminescence detection for food and environmental analysis: a review, Anal Lett 44 (1–3) (2011) 176–215.

[76] M. Lee, Basic skills in interpreting laboratory data, American Society of Health-System Pharmacists, USA, 2013.

[77] L.J. Kricka, Chemiluminescent and bioluminescent techniques, Clin Chem 37 (9) (1991) 1472–1481.

[78] L. Gámiz-Gracia, et al., Analysis of pesticides by chemiluminescence detection in the liquid phase, TrAC Trends Anal Chem 24 (11) (2005) 927–942.

[79] W. Zhao, K. Sakurai, Seeing elements by visible-light digital camera, Sci Rep 7 (2017) 45472.

[80] M.K. Khoury, I. Parker, D.W. Aswad, Acquisition of chemiluminescent signals from immunoblots with a digital single-lens reflex camera, Anal Biochem 397 (1) (2010) 129–131.

[81] J. Wang, et al., Surface plasmon resonance sensors on raman and fluorescence spectroscopy, Sensors 17 (12) (2017) 2719.

[82] S. Bouguelia, et al., On-chip microbial culture for the specific detection of very low levels of bacteria, Lab Chip 13 (20) (2013) 4024–4032.

[83] V. Koubová, et al., Detection of foodborne pathogens using surface plasmon resonance biosensors, Sensors Actuators B Chem 74 (1) (2001) 100–105.

[84] R. D'Agata, G. Spoto, Artificial DNA and surface plasmon resonance, Artif DNA PNA XNA 3 (2) (2012) 45–52.

[85] M. Rusnati, et al., Speeding up the identification of cystic fibrosis transmembrane conductance regulator-targeted drugs: an approach based on bioinformatics strategies and surface plasmon resonance, Molecules 23 (1) (2018) 120.

[86] P.P. Vachali, et al., Surface plasmon resonance (SPR)-based biosensor technology for the quantitative characterization of protein-carotenoid interactions, Arch Biochem Biophys 572 (2015) 66–72.

[87] A.H.-P. Ho, et al., SPR biosensors, in: A.H.P. Ho, D. Kim, M.G. Somekh (Eds.), Handbook of photonics for biomedical engineering, Springer Netherlands, Dordrecht, 2014, pp. 1–19.

[88] A. Abbas, M.J. Linman, Q. Cheng, Sensitivity comparison of surface plasmon resonance and plasmon-waveguide resonance biosensors, Sensors Actuators B Chem 156 (1) (2011) 169–175.

[89] J. Hu, K. Fu, P.W. Bohn, Whole-cell Pseudomonas aeruginosa localized surface plasmon resonance aptasensor, Anal Chem 90 (3) (2018) 2326–2332.

[90] J. Hu, et al., Whole-cell biosensing by siderophore-based molecular recognition and localized surface plasmon resonance, Anal Methods 11 (3) (2019) 296–302.

[91] M. Piliarik, J. Homola, Surface plasmon resonance (SPR) sensors: approaching their limits? Opt Express 17 (19) (2009) 16505–16517.

[92] L. Niu, et al., Integrating plasmonic diagnostics and microfluidics, Biomicrofluidics 9 (5) (2015) 052611.

[93] H. Gai, Y. Li, E.S. Yeung, Optical detection systems on microfluidic chips, Top Curr Chem 304 (2011) 171–201.

[94] O. Tokel, et al., Portable microfluidic integrated plasmonic platform for pathogen detection, Sci Rep 5 (2015) 9152.

[95] M.D. Zordan, et al., Detection of pathogenic E. coli O157:H7 by a hybrid microfluidic SPR and molecular imaging cytometry device, Cytometry A 75 (2) (2009) 155–162.

[96] S.-Y. Ding, et al., Electromagnetic theories of surface-enhanced Raman spectroscopy, Chem Soc Rev 46 (13) (2017) 4042–4076.

[97] A.M. Polubotko, Dipole-quadrupole theory of surface enhanced infrared absorption and appearance of forbidden lines in the spectra of symmetrical molecules, Opt Spectrosc 114 (5) (2013) 696–703.

[98] Z.-Q. Tian, et al., Expanding generality of surface-enhanced Raman spectroscopy with borrowing SERS activity strategy, Chem Commun (34) (2007) 3514–3534.

[99] M. Fleischmann, P.J. Hendra, A.J. McQuillan, Raman spectra of pyridine adsorbed at a silver electrode, Chem Phys Lett 26 (2) (1974) 163–166.

[100] C. Wang, et al., Detection of extremely low concentration waterborne pathogen using a multiplexing self-referencing SERS microfluidic biosensor, J Biol Eng 11 (1) (2017) 9.

[101] S.H. Lim, et al., Bacterial culture detection and identification in blood agar plates with an optoelectronic nose, Analyst 141 (3) (2016) 918–925.

[102] S. Jongjinakool, et al., Gold nanoparticles-based colorimetric sensor for cysteine detection, Energy Procedia 56 (2014) 10–18.

[103] H. Aldewachi, et al., Gold nanoparticle-based colorimetric biosensors, Nanoscale 10 (1) (2018) 18–33.

[104] M. Retout, et al., Rapid and selective detection of proteins by dual trapping using gold nanoparticles functionalized with peptide aptamers, ACS Sens 1 (7) (2016) 929–933.

[105] L. Zheng, et al., A microfluidic colorimetric biosensor for rapid detection of Escherichia coli O157:H7 using gold nanoparticle aggregation and smart phone imaging, Biosens Bioelectron 124–125 (2019) 143–149.

[106] J. Noiphung, W. Laiwattanapaisal, Multifunctional paper-based analytical device for in situ cultivation and screening of Escherichia coli infections, Sci Rep 9 (1) (2019) 1555.

[107] A. Abdollahi-Aghdam, M.R. Majidi, Y. Omidi, Microfluidic paper-based analytical devices (μPADs) for fast and ultrasensitive sensing of biomarkers and monitoring of diseases, Bioimpacts 8 (4) (2018) 237–240.

[108] A.W. Martinez, et al., Patterned paper as a platform for inexpensive, low-volume, portable bioassays, Angew Chem Int Ed 46 (8) (2007) 1318–1320.

[109] M. Sher, et al., Paper-based analytical devices for clinical diagnosis: recent advances in the fabrication techniques and sensing mechanisms, Expert Rev Mol Diagn 17 (4) (2017) 351–366.

[110] A.W. Martinez, et al., Simple telemedicine for developing regions: camera phones and paper-based microfluidic devices for real-time, off-site diagnosis, Anal Chem 80 (10) (2008) 3699–3707.

[111] G.G. Morbioli, et al., Technical aspects and challenges of colorimetric detection with microfluidic paper-based analytical devices (muPADs)—a review, Anal Chim Acta 970 (2017) 1–22.

[112] J.-Y. Kim, M.-K. Yeo, A fabricated microfluidic paper-based analytical device (μPAD) for in situ rapid colorimetric detection of microorganisms in environmental water samples, Mol Cell Toxicol 12 (1) (2016) 101–109.

[113] N.M. Rodriguez, et al., A fully integrated paperfluidic molecular diagnostic chip for the extraction, amplification, and detection of nucleic acids from clinical samples, Lab Chip 16 (4) (2016) 753–763.

[114] H. Shafiee, et al., Paper and flexible substrates as materials for biosensing platforms to detect multiple biotargets, Sci Rep 5 (2015) 8719.

[115] T. Lam, et al., A chemically patterned microfluidic paper-based analytical device (C-microPAD) for point-of-care diagnostics, Sci Rep 7 (1) (2017) 017-01343.

[116] L. Yu, Z.Z. Shi, Microfluidic paper-based analytical devices fabricated by low-cost photolithography and embossing of Parafilm®, Lab Chip 15 (7) (2015) 1642–1645.

[117] R. Ghosh, et al., Fabrication of laser printed microfluidic paper-based analytical devices (LP-μPADs) for point-of-care applications, Sci Rep 9 (1) (2019) 7896.

[118] A.K. Yetisen, M.S. Akram, C.R. Lowe, Paper-based microfluidic point-of-care diagnostic devices, Lab Chip 13 (12) (2013) 2210–2251.

[119] J. Alamán, et al., Inkjet printing of functional materials for optical and photonic applications, Materials 9 (11) (2016) 910.

[120] G. Hernandez-Vargas, et al., Electrochemical biosensors: a solution to pollution detection with reference to environmental contaminants, Biosensors 8 (2) (2018) 29.

[121] D.W. Kimmel, et al., Electrochemical sensors and biosensors, Anal Chem 84 (2) (2012) 685–707.
[122] A. Florea, et al., Electrochemical biosensors as potential diagnostic devices for autoimmune diseases, Biosensors 9 (1) (2019) 38.
[123] G.K. Mishra, et al., Food safety analysis using electrochemical biosensors, Foods 7 (9) (2018) 141.
[124] M. Majdinasab, et al., An overview on recent progress in electrochemical biosensors for antimicrobial drug residues in animal-derived food, Sensors 17 (9) (2017) 1947.
[125] G. Lee, et al., Single microfluidic electrochemical sensor system for simultaneous multi-pulmonary hypertension biomarker analyses, Sci Rep 7 (1) (2017) 017-06144.
[126] A.A. Zuber, E. Klantsataya, A. Bachhuka, 3.06—Biosensing, in: D.L. Andrews, R.H. Lipson, T. Nann (Eds.), Comprehensive nanoscience and nanotechnology, second ed., Academic Press, Oxford, 2019, pp. 105–126.
[127] N.R. Stradiotto, H. Yamanaka, M.V.B. Zanoni, Electrochemical sensors: a powerful tool in analytical chemistry, J Braz Chem Soc 14 (2003) 159–173.
[128] X. Wu, et al., Chapter 12—application of novel nanomaterials for chemo- and biosensing of algal toxins in shellfish and water, in: X. Wang, X. Chen (Eds.), Novel nanomaterials for biomedical, environmental and energy applications, Elsevier, USA, 2019, pp. 353–414.
[129] J.F. van der Bent, et al., Improving the limits of detection in potentiometric sensors, Meas Sci Technol 26 (12) (2015) 125104.
[130] J.R. Stetter, J. Li, Amperometric gas sensors—a review, Chem Rev 108 (2) (2008) 352–366.
[131] M. Govindhan, B.-R. Adhikari, A. Chen, Nanomaterials-based electrochemical detection of chemical contaminants, RSC Adv 4 (109) (2014) 63741–63760.
[132] C. van der Horst, et al., Stripping voltammetric determination of palladium, platinum and rhodium in freshwater and sediment samples from South African water resources, J Environ Sci Health A Tox Hazard Subst Environ Eng 47 (13) (2012) 2084–2093.
[133] Z. Altintas, et al., A fully automated microfluidic-based electrochemical sensor for real-time bacteria detection, Biosens Bioelectron 100 (2018) 541–548.
[134] S. Ghosh Dastider, et al., Low concentration E. coli O157:H7 bacteria sensing using microfluidic MEMS biosensor, Rev Sci Instrum 89 (12) (2018) 5043424.
[135] S. Jin, et al., A novel impedimetric microfluidic analysis system for transgenic protein Cry1Ab detection, Sci Rep 7 (2017) 43175.
[136] Y.H. Chuang, et al., Electrical impedimetric biosensors for liver function detection, Biosens Bioelectron 28 (1) (2011) 368–372.
[137] J. Liu, et al., An integrated impedance biosensor platform for detection of pathogens in poultry products, Sci Rep 8 (1) (2018) 16109.
[138] Q. Chen, et al., A sensitive impedance biosensor based on immunomagnetic separation and urease catalysis for rapid detection of Listeria monocytogenes using an immobilization-free interdigitated array microelectrode, Biosens Bioelectron 74 (2015) 504–511.
[139] S. Ghosh Dastider, et al., Efficient and rapid detection of Salmonella using microfluidic impedance based sensing, J Sens 2015 (2015) 8.
[140] R. Wang, et al., Impedimetric detection of bacteria by using a microfluidic chip and silver nanoparticle based signal enhancement, Microchim Acta 185 (3) (2018) 184.
[141] J. Liu, et al., A microfluidic based biosensor for rapid detection of Salmonella in food products, PLoS One 14 (5) (2019), e0216873.

[142] G.G. Guilbault, J.G. Montalvo Jr., A urea-specific enzyme electrode, J Am Chem Soc 91 (8) (1969) 2164–2165.
[143] X.W. Huijsdens, et al., Detection of Helicobacter species DNA by quantitative PCR in the gastrointestinal tract of healthy individuals and of patients with inflammatory bowel disease, Pathog Dis 41 (1) (2004) 79–84.
[144] J.L. Holland, et al., PCR detection of Escherichia coli O157:H7 directly from stools: evaluation of commercial extraction methods for purifying fecal DNA, J Clin Microbiol 38 (11) (2000) 4108–4113.
[145] G. Huang, et al., A rapid, low-cost, and microfluidic chip-based system for parallel identification of multiple pathogens related to clinical pneumonia, Sci Rep 7 (1) (2017) 6441.
[146] M.U. Kopp, A.J. Mello, A. Manz, Chemical amplification: continuous-flow PCR on a chip, Science 280 (5366) (1998) 1046–1048.
[147] C.D. Ahrberg, A. Manz, B.G. Chung, Polymerase chain reaction in microfluidic devices, Lab Chip 16 (20) (2016) 3866–3884.
[148] K.J. Shaw, et al., Rapid PCR amplification using a microfluidic device with integrated microwave heating and air impingement cooling, Lab Chip 10 (13) (2010) 1725–1728.
[149] Y. Zhang, H.-R. Jiang, A review on continuous-flow microfluidic PCR in droplets: advances, challenges and future, Anal Chim Acta 914 (2016) 7–16.
[150] C.J. Easley, et al., A fully integrated microfluidic genetic analysis system with sample-in-answer-out capability, Proc Natl Acad Sci USA 103 (51) (2006) 19272–19277.
[151] J. Chen, et al., Electrokinetically synchronized polymerase chain reaction microchip fabricated in polycarbonate, Anal Chem 77 (2) (2005) 658–666.
[152] J.Y. Cheng, et al., Performing microchannel temperature cycling reactions using reciprocating reagent shuttling along a radial temperature gradient, Analyst 130 (6) (2005) 931–940.
[153] N.C. Cady, et al., Real-time PCR detection of Listeria monocytogenes using an integrated microfluidics platform, Sensors Actuators B Chem 107 (1) (2005) 332–341.
[154] C.R. Poulsen, et al., Detection of a putative virulence cadf gene of Campylobacter jejuni obtained from different sources using a microfabricated PCR chip, J Rapid Methods Autom Microbiol 13 (2) (2005) 111–126.
[155] Z. Guttenberg, et al., Planar chip device for PCR and hybridization with surface acoustic wave pump, Lab Chip 5 (3) (2005) 308–317.
[156] C.D. Ahberg, A. Manz, P. Neuzil, Single fluorescence channel-based multiplex detection of avian influenza virus by quantitative PCR with intercalating dye, Sci Rep 5 (2015) 11479.
[157] T. Tangchaikeeree, et al., Combination of PCR and dual nanoparticles for detection of Plasmodium falciparum, Colloids Surf B: Biointerfaces 159 (2017) 888–897.
[158] M.A. Northrup, et al., DNA amplification with a microfabricated reaction chamber Transducer, in: The 7th international conference on solid-state sensors and actuators, Yokohama, Japan, 1993, pp. 924–926.
[159] C. Zhang, D. Xing, Miniaturized PCR chips for nucleic acid amplification and analysis: latest advances and future trends, Nucleic Acids Res 35 (13) (2007) 4223–4237.
[160] S. Li, et al., A continuous-flow polymerase chain reaction microchip with regional velocity control, J Microelectromech Syst 15 (1) (2006) 223–236.
[161] C.F. Chou, et al., A miniaturized cyclic PCR device, in: Micro total analysis systems 2001, Springer Netherlands, Dordrecht, 2001.
[162] Y. Zhang, P. Ozdemir, Microfluidic DNA amplification—a review, Anal Chim Acta 638 (2) (2009) 115–125.

[163] A. Naghdloo, E. Ghazimirsaeed, A. Shamloo, Numerical simulation of mixing and heat transfer in an integrated centrifugal microfluidic system for nested-PCR amplification and gene detection, Sensors Actuators B Chem 283 (2019) 831–841.

[164] M. Oshiki, et al., Microfluidic PCR amplification and miseq amplicon sequencing techniques for high-throughput detection and genotyping of human pathogenic RNA viruses in human feces, sewage, and oysters, Front Microbiol 9 (2018) 830.

[165] B. Shu, C. Zhang, D. Xing, Highly sensitive identification of foodborne pathogenic Listeria monocytogenes using single-phase continuous-flow nested PCR microfluidics with on-line fluorescence detection, Microfluid Nanofluid 15 (2) (2013) 161–172.

[166] W.-L. Chou, et al., Recent advances in applications of droplet microfluidics, Micromachines 6 (9) (2015) 1249–1271.

[167] L. Shang, Y. Cheng, Y. Zhao, Emerging droplet microfluidics, Chem Rev 117 (12) (2017) 7964–8040.

[168] W.W. Liu, et al., Droplet-based multivolume digital polymerase chain reaction by a surface-assisted multifactor fluid segmentation approach, Anal Chem 89 (1) (2017) 822–829.

[169] X. Bian, et al., A microfluidic droplet digital PCR for simultaneous detection of pathogenic Escherichia coli O157 and Listeria monocytogenes, Biosens Bioelectron 74 (2015) 770–777.

[170] G. Seyrig, et al., Using LAMP for low-cost screening of multiple waterborne pathogens, Environ Microbiol Curr Technol Water Appl 4 (2011) 103–125.

[171] M. Azizi, et al., Pathogenic bacteria detection using RNA-based loop-mediated isothermal-amplification-assisted nucleic acid amplification via droplet microfluidics, ACS Sens 4 (4) (2019) 841–848.

[172] A. Salman, et al., Shunting microfluidic PCR device for rapid bacterial detection, Talanta 207 (2020) 120303.

[173] S.L. Spurgeon, R.C. Jones, R. Ramakrishnan, High throughput gene expression measurement with real time PCR in a microfluidic dynamic array, PLoS One 3 (2) (2008) 0001662.

[174] K.J. Bosman, et al., Comparison of digital PCR platforms and semi-nested qPCR as a tool to determine the size of the HIV reservoir, Sci Rep 5 (2015) 13811.

[175] W.W.A. Niessen, Chromatography-MS, methods, in: J.C. Lindon (Ed.), Encyclopedia of spectroscopy and spectrometry, second ed., Academic Press, Oxford, 1999, pp. 309–316.

[176] X. Wang, et al., Microfluidics-to-mass spectrometry: a review of coupling methods and applications, J Chromatogr A 1382 (2015) 98–116.

[177] X. Bian, et al., Microfluidic air sampler for highly efficient bacterial aerosol collection and identification, Anal Chem 88 (23) (2016) 11504–11512.

[178] L. Rodríguez-Lorenzo, et al., Gold nanostars for the detection of foodborne pathogens via surface-enhanced raman scattering combined with microfluidics, ACS Appl Nano Mater 2 (10) (2019) 6081–6086.

[179] I.F. Cheng, et al., Rapid (<5min) identification of pathogen in human blood by electrokinetic concentration and surface-enhanced raman spectroscopy, Sci Rep 3 (2013) 2365.

[180] K.A. Mitchell, B. Chua, A. Son, Development of first generation in-situ pathogen detection system (Gen1-IPDS) based on NanoGene assay for near real time E. coli O157:H7 detection, Biosens Bioelectron 54 (2014) 229–236.

[181] X. Li, et al., Microfluidic system for rapid detection of airborne pathogenic fungal spores, ACS Sens 3 (10) (2018) 2095–2103.
[182] M. Yang, et al., Lab-on-a-chip for carbon nanotubes based immunoassay detection of Staphylococcal Enterotoxin B (SEB), Lab Chip 10 (8) (2010) 1011–1017.
[183] F. Tan, et al., A PDMS microfluidic impedance immunosensor for E. coli O157:H7 and Staphylococcus aureus detection via antibody-immobilized nanoporous membrane, Sensors Actuators B Chem 159 (1) (2011) 328–335.
[184] A. Sayad, et al., A microdevice for rapid, monoplex and colorimetric detection of food-borne pathogens using a centrifugal microfluidic platform, Biosens Bioelectron 100 (2018) 96–104.
[185] R. Singh, S. Hong, J. Jang, Label-free detection of influenza viruses using a reduced graphene oxide-based electrochemical immunosensor integrated with a microfluidic platform, Sci Rep 7 (2017) 42771.
[186] J. Luo, et al., A real-time microfluidic multiplex electrochemical loop-mediated isothermal amplification chip for differentiating bacteria, Biosens Bioelectron 60 (2014) 84–91.
[187] C. Zhao, X. Liu, A portable paper-based microfluidic platform for multiplexed electrochemical detection of human immunodeficiency virus and hepatitis C virus antibodies in serum, Biomicrofluidics 10 (2) (2016) 024119.
[188] B.L. Fernandez-Carballo, et al., Continuous-flow, microfluidic, qRT-PCR system for RNA virus detection, Anal Bioanal Chem 410 (1) (2018) 33–43.
[189] R. Prakash, et al., Multiplex, quantitative, reverse transcription PCR detection of influenza viruses using droplet microfluidic technology, Micromachines 6 (2015) 1.
[190] B. Pang, et al., Rapid and quantitative detection of Vibrio parahemolyticus by the mixed-dye-based loop-mediated isothermal amplification assay on a self-priming compartmentalization microfluidic chip, J Agric Food Chem 65 (51) (2017) 11312–11319.
[191] X. Jiang, et al., A continuous-flow high-throughput microfluidic device for airborne bacteria PCR detection, Lab Chip 14 (4) (2014) 671–676.
[192] S. Kalsi, et al., Rapid and sensitive detection of antibiotic resistance on a programmable digital microfluidic platform, Lab Chip 15 (14) (2015) 3065–3075.

CHAPTER

Microfluidic devices and drug delivery systems

7

Mohammad Rabiee[a,*], Negar Namaei Ghasemnia[a], Navid Rabiee[b], and Mojtaba Bagherzadeh[b]

[a]Biomaterials Group, Department of Biomedical Engineering, Amirkabir University of Technology, Tehran, Iran

[b]Department of Chemistry, Sharif University of Technology, Tehran, Iran

**Corresponding author. E-mail: mrabiee@aut.ac.ir*

In this chapter, the role of microfluidic technologies in the field of drug delivery systems is discussed. Studies have demonstrated that microfluidic systems can be used to study and improve drug delivery systems. The purpose of this chapter is to introduce microfluidic technology and its advantages in comparison to conventional approaches and highlight the advances and advantages of employing this technology in drug delivery systems. Moreover, the challenges and future perspectives of incorporating microfluidic systems in the field of drug delivery are discussed.

7.1 Introduction to microfluidics

In the past few decades, microelectromechanical systems (MEMS) have been developed for various applications in biomedical sciences [1]. Developments in microfabrication including micromachining, have advanced the use of MEMS with an emphasis on reducing the costs of providing a biochemical laboratory on a small chip, by using microfluidic systems. These systems can be used in different applications such as drug delivery and neural prosthetics [1, 2]. The advantages of microfluidics include smaller dimensions and compact size, consumption of small quantities of samples and reagents, improved functionality, high-throughput screening, more sensitivity, lower cost, rapid analysis, precise control, and improved reliability. Miniaturized devices can combine sensing, the ability to carry out reactions on the same or another substrate, and signal transduction much more efficiently in comparison to other devices fabricated by traditional methods [2–4].

Microfluidics or lab-on-a-chip (LOC) technology has attracted increasing interest. It involves the fabrication of devices at the micron-scale containing valves, pumps, mixers, microchannels, and microchambers, which have dimensions in the

Biomedical Applications of Microfluidic Devices. https://doi.org/10.1016/B978-0-12-818791-3.00013-9

range of tens to hundreds of micrometers, and can control the flow behavior of small volumes of fluids [3, 5].

Microfluidics involve the design, fabrication, and formulation of devices that can manipulate and control tiny volumes of fluids, microparticles, or nanoparticles for special purposes [1]. In a simple design of a typical microfluidic device, the fluid enters into microscale-diameter channels via the inlets and passes through these microchannels via a pressure-driven force applied by a syringe pump or by an electric field across the outlet [3].

In the early stage of the development of microfluidic devices, existing techniques employing microelectronics, photolithography, or etching of a silicon substrate played an important role. However, the cost of these technologies and the requirement for a clean-room environment led to the search for more efficient approaches. McDonald *et al.* suggested employing the soft lithography technique in order to produce low-cost poly(dimethylsiloxane) (PDMS) microfluidic chips rapidly. PDMS has some advantages for this goal, for example, it is flexible and nontoxic and is optically transparent with the ability to be sealed reversibly and irreversibly. Soft lithography is an easy technique for fabricating microdevices with planar geometries [6].

Microfluidic technology involves the combination of different scientific fields including engineering, biochemistry, nanotechnology, physics, and biotechnology [5, 7]. The applications of microfluidic systems are many and various, and are not only limited to chemical and biochemical analysis [1], but are used for chemical synthesis [8], sensors [9], cell capture and counting, micropumps, actuators, and high-throughput screening assays [1, 10].

Soft lithography techniques have become a well-standardized method for the fabrication of microfluidic devices [11].

To understand interfacial phenomena, microscale studying is necessary. In this field, the effect of viscosity, interfacial tension, and pressure drop are more important than the effect of gravity [3].

Microscale flows are generally laminar because they are short in length scale so in microfluidics, controlling the concentration of the molecules in microchannels is possible [3, 4].

In summary, development of microfluidic technologies that can precisely control and manipulate fluid flows and particles at micron and submicron dimensions offer many benefits compared with the traditional macroscale platforms that are listed below:

(1) decreasing the consumption of reagent/sample volumes down to picoliter volumes;
(2) decreasing waste products due to using low amounts of components and precise control of the fluid flow;
(3) reducing the costs;
(4) possibility of controlling and rapid cycling of the temperature;
(5) enabling the modeling of physiological conditions for 3D cell-culture or cell-based assays;
(6) enabling faster diffusion, mass, and heat transfer;

(7) reducing the analysis and reaction times to shorter than a few seconds;
(8) reducing waste production;
(9) allowing continuous supply of oxygen and nutrients;
(10) providing the integration of several steps, including cell culture, cell capture, cell lysis, and mixing;
(11) high accuracy, efficiency, and sensitivity

Currently, microfluidics have applications in different fields such as biology, medicine, chemistry, and environmental science [5, 12, 13].

7.2 Fabrication of the microfluidic device

7.2.1 Geometry

In the design of microfluidic systems, T-junctions, co-flowing, and flow-focusing are the three types of basic geometric configurations [13, 14]. The geometry of the channels directly affects the droplet generation [6]. A microfluidic device can be fabricated with multiple geometries. In the T-junction geometry, there is a "T" shaped intersection in which two immiscible fluids meet each other and then the resulting droplets of these two phases move in a single direction. In the co-flowing state, there is one microchannel inside another microchannel and both phases move in the same direction. The discontinuous phase moves in the central channel and the continuous phase flows between two microchannels [13]. In flow-focusing geometry, phases move in different directions. The continuous phase flows through two side channels and when it encounters the discontinuous phase at the intersection, it leads to the formation of droplets including both the discontinuous phase and the continuous phase [15].

7.2.2 Materials

In addition to the geometry, the material that is used is important. Different types of materials have been employed such as PDMS [16], polycarbonate (PC) [17], polymethyl methacrylate (PMMA) [18, 19], polyether ether ketone (PEEK) [20], cyclic olefin copolymer (COC) [21, 22], polyimide plastic resin (PIPR) [23], silicon [24], glass [25, 26], quartzose (SiO_2) [27], or combinations of these materials, for example PMMA and PC [28], or PDMS and PC [29].

Glass and silicon are two suitable materials, which can undergo micromachining and MEMS for transducing applications such as gyroscopes or accelerometers, due to their appropriate mechanical properties. However, most biomedical devices are made from polymeric materials that can exist in a glassy or rubbery state, which provides different structures compared to silicon or glass. Also, polymeric materials provide a better interface with biological substances [2].

PMMA and PDMS are polymeric materials, which are commonly used for the fabrication of microfluidic devices using the soft-lithography technique [30, 31].

One of the limitations of these two polymers is their swelling after exposure to strong solvents like acetone. When swelling occurs in the microchannels of a microfluidic device, the fluid flow changes, thus the control over the processes decreases. This problem can be solved by using other polymers, for instance, PTFE or COC that are resistant against strong solvents. Fabrication of microfluidic devices from these chemical resistant polymers can be accomplished using the hot-embossing technique [5].

7.3 Applications of microfluidic devices

Microfluidic devices can be used for many applications, for instance, generating reproducible and monodisperse gene/drug microcarriers or nanocarriers with appropriate physical properties such as size and shape. Microfluidic systems can also be used as in situ platforms for high-throughput multiplexed screening of drugs in various formats such as cell-on-a-chip, organ-on-a-chip, and also human-on-a-chip platforms to evaluate drug responses, side effects, and to partially replace animals in research studies. In designing microfluidic devices, there are some factors that should be considered that affect the results. For example, the materials which are chosen to produce the device, compatibility of the materials with different solvents, the types of mixing elements, the number of inlets, and the design of the channels and their dimensions [5].

In medical treatment, researchers are always trying to develop novel approaches to enhance the effectiveness of drugs by better targeting of the drugs to the tissues. The motivation for this aim includes minimizing negative side effects and reducing drug cytotoxicity [32–34].

Prognosis and monitoring of disease treatment are becoming ever more important. Sensitive and frequent testing is becoming essential for personalized healthcare. Therefore, innovation and progression in the fields of biomedicine and microfluidics can allow the development of improved bioassays for monitoring patient response to treatment and home testing assays to check biomarkers which may be significant for early disease detection [4].

In the pharmaceutical industry, there are some critical requirements for novel techniques and devices to direct the drug discovery and development and to predict the response of cells and humans to newly discovered drugs.

Microfluidic systems can play a key role in the pharmaceutical industry. Some applications of microfluidic techniques in the production and use of biopharmaceuticals are straightforward, such as analytical systems used for monitoring the production of protein-based drugs, such as therapeutic antibodies. But other applications of this technique need more complicated technical designs. For example, tests that rely on human cells to predict the performance in human clinical treatments. High levels of reproducibility and easy manipulation are important properties for these applications [4].

7.4 Microfluidic devices in drug delivery systems

Drug delivery systems have recently gained much attention. Improving the tolerability and efficacy of the patients, increasing the specificity, bioavailability, and efficiency of the drugs are important issues, besides reducing toxicity and side effects [13]. It should be considered that conventional bulk methods for the fabrication of drug and gene delivery systems, have some disadvantages, like requiring a large amount of drugs or chemicals which are expensive or not available on a large scale, the impossibility of producing carriers loaded with multiple therapeutic factors, generating particles with different sizes to tailor the release profile. There are difficulties associated with drug delivery and to examine the effects of the drugs in terms of their toxicity and therapeutic efficiency in vivo that rely on testing many animals [5, 35, 36].

Many studies have focused on eliminating the disadvantages of conventional delivery methods, including improving solubility and permeability, decreasing toxicity resulting from the incorrect dosage, preventing degradation by enzymes and interactions with foods, and preventing inflammation and irregular absorption. In these studies, novel technologies, such as microfluidic systems have recently been employed. Microfluidics have lower fabrication costs, and high functionality and reliability have caused a revolution in the chemical and biological research fields. The use of miniaturized chip-scale devices will have a significant impact on drug delivery systems [13].

These days, genomics, proteomics, and drug discovery are important topics, so microfluidic systems which allow the transport of fluids in the microscale with high precision have attracted attention [37]. Microfluidics have been used in different fields such as biology, drug discovery, gene expression, tissue engineering, and clinical diagnostics [38–42].

As mentioned above, the applications of microfluidic systems are very broad. They can be used in DNA sequencing, cell culture, single-cell manipulation, cell separation, chemical screening, and electrophoretic separation [43]. In the drug delivery field, microfluidics can be employed for delivering peptides, proteins, and DNA-based drugs that may be degraded by enzymes [44]. On the other hand, there is a possibility of mobile applications in chemical analysis and producing drugs using portable miniaturized microfluidic devices. Microarray platforms have greater importance in comparison with bulk volume-based techniques for the examination of a wide range of novel medicines on the micro and nanoscale, and surface phenomena [13].

It is advantageous to have the same order of size between the structure to be analyzed and the device to carry out the analysis. For instance, cells, microparticles, and large proteins have sizes similar to micromachined structures, so that biochemical and biophysical analyses of a single cell may be possible [37].

For instance, the controlled release of the drug dexamethasone from microfibers prepared as an amphiphilic derivative of hyaluronic acid was reported using microfluidic technology [45]. Another report from Cardoso et al. described the synthesis of microstructures from vinylidene fluoride-co-chlorotrifluoroethylene with desired architecture, morphology, and wettability, using a cheap and reproducible method based on microfluidic technology [46].

The main important reasons for the growth of microfluidic technology in drug delivery systems include the high efficiency of drug encapsulation requiring only small amounts of reagents and drugs, and the ability to produce uniform particles with a lower size distribution [47, 48].

The ability to mix an active component into the discontinuous phase that will then be automatically encapsulated in the next level increases the efficiency of the drug encapsulation process. The viscosity of the fluid, the Reynolds number, and the capillary liquid properties are the important parameters that should be optimized to obtain the microparticles and nanoparticles with the desired morphology, size, and shape. Paying attention to the flow rate of fluids and the geometry of the device is also important for this purpose [13].

It has been shown that using microfluidic systems provides the ability to encapsulate several hydrophilic or hydrophobic drugs in a single type of particle and also improve the drug loading capacity [49, 50].

7.5 Microfluidics in the fabrication of drug delivery carriers

To improve medical therapies, one significant issue is the delivery of drugs and genes into living cells effectively. The techniques to improve gene delivery into cells, are virus transfection, calcium phosphate-mediated transfection, liposome-mediated transfection, particle bombardment, and direct injection [37].

In the case of drug delivery, drug carriers play a significant role because they affect the bioavailability, release rate, and side effects of the drugs. Also, improving the absorption of unstable and poorly soluble drugs is an important point. In drug delivery systems, the accuracy and reliability of drug release profiles depend on the size, uniformity, composition, and shape of the drug carriers [51, 52]. For example, in the case of oral drug carrier formulations, stability in the acidic condition of the stomach, availability to pass through the intestinal mucosal membrane, and entering the bloodstream are necessary [13, 52]. Also, rapid filtering out in the kidneys occurs for nanoparticles which are smaller than 10 nm in diameter. In contrast, large particles can be removed by phagocytosis after recognition via the immune system [53, 54]. Thus, the development of efficient drug carriers is a considerable issue in drug delivery studies.

Microfluidic systems can be employed to better control the fabrication process of drug delivery systems, in order to produce carriers with more precise composition, size, and specific properties. The results of this controllable process are predictable and allow preprogramed drug delivery, release, distribution, and removal with the aim of improving the overall therapeutic response [55, 56].

In this section, the production of self-assembled, droplet-based, and nonspherical carriers employing microfluidic technology is discussed.

7.5.1 Self-assembled drug carriers

Microscale and nanoscale drug carriers can be produced by a self-assembly process that takes place in microfluidic platforms. This occurs by the interaction of two or more components at the interfacial layer leading to the creation of the particles. The processes include hydrodynamic flow focusing (HFF), and passive or active mixing leading to self-assembly reactions. The basis of this process is the formation of a carrier solution consisting of a surfactant in the center of a microchannel surrounded by a miscible buffer (Fig. 7.1A) [52]. In the microfluidic platforms, which rely on hydrodynamic flow focusing, because of the short diffusion distance, the narrow width of the core flow leads to rapid mixing [57]. The use of micromixers to produce nanoparticles causes a reduction in the time for the mixing and enhances the self-assembly process [58]. There are two types of microfluidic mixers, passive and active systems. In passive mixers, mixing of the interfaced flows is performed without using any external forces (such as are used in active mixing) and just by introducing surface microarchitectural features or sudden changes in the stream structure (Fig. 7.1B). For example, lipid nanoparticles (LNPs) containing small-interfering RNA (siRNA), were fabricated using a passive microfluidic mixer, leading to their rapid preparation and improved gene silencing efficiency [59]. It should be noted that for generating multilayer carriers for the sequential delivery of multiple agents, single-step HFF and micromixers cannot be used. So, for this aim diffusion-based microfluidic platforms with consecutive steps taking place in a solution can be used (Fig. 7.1C) [60].

The size of the synthesized carriers can be controlled by changing the mixing rates of different flows, which depends on the configuration of the channels, the diffusion coefficient, and flow rates of the various miscible fluids. Mixing-based microfluidic systems have been employed to allow the self-assembly of lipid and polymeric nanoparticles in a precise manner, followed by immobilization or encapsulation of drugs in these carriers [52]. The resulting self-assembled particles are generally smaller than 1 μm in diameter. This size is desirable for both minimizing the chance of recognition by phagocytes and facilitating the transport of the carriers across physiological barriers [54].

Liposomes have been investigated in many pharmaceutical, biological, and also in some industrial applications. For instance, in biological systems, liposomes can be used for delivering drugs, genes, and deoxyribonucleic acid (DNA) vectors or other therapeutic agents. The most common liposome preparation procedure is the bulk hydration of lipids in aqueous mediate. The resulted liposomes are large in size, polydisperse, and multilamellar. Film hydration, normal phase integration, reversed-phase evaporation, pH adjustment, freeze-thaw cycling, and detergent depletion are some methods that work based on mixing of bulk phases which can create unpredictable conditions affecting the formation of liposomes. Therefore, these methods can also produce polydisperse and multilamellar liposomes. After the preparation of liposomes using most of the methods, additional post-processing steps are required in order to obtain suitable and homogenous liposomes with the desired size [61].

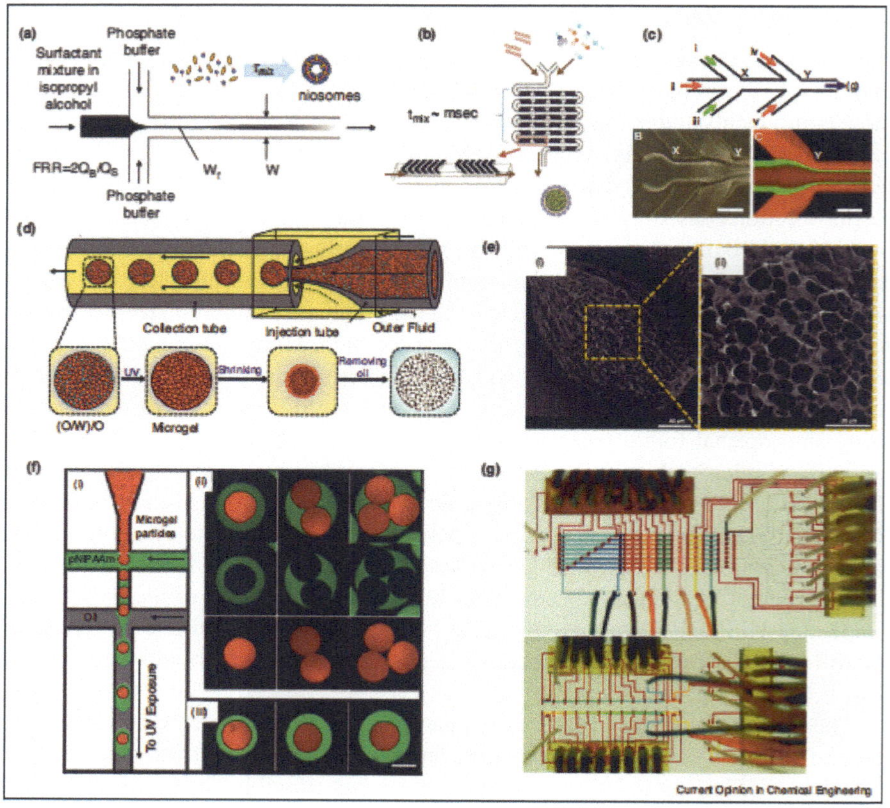

FIG. 7.1

Producing gene and drug carriers using microfluidic systems. (A) Schematic of a diffusion-based microfluidic mixer and niosome self-assembly by HFF (10 nm < Dp < 100 nm). (B) Production of a lipid nanoparticle (LNP) small interfering RNA (siRNA) formulation using the staggered herringbone micromixer (20 nm < Dp < 100 nm). (C) Fabrication of Bcl-2 antisense deoxyoligonucleotide loaded lipopolyplex with multiinlet microfluidic HFF system (100 nm < Dp < 300 nm). (D) Droplet-based microfluidic system for open-cell porous poly(N-isopropylacrylamide) (PNIPAM) microgel generation (150 mm < Dp < 450 mm), (E) SEM images of produced PNIPAM microgels with open-cell porous structure. (F) Production of microgel capsules composed of two miscible yet distinct layers employing a double emulsion format within a droplet-based microfluidic system (20 mm < Dp < 100 mm). (G) Programmed microfluidic platform for generating a combinatorial library of DNA loaded supramolecular particles (40 nm < Dp < 200 mm).

Reprinted with permission from Riahi R, et al. Microfluidics for advanced drug delivery systems. Curr Opin Chem Eng 2015;7:101–12, Elsevier.

The size of the liposomes and the size distribution are key factors for in vivo applications, since the dosage of the drug, targeting and rate of the elimination from the body are related to the liposome size. There is the possibility of encapsulating both hydrophilic substances inside the aqueous core, and lipophilic substances within the lipid bilayer. In drug delivery applications, liposomes can be used as drug transporters so that small size and monodispersity of the liposomes are important. Recognition and elimination of liposomes by the renal system depend on their size besides other factors such as coatings. In general, the elimination of larger liposomes is more rapid than smaller liposomes. The curvature of the liposomes is an important factor in recognition by the complement system. By reducing the size of the liposomes the curvature increases which inversely affects the number of detection sites. Thus, decreasing the size results in decreasing the clearance rate via the complement system. By hydrodynamic focusing, fabrication of liposomes with controlled size in the range of 50 to 150 nm is achievable, which are desirable for drug delivery applications due to their low elimination rate. The lifetime of liposomes in biological environments before their internal components begin to leak, restricts their potential use for encapsulating therapeutic agents. Employing techniques with the ability to control the size of the liposomes during their preparation without requiring extra steps, allows simple preparation of liposomes enhancing their applicability. Using microfluidic techniques to fabricate liposomes results in producing monodisperse distributions with desired sizes by controlling the flow rates of the fluids in the microfluidic device. As mentioned previously, microfluidic devices allow exact mixing control by adjusting molecular diffusion and fluid forces on the micrometer scale [61].

Liposomes can be employed in order to decrease the toxicity of drugs. Liposome-encapsulated drugs can be fabricated via microfluidic systems, in which two aqueous streams focus a flow of lipids dissolved in alcohol into a microfluidic channel. By setting the alcohol and aqueous flow rates, particles with diameters 50–150 nm in size can be produced [61, 62].

Abhay et al. studied the generation of monodisperse self-assembled liposomes using a hydrodynamic flow-focusing microfluidic approach and examined the relationship between the cellular uptake mechanisms and the size of the liposomes [63]. In another study, the fabrication of docetaxel-loaded homogeneous nanoparticles using a polylactic-*co*-glycolic acid-polyethylene glycol (PLGA-PEG) copolymer employing microfluidic nanoprecipitation was reported. This method produced particles with a size of 20–25 nm, which were smaller than the particles produced by bulk emulsion precipitation methods that gave a size of 30–100 nm. Furthermore, the half-life of these particles obtained via the microfluidic technology was almost twice as long as the particles fabricated using the bulk method [57].

7.5.2 Droplet-based carriers

Emulsions have suitable encapsulation properties that have long been utilized in many industries, for instance, food, cosmetics, chemistry, and pharmaceuticals [64, 65]. These days, the generation of complex microparticles that can be used as drug carriers or agents for sorting DNA or proteins, has been made possible using emulsion technology [66]. One issue that should be considered for extending the use of emulsions for the fabrication of microparticles is the high efficiency of producing stable monodisperse emulsions. The monodispersity of emulsions enhances the signal-to-noise ratio in many assays and allows better standardization [67].

For emulsion generation, classical methods including mixers, colloid mills, and sonicators can be applied. Although these approaches may allow high-throughput emulsion production, the lack of control over the size of the droplets and their size distribution is the main problem [15].

In single emulsions, there are two immiscible liquids. The nature of the particles is determined based on the selection of the solutions in the discontinuous and continuous phases, where a continuous phase surrounds the dispersed phase. These phases can have different properties ranging from hydrophilic to hydrophobic. For the encapsulation of hydrophobic agents or drugs, oil-in-water (O/W) emulsions are employed. In multiple emulsions, three phases exist. There is one emulsion that consists of several drops immersed into a second phase, which then enters into a third phase. Water-in-oil-in-water ($W_1/O/W_2$) and oil-in-water-in-oil ($O_1/W/O_2$) are two kinds of multiple emulsions that have been explored. Multiple emulsions can be categorized into double, triple, and quadruple emulsions, representing the number of different phases. Double emulsions are more often used because the production of controlled droplets with the desired characteristics is less complicated, and using the droplets as a template for further microcapsules is possible. The ability for encapsulating polar and nonpolar molecules in double emulsions may provide better-controlled release due to the excess barrier produced. Multiple emulsions have applications in drug encapsulation for pharmaceutical purposes [13].

An important point in drug delivery systems is a well-shaped and uniform capsule for immobilizing drugs into micro or nanoparticles. Many techniques have been used to produce nanoparticles [68]. Several of them require the use of materials that have a significant level of toxicity or biological hazards [69]. On the other hand, in the field of drug encapsulation using nanoparticles, physical characteristics such as size distribution, shape, and encapsulation efficiency are the key factors. Therefore, it is necessary to choose the best methods for generating micro or nanoparticles to produce uniform and homogenous particles for drug encapsulation. In this respect, microfluidics can be a suitable technique for the fabrication of particles with intended physical characteristics using single or multiple emulsions [13].

One of the recent achievements of microfluidic systems is the synthesis of niosomes, which are nonionic surfactant based vesicles. These are self-assembled membranes formed by a combination of diacetyl phosphate and cholesterol. The microfluidic device that was applied for this aim, resulted in the rapid mixing of two miscible fluids in the channels. The niosomes produced were significantly reduced in size compared to bulk methods [13, 53].

This technology is known as droplet microfluidics. There is a possibility for controlling the droplet size to generate monodisperse microparticles. Generally, the yield in microfluidic emulsifier systems is low and these systems are markedly slower in comparison to conventional emulsification methods [70]. To increase the productivity level of such devices, scaling-up can be employed [71].

Droplet-based microfluidic systems can provide the ability to synthesize carriers in a highly reproducible manner. Homogeneous drug-loaded particles, microbubbles, microcapsules, and microgels can be fabricated using this popular method (Fig. 7.1D–F) [4, 52]. The interfacial tension between the immiscible fluids combined with the shear stress leads to the production of droplets. The flow rates, solution viscosity, and surface tension all affect the size of the particles. The main difference between this method and the self-assembly method is the size of the resulting particles. In general, self-assembled approaches are employed to produce nanoparticles. Particles that are synthesized via droplet-based microfluidic platforms have sizes in the range of microns. These microcarriers have some benefits like the possibility of high-dose drug loading and maintaining sustained drug release for a longer time. Droplet-based microfluidic methods for the generation of single and multiple emulsion-based carriers can be carried out by using combination geometries like flow focusing, cross-flow, and co-flow. Computer-controlled microfluidic systems with integrated microvalves and micropumps have been designed to control the composition, shape, and size of the particles that can be loaded with genes or drugs (Fig. 7.1G) [52].

Droplet-based microfluidic systems are useful for the generation of multifunctional drug carriers with controllable size and drug release profiles [52].

7.5.3 Nonspherical carriers and particles

Two methods can be used to generate spherical particles. Recent studies demonstrated that the shape of the particles affects their blood circulation time within the human body, the in vivo biodistribution, and uptake mechanisms [72]. Thus, in drug delivery systems, non-spherical particles have been investigated. Using this method, mimicking the properties of natural entities like red blood cells is possible. Also, their high surface-to-volume ratio improves cell membrane attachment for drug delivery. Kolhar et al. fabricated needle-shaped nanoparticles for delivery of siRNA to the vascular endothelium to carry out gene silencing [73]. Self-assembly and coalescence of droplets generated by emulsion-based platforms, flow lithography, deforming and stretching droplets in channels before or within solidification, can be used for the fabrication of non-spherical particles (Fig. 7.2A) [52]. Disk-like, cylindrical, and rod-like particles can be fabricated via self-assembly and coalescence of droplets [74, 75]. Anisotropic particles can be produced via stretching or deformation of the generated emulsion droplets. Fabrication of toroids can be achieved using this method by controlling the solvent diffusion rate as well as the flow rate (Fig. 7.2B) [52]. In flow lithography, particles can be formed by exposing a flow of photocross-linkable polymer solution to light [76]. The use of a photomask allows for the fabrication of particles with a predefined shape. Flow lithography has two types, which are continuous flow and stop-flow lithography. In the stop-flow method, first, the pre-polymer solution fills the microchannel, then the light is delivered in the microchannel with stopped-flow to produce the particles (Fig. 7.2C) [52]. In continuous flow

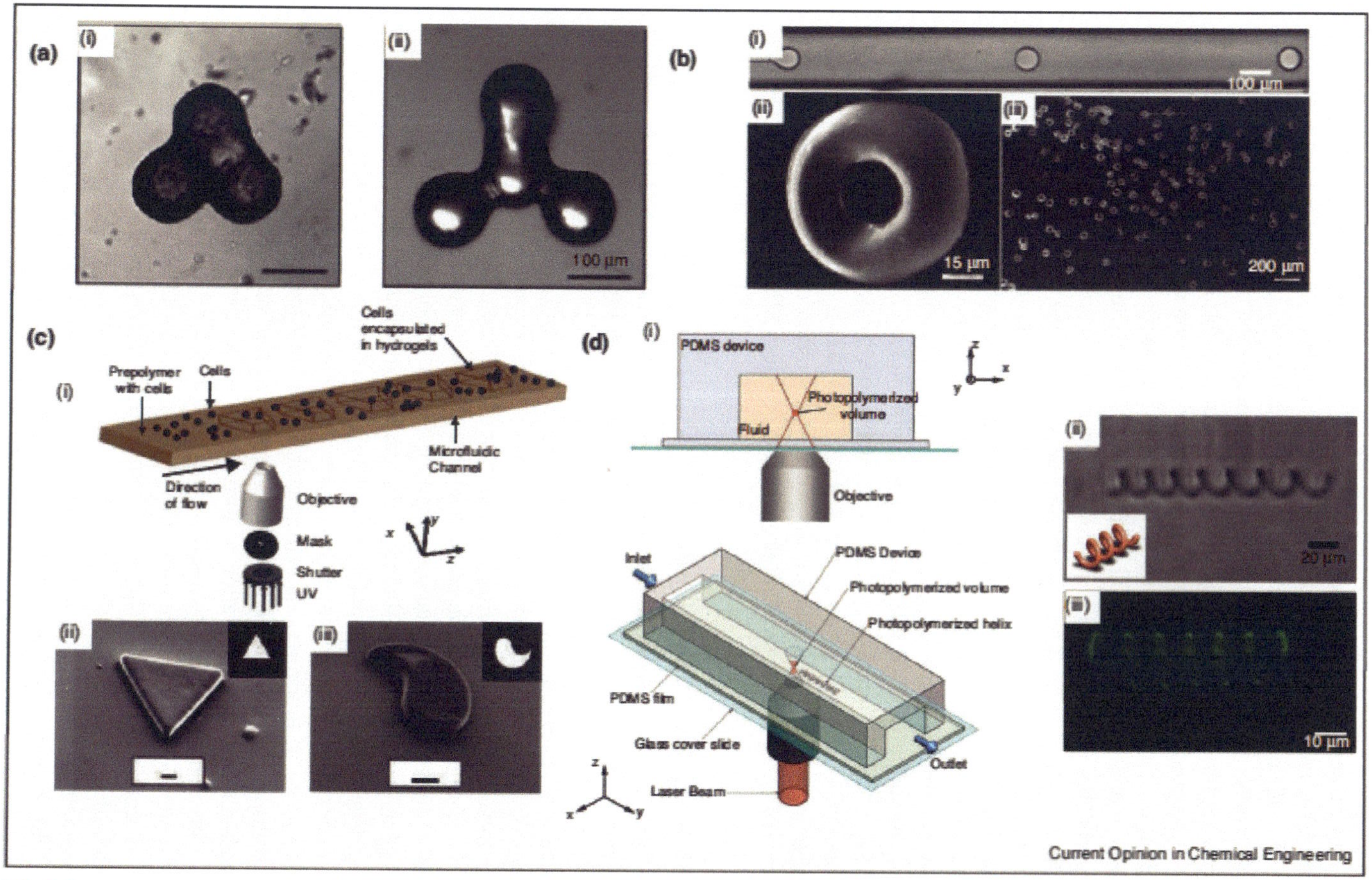

FIG. 7.2

Microfluidic platforms for producing carriers and non-spherical particles. (A) The coalescence of spherical particles results in non-spherical particle generation. (B) Toroid-like particles produced by microfluidic emulsion with subsequent precise solvent evaporation. (C) Generation of planar particles using stop-flow lithography. (i) Schematic of the device, (ii, iii) generated planar particles employing flow lithography. (D) Producing of 3D particles using a two-photon continuous flow lithography method. (i) Schematic of the method, (ii, iii) bright field and fluorescent images of thr generated helical structure.

Reprinted with permission from Riahi R, et al. Microfluidics for advanced drug delivery systems. Curr Opin Chem Eng 2015;7:101–12, Elsevier.

lithography, turning the light illumination system on and off repeatedly is used to fabricate the particles [77]. In comparison to these two techniques, stop-flow lithography shows lower efficiency than continuous flow systems. For instance, fabrication rates of 100 particles per second can be achieved in continues flow lithography. In both continuous flow and stop-flow lithography systems, the fabrication of planar particles is possible. For generating 3D particles, a kind of microfluidic platform combined with a two-photon polymerization system can be used (Fig. 7.2D). This method is not very applicable in drug delivery due to its relatively low throughput. However, flow lithography methods can be used for fabrication of both spherical and nonspherical particles, its main limitation is low throughput. Operation of flow lithography microfluidic platforms is easier in comparison to droplet-based systems, due to the presence of only a single phase in the microchannel. But it should be mentioned that this method cannot be used for light-sensitive drugs. The size of the particles in flow lithography platforms depends on the resolution of the illumination system. So, the generation of particles with submicron sizes is a limitation [52].

7.6 Effective parameters for the production of carriers

Efficacy of the production of drug and gene carriers depends on the microfluidic fabricators, including droplet generator, chaotic mixer, diffusion-based mixer, or automated microfluidic systems. Among the mentioned fabricators, the microfluidic diffusion-based mixer is most commonly used. It has several inlets and only one outlet. In this kind of fabricator, the length of the channel and the stream rate are the key factors in the reaction between molecules and the carrier material. It should be taken into consideration that mixing methods may cause a large content of unreacted materials since these methods depend on the diffusion between different flows under a continuous stream process in the boundary. The presence of unreacted materials can result in increased cytotoxicity and lower the drug transport rate. On the other hand, droplet generation methods can be used as alternative approaches where reactions are independently performed in the droplets. These systems enable precise control of many parameters such as the ratio between molecules that react with each other in the microchannels, the reaction rate, the size, and the total volume besides avoiding contamination problems [78, 79].

7.7 Carrier materials

Extensive studies have been devoted to drug carriers employing biomaterials with controllable drug release, or employing antibodies with a specific site of action. For instance, carriers with the ability to respond to temperature or pH can release loaded drugs on demand that have been synthesized using bulk methods [80, 81]. Employing conventional methods such as emulsification is not precise enough to generate reproducible results. However, it becomes more difficult to control multiple release profiles while using different drugs, because using bulk methods, we do not have exact control over the composition of the carriers. Moreover, in bulk methods, large amounts of drugs may be required for the desired result which may not be economical [52].

There are two main purposes for the encapsulation of drugs. One is to protect the drugs from enzymatic degradation, while the other is to reduce their toxicity [13].

Phospholipid nanoparticles can also be prepared using a microfluidic system instead of the standard thin-film hydration technique because it is simpler and faster and has no negative effects on the encapsulation efficiency. It was demonstrated that protein microencapsulation via the emulsion technique using a microfluidic device had a high efficiency of about 84% and stability for up to 4 weeks [82]. These favorable results underline the importance of microfluidic systems in drug delivery.

Microparticles and nanoparticles for use as carriers in drug delivery systems should be fabricated from biodegradable, nontoxic, and biocompatible materials. In this case, mesoporous materials have gained attention due to their appropriate sites for encapsulating drugs, proteins, and bioactive compounds, and also a uniformly porous surface that allows functionalization with other materials. MCM-41, MCF, and SBA-15 are some examples of mesoporous materials [13]. Also, magnetic particles because of their ability to target specific cells using external magnetic fields have been explored. In this regard, magnetite (Fe_3O_4) and maghemite (γ-Fe_2O_3) because of their properties such as low toxicity and stability are important [83]. Moreover, gold, silver, platinum, aluminum, and titanium dioxide are metallic materials that have been used as drug delivery carriers [84]. In microfluidic systems, polymeric materials such as poly(caprolactone) (PCL), poly(vinyl alcohol) (PVA), PEG, polylactide (PLA), and PLGA are suitable for the immobilization of bioactive compounds [13]. Carriers produced using these polymeric materials have good biocompatibility, biodegradability, low toxicity, and can provide sustained and controlled drug release over long periods. Furthermore, the possibility of modification of these polymers means they can be tailored for special purposes [85]. One example of using polymeric materials as drug delivery carriers is the microencapsulation of an anticancer drug like camptothecin into PLGA and PLA carriers [86].

In one of the studies, microencapsulation of rifampicin, a drug used for treating tuberculosis, into PLGA was carried out by a microchannel emulsification-solvent evaporation method. Also, PLGA has been used as a drug delivery carrier in the field of psychiatry where haloperidol, a dopamine antagonist, was encapsulated into these carriers using the cross-flow membrane emulsification (XME) process, which is a modified membrane encapsulation method [87].

In membrane emulsification, the discontinuous phase passes through the pores of a microporous membrane and enters into the continuous phase. This technique has been studied in combination with a cross-linking process in order to encapsulate peptides and proteins. Wang *et al.* succeeded in producing insulin-loaded chitosan microspheres with good efficiency and chemical stability. These examples show the versatility and modifiability of microencapsulation to improve the properties of drugs such as their solubility and bioavailability [13].

7.8 Examples of immobilization of drugs using microfluidic technology for drug delivery

Drug encapsulation can be performed using either single or multiple emulsions which are based on the number of phases. For this purpose, first, the drug should be mixed with one of the phases. With regard to the geometry of the microfluidic device, when the dispersed phase containing the drug encounters the continuous phase, particles form due to the shear stress caused by the fluid flow. Generally, hydrophilic and hydrophobic drugs are encapsulated via water-in-oil (W/O) and oil-in-water (O/W) emulsions, respectively [13].

One of the studies in this area concerned the encapsulation of doxorubicin (DOXO) into human serum albumin (HSA) microparticles via a microfluidic system. These microparticles have applications in the transcatheter arterial chemoembolization (TACE) approach to treat hepatic cancer. Glass was chosen as a material to fabricate the device with co-flow geometry. The oil phase consisted of medium-chain triglyceride oil, Span 80, and glutaraldehyde as a cross-linking agent, and the aqueous phase included HSA solution with a specific amount of DOXO and Tween 80. The flow rates of these two phases were adjusted. The study showed that the size of the resulting particles is related to the ratio of the oil phase and the aqueous phase, and also to the flow rates of these phases. In vitro tests found rapid drug release on the first day (about 10% of the loaded drug). In the next 30 days, a sustained drug release was observed (16% of the total loaded drug). In vivo studies showed that this method led to inhibition of tumor growth [88].

In another study, echogenic liposomes were prepared and loaded with recombinant tissue-type plasminogen activator (rt-PA), a drug for the treatment of ischemic stroke. The microfluidic system was constructed from PDMS with complex flow-focusing geometry. The oily phase and rt-PA were streamed in the outer and inner channels, respectively. The average size of the particles was about 5 μm and the encapsulation efficiency was estimated at 69%. The particles were not stable for more than 30 min so a surfactant, Pluronic F-127, was used to reduce particle aggregation and improve their stability. It was observed that at a constant drug flow, the particle size was reduced by increasing the lipid flow. It was realized that the loading efficiency of rt-PA in liposomes via the microfluidic system was lower than conventional methods. For this purpose, future research is required to solve the problems and drawbacks, such as particle stability and aggregation [89].

Xi *et al.* worked on a simple method for the entrapment of two anticancer drugs using PLGA polymer and a fluidic nanoprecipitation system. They investigated two types of drugs, paclitaxel (hydrophobic) and doxorubicin hydrochloride (hydrophilic). Their system allowed the simultaneous loading of different compounds by the emulsification of hydrophilic drugs and the nanoprecipitation of hydrophobic drugs [90].

In the case of the use of microfluidic techniques for synthesizing homogenous drug delivery carriers, Wu *et al.* employed a microfluidic system to examine the correlation between the amount of the released drug from PLGA microspheres and their microstructure in terms of size. Their kinetic analysis showed that the monodisperse particles fabricated by the microfluidic system displayed slower drug release profiles compared to those generated by conventional methods with the same average size. This was related to the drug distribution inside the particles, where the drug distribution was more uniform with the microfluidic technique [91, 92].

As mentioned above, one of the advantages of using microfluidic systems is the ability to encapsulate multiple drugs at the same time. In this case, Khan et al. investigated the loading of ketoprofen and ranitidine HCl into a core-shell microparticle. The core and the shell were made of poly(methyl acrylate) and poly(acrylamide), respectively. Ketoprofen was entrapped into the core while ranitidine HCl was encapsulated into the shell of the particles. These core-shell microparticles had an average size between 100 and 151 μm. A T-geometry was used to design this microfluidic device. There was one oily phase as the continuous phase and the discontinuous phases included ranitidine-shell and ketoprofen-core. The polymerization of the particles occurred after the T-junction via UV irradiation. Encapsulation efficiency and the release rate of these two drugs differed from each other because the ketoprofen loading was higher than ranitidine HCl. The encapsulation efficiencies of ketoprofen and ranitidine HCl were almost 80% and 50%, respectively and the ketoprofen release was slower than ranitidine HCl [49].

Dhar *et al.* reported an approach to treat prostate cancer using drug-loaded nanoparticles, which were fabricated using a microfluidic channel. Two types of drugs, cisplatin, and docetaxel were encapsulated in nanoparticles using this protocol. The nanoparticles showed a good loading efficiency of both hydrophobic and hydrophilic drugs. The functional mechanism of these targeted nanoparticles was by attaching to the membrane prostate-specific antigen on prostate cancer cells, followed by internalization via endocytosis which was investigated using a fluorescent dye [93].

7.9 Benefits of using microfluidics in drug delivery systems

Some of the main advantages of microfluidics in drug delivery are control of dosage, targeted delivery, controlled drug release, ability for multiple dosing, and negligible side effects. Microfluidics have been confirmed as a technology for the fabrication of direct drug delivery systems and drug carriers, and also for high-throughput screening and studies on the immobilization of drugs [13].

Microfluidic systems can improve the effectiveness of drugs, which have a short half-life in vivo or may have negative side-effects after systemic administration. The fabrication of microneedles and also needle-free injection systems is another achievement of the use of microtechnologies [52].

The integration of biosensing platforms and microfluidics results in novel drug delivery systems that can monitor and analyze treatment results [94].

Mimicking the in vivo microenvironment by using microfluidic techniques and tissue engineering can help us to study the efficacy of drug delivery approaches [52].

To evaluate the toxicological and pharmacological effects of drugs, in vitro and in vivo assays are essential. For toxicological studies, a microfluidic device can be used to test the effects of a drug or of multiple drugs. This could be in the form of cell-on-a-chip, organ-on-a-chip, or human-on-a-chip platforms. These techniques have partially replaced animals in biomedical research [5, 13].

7.10 Direct drug delivery via microfluidic systems

The utilization of microfluidic devices for generating complex drug carriers was discussed above. Another application for microfluidic systems is the direct transport or delivery of active molecules and drugs. In these systems, targeted drug delivery is achievable. Delivering drugs to a chosen anatomical site can lead to the enhancement of the local bioavailability of the drug, and also has an important role in decreasing negative side effects that result from drug interactions with other distant organs. Furthermore, in the case of transdermal drug delivery, microfluidic systems have led to outstanding achievements. The main purpose of these systems employing a single needle or an array of microneedles to deliver drugs across the skin is overcoming the barrier of the stratum corneum (SC) in the top layer of the skin [52]. In this part, the use of microfluidic systems for localized and transdermal drug delivery is discussed.

7.10.1 Localized drug delivery

Microfluidic implantable devices and drug-loaded polymeric particles are some of the techniques that have been used for localized drug delivery [95]. In comparison to other diffusion-based local delivery systems with non-uniform and continuous release profiles, microfluidic devices can prepare on-demand drug release systems that employ convective forces. This ability allows suitable control over the release profile. Microfluidic systems used for transporting drugs generally have a drug reservoir, a pump or actuator, a valve, and also a membrane for adjusting the release rate. The easiest way to release the drug is to physically compress the drug reservoir [52]. Lo et al. designed a microfluidic drug delivery platform with a rechargeable drug reservoir to treat ocular diseases. In this system, there was a PDMS-based check valve for controlling the drug release rate after manual pressurizing of the reservoir (Fig. 7.3A and B). The rate of the drug release could be changed from 0.61 to 1.57 mL/s with 250 and 500 mmHg of applied pressure, respectively. The variation in the release rate of the drug in response to the applied pressure was the main limitation of this system, particularly if the device was finger actuated [96]. On the other hand, compressing the drug reservoir of implantable devices is challenging, and to achieve this goal, researchers have attempted to find simple mechanism. For example, Chung et al. designed a drug reservoir covered with a membrane with two electrodes embedded at the top and bottom of its surface (Fig. 7.3C). By applying an electrical potential between these two electrodes, the drug was released due to a chemical reaction which caused gas bubble formation leading to breaking of the membrane [97].

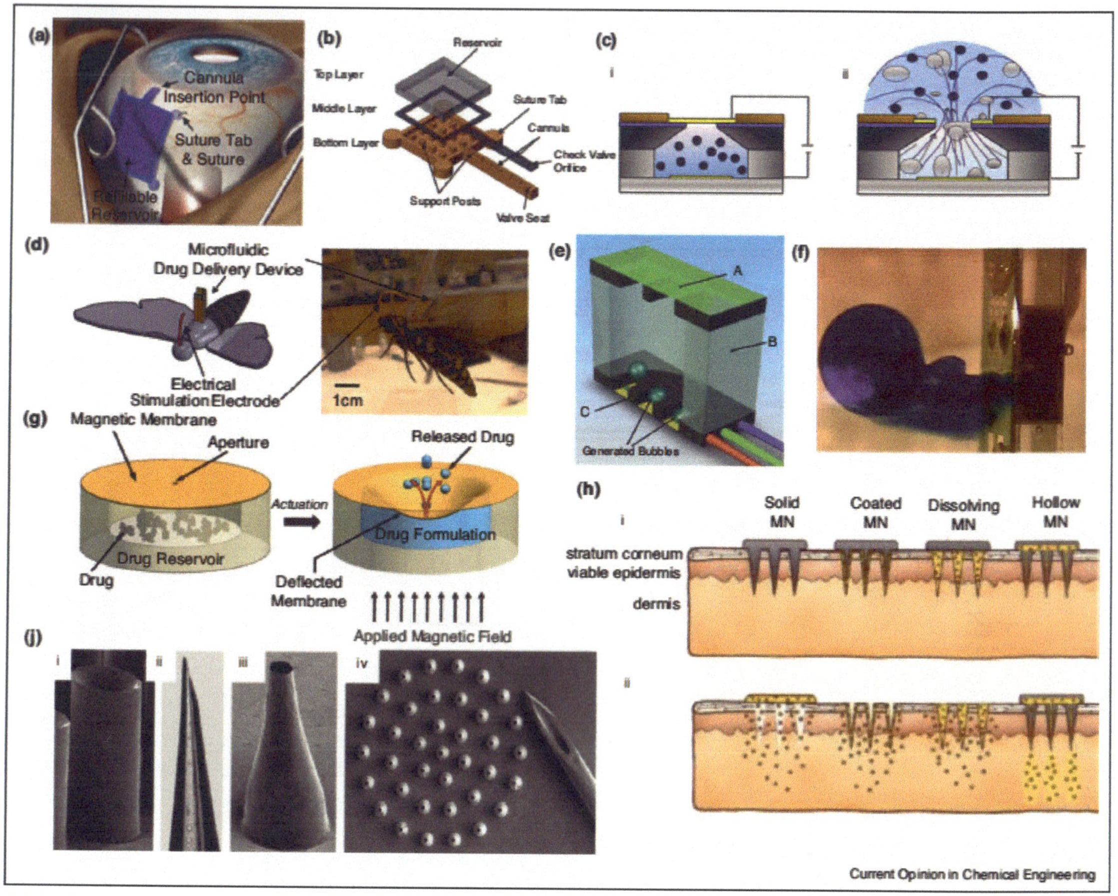

FIG. 7.3

Microfluidic systems for direct drug delivery. (A) Implantation of a microfluidic drug delivery platform for ocular applications, where the drug reservoir was sutured to the sclera and placed underneath the conjunctiva. (B) Components of the employed drug delivery platform. (C) Drug delivery platform where the application of an electrical field between the top and bottom electrodes introduced bubbles in the chamber which led to drug release. (D) A schematic image of a wireless microfluidic system for controlling the flight of Manduca sexta. (E) Microfluidic drug delivery in which heaters generated bubbles to break the membrane and release the drug. (F) Side view of the device illustrating methylene blue release. (G) Principle of operation of a magnetically actuated drug delivery system. (H) Various types of microneedle arrays. (J) SEM images of hollow metal (i, iii) and glass (ii) microneedles. (iv) An array of 500 mm long tapered metal microneedles next to a 26-gauge needle.

Reprinted with permission from Riahi R, et al. Microfluidics for advanced drug delivery systems. Curr Opin Chem Eng 2015;7:101–12, Elsevier.

A similar device was implanted into a kind of moth to control its behavior through chemical delivery (Fig. 7.3D) [98]. Elman et al. utilized a microfluidic system with a reservoir covered by a silicon nitride membrane (Fig. 7.3E and F). The reservoir consisted of a heating module that caused the rupture of the brittle membrane in a defined manner and thereby released the drug [99]. The mentioned system led to rapid delivery and could be employed in an emergency scenario. It should be noted that thermally unstable drugs and growth factors cannot be delivered using this kind of system, due to the generated heat. Also employing this device for sustained drug delivery over the long term is not possible [52]. Also, drug delivery systems using magnetic actuation can be used for localized drug delivery because of the ability of a magnetic field to penetrate the body. Pirmoradi et al. fabricated a microfluidic device that consisted of a drug reservoir that was sealed by an iron oxide doped PDMS membrane (Fig. 7.3G). There was an aperture on the membrane that allowed the drug to exit. The membrane responded and was deformed by applying a magnetic field that caused the extrusion of the drug from the aperture of the membrane. In cyclic drug delivery, the inconsistency of the release rate in each cycle is the main challenge for magnetic actuation systems [100].

It should be noted that after their successful operation, implanted platforms must be degraded or resorbed without any secondary surgery needed for removal. In addition, the mechanical characteristics of these implantable systems should be similar to the surrounding tissue in order not to interfere with tissue function. Developing a platform with an easy actuation mechanism and subnanoliter scale flow resulting in long term drug delivery has received plenty of attention. In designing such long-lasting drug delivery systems, their interaction with tissue, and possible immune and inflammatory responses are important factors. Inflammation has an influence on the function of the device and may eventually cause device rejection. Fibrosis also has a significant effect on the device performance, because when fibrosis occurs, the nozzles become blocked and the movement of mechanical components will face problems. So, coating the device with antifibrotic factors may help to overcome this problem [52].

7.10.2 Skin anatomy and transdermal drug delivery

Advances in new active pharmaceutical components have led to research into novel and efficient functional delivery systems. The most common routes for the administration of drugs are the oral, parenteral, ophthalmic, and transdermal routes. In addition, less well-investigated routes like nasal, pulmonary, or buccal are possible [101]. It should be noted that each of these routes has its particular characteristics, advantages, and disadvantages. For instance, the merits of oral drug delivery systems are patient compliance, low cost, absorption via a large surface area with a rich blood supply, and the possibility for engineering and controlling the drug release within the digestive system. But besides these advantages, there are some limitations such as drug degradation in the gastrointestinal tract, local irritation, first-pass metabolism, insignificant absorption and also, variation in absorption levels because of parameters such as pH, mucus layer, motility, and other factors. In the parenteral route, rapid onset of action, continuous drug delivery by infusion, and precise drug delivery are advantages. However, the problems of this route include pain upon injection, the requirement for clinical expertise to deliver the drugs, and also the risk of infection and problems in attaining continuous drug delivery. In drug delivery studies one of the main topics is transdermal drug delivery systems because of their advantages over parenteral and oral drug delivery systems [102].

The properties and physicochemical characteristics of drugs are important factors for delivery via transdermal patches. Conventional transdermal patches can be classified into two types based on their physical structure. These two groups are reservoir-based and matrix-based patches [102]. Transdermal drug delivery is noninvasive and can be self-administered offering several benefits such as good patient compliance, large surface area of skin for delivering the drugs, releasing drugs over long periods of time (up to a week), avoidance of first-pass metabolism, rapid termination of dosing after patch removal, etc. It worth mentioning that transdermal delivery is used when there is a large first-pass effect in the liver which causes premature removal of drugs from circulation. In addition, transdermal routes offer safer drug delivery, compared to painful hypodermic injections that may be problematic especially in developing countries, the creation of hazardous medical waste, and the risk of transmitting disease by reuse of needles.

Only a limited number of drug products have been successfully marketed using transdermal delivery because of the resistance of the outer layer of the skin, stratum corneum, preventing the transport of drugs. These problems can be solved by developing micron-sized needles to deliver the drug painlessly across the skin layer [102, 103].

Compared to other delivery approaches, successful transdermal drugs only need doses of milligrams per day or less. The drugs generally have molecular weights only up to a few hundred Daltons, with high octanol-water partition coefficients meaning they are lipid-soluble. Employing the transdermal method for delivering hydrophilic drugs has challenges. For example, the transdermal delivery of macromolecules and peptides faces particular difficulties as well as genetic treatments exploiting DNA molecules or siRNA.

In addition, compared to the hypodermic delivery route, the delivery of vaccines via the transdermal route can lead to improved immune responses by targeting them to highly immunogenic Langerhans cells within the skin [103].

The skin is composed of three regions called from the outer layer to the inner layer: epidermis, dermis, and hypodermis, respectively [104]. The epidermis layer has a thickness of about 150–200 μm. The outermost layer of the epidermis, which is about 10–20 μm thick and consists of dead keratinocyte cells embedded within lipid, is called the SC. This thin layer acts as a barrier and restricts the transport of drugs in transdermal delivery [37, 105]. The inner layer is the viable epidermis (VE) about 50–100 μm thick and consists of living keratinocytes and a few nerves. In this layer, drug absorption can occur by entering blood vessels [37]. The mechanical strength of the skin is due to the dermis layer because of its fibroelastic structure. This middle layer (dermis) contains an abundant nervous and vascular network and is the reason for the pain occurring during injections because of the possible disruption of nerve endings within the dermis. One of the main challenges in delivering drugs across the skin is to cross the intact SC layer without any damage to underlying nerve endings. Just a few types of drug molecules with low molecular weight (less than 500 *Da*) and high lipophilicity can be delivered directly through the skin by passive diffusion [106, 107].

In order to increase drug penetration across the skin, different physical and chemical methods have been explored. In chemical approaches, the use of penetration enhancers, such as surfactants, fatty acids/esters, and solvents with the aim of partially dissolving the SC lipids or improving the solubility of drugs have been investigated. On the other hand, it has been demonstrated that electroporation, iontophoresis, sonophoresis, photoacoustic and magnetophoresis that are categorized as physical methods, could be used to create pathways for passing only a few drugs across the skin [37, 102].

It is worth mentioning that each of these methods has its own disadvantages. Generally, chemical methods are applicable only for small drug molecules and often lead to skin irritation while physical approaches increase the cost and complexity due to requiring equipment like devices using a power supply [108, 109].

Micromachining technology provides many opportunities in the field of biomedical instrumentation. The needle is one of the simplest biomedical instruments. Using hypodermic needles for delivering drugs or aspirating body fluid through the human skin is standard medical practice. However, the smallest diameter of these needles that can be fabricated by conventional machining methods is about 160 μm (34 gauge). This diameter is relatively large and in addition to causing pain, can reduce or eliminate precision delivery. On the other hand, in biotechnology, delivering molecules on the nanometer scale with micron precision is necessary and since common and simple hypodermic needles cannot meet these requirements, micromachining technology makes the fabrication of smaller needles possible. Microneedles due to their small size have several applications for painless drug delivery through the skin (transdermal or intradermal), cell manipulation, closed-loop chemical stimulation of tissues, sample collection, and delivery in chemical and biochemical analysis, and interconnection between microscopic and macroscopic fluidic systems [37].

The concept of microneedle was first introduced in 1976, but the required technology for fabrication of these micron-sized needles was not widely available until the 2000s [110]. Microneedles have been made of metals, silicon, and other materials using low-cost mass production microelectronics industry tools. The external diameter of the microneedles is less than 300 μm and their length is about 50–900 μm [111]. The dimension of the microneedles is designed in a way that penetrate through the epidermis up to a depth of 70–200 μm so because they do not penetrate the dermis layer that contains the nerves, no pain is felt [112, 113].

The enhancement of drug delivery across the skin using microneedles is a rapidly increasing field compared with other transdermal delivery approaches [102].

7.10.2.1 Microneedles

In direct injection, drugs are delivered through the skin, but other methods create submicron pores in the SC layer, thus increasing the transport rate of the drugs. One way to accomplish this goal is the use of microneedles. These micron-sized pores are large enough to provide high drug transport rates, while they are too small to cause lasting damage to the skin [37].

Microneedles can be classified into different groups shown below:

1. Solid microneedles that disrupt the skin barrier
2. Drug-coated microneedles
3. Dissolvable microneedles with the ability to release the drug at a steady rate
4. Hollow microneedles providing convective drug delivery across the epidermis barrier (Fig. 7.3H) [52].

These microneedles can be fabricated using MEMS and made of metals, silicon, polymers, or polysaccharides. Solid coated microneedles can be used for drug delivery purposes, and after puncturing the superficial layer of the skin, transport of the drug begins [102].

Advancements in microneedle design have led to the creation of degradable and hollow microneedles to deliver higher doses of drugs and control the drug release. In the case of hollow microneedles, additional methods such as electrophoresis, iontophoresis, and sonophoresis can be employed to modify the drug transport. Macromolecules like insulin, immunobiologicals, growth hormones, proteins, and peptides can be delivered via microneedles. Also, the delivery of cosmeceuticals for treatment of skin problems such as scars, pigmentation, acne, and wrinkles is possible, as well as for skin tone improvement [102].

There is a possibility for transdermal drug delivery by the fabrication of microneedles contained within a patch. Patches containing microneedles can be used for the delivery of drugs, vaccines, biopharmaceuticals, etc. The rapid response in this delivery method is due to the disruption of the SC by the microneedles [114].

McAllister *et al.* fabricated tapered microneedles using different materials such as silicon, metals, or glass (Fig. 7.3J). They used these microneedles in order to deliver insulin and suggested that this delivery method could be an effective approach to decrease blood sugar levels [115]. Yu *et al.* produced silicon microneedles for the purpose of electrocardiography (ECG). The microneedles penetrated through the skin and led to reducing the impedance of the electrode-skin-electrode junction. Furthermore, the injection of NaCl solution as an electrolyte can be done through microneedles. They demonstrated that the signal-to-noise ratio of ECG measurement by electrodes equipped with microneedles was improved in comparison to electrodes with a flat surface [116].

Transdermal microfluidic drug delivery systems based on microneedles are an alternative to hypodermic needles and they can be used as multifunctional platforms by integration with sensing systems. So, by combining micromachining technology with microelectronics many functions can be integrated into the needles. The integration of sensors into microneedles can be used to measure the reaction of cells and tissues to applied drugs. Also, the response signal from the sensor caused by the chemical stimulation by the drug allows closed-loop controlled cell stimulation. In addition to examining single-cell responses using microneedles, there is also a possibility to manipulate the response. Furthermore, precise and controlled fluid sampling can be performed for chemical and biochemical tests using microneedles [37, 52]. It should be noted that needle clogging and tissue fibrosis can also occur with these systems and will affect their performance. Moreover, bacterial infection is another problem that may limit the use of transdermal drug delivery systems for long-term treatment and it is due to the breach that is created in the skin barrier for the duration of their use. Therefore, particular consideration should be given to the design of such systems [52].

Two significant success stories have been, microneedles embedded in the skin for delivering insulin which significantly reduced blood glucose levels, and solid microneedles coated with vaccines resulting in a good antibody response [37]. For instance, there was a report of microneedle patches, which included 57 coated microneedles. Also, electrodes fabricated using polymeric microneedles could be used to measure the level of glucose and lactic acid in solution by enzyme reaction with these reagents with the glucose oxidase and lactose oxidase enzymes. The detection limit of this biosensor was up to 1 μM for both glucose and lactate [117]. Recently, platforms based on the microneedles technique have been used for vaccination. It has proved that better and deeper penetration of vaccines using microneedles caused a higher immunoglobulin G2 (igG2) titer compared to a commercial tetanus toxoid vaccine [118].

7.11 Microfluidics for drug delivery: Cellular and organ level

The first step in drug discovery is the choice of the target protein or gene that the drug is designed to affect or interact with. This process is followed by the technical or commercial optimization of the drug and then clinical trials are undertaken. In comparison with the usual drug manufacturing techniques, microfluidic systems offer some benefits, such as the precise control of fluids, requiring minimal reagents, and rapid reaction times. The applications of these systems include preclinical investigations, the creation of dosage formulations, cytotoxicity experiments, target selection, and validation [62]. In the field of drug-delivery systems, microfluidic devices can be used in the manufacture of drug carriers, high-throughput screening, on-site analysis, compound generation, protein crystallization, and organ-on-a-chip setups, some of which are discussed in the following section [13].

7.11.1 On-site analysis

The concept of on-site analysis includes the measurement of protein content, protein separation, or single amino acid evaluation in a lysed cell preparation using a microfluidic system. One study by Huang *et al.* described a system that could lyse, separate, and measure the amount of protein within a single cell. The protein labeling was done via fluorescent-antibody binding and the molecular composition was examined via optical methods [119]. Some microfluidic chip-capillary electrophoresis devices have been studied for on-site analysis. These devices work based on the quantification of an appropriate range of biomarkers such as proteins or electrolytes in a small amount of sample [120]. Also, Chenouard *et al.* in order to discover and analyze mutations to distinguish between genome-edited and wild-type animals, developed a heteroduplex mobility assay [121]. In another study, an electrode with a composite structure was fabricated using carbon-polydimethylsiloxane and used to measure the components in a traditional Chinese herbal medicine called *Rhizoma chuanxiong*. By coupling this device with capillary electrophoresis, separation and detection of metabolites, for example, vanillin acid, caffeic acid, and ferulic acid were possible [122].

Separation of particles with different sizes is possible, based on inertia, or hydrodynamic effects like elasticity. Particle separation based on viscoelasticity has especially studied because this technique can be used with a wide range of flow rates. In this case, separation occurs by pushing larger particles downstream in a straight channel depending on elasto-inertial mechanisms. It should be noted that with a high particle concentration, a decrease in the purity of the particles is observed [123]. Liu et al. accomplished particle separation based on size with low efficiency and tested the system for cell separation using *E. coli* and red blood cells [124]. The use of a two-stage microfluidic system may improve the particle separation. The two stage-mechanism first concentrates the particles in the internal channel within a size range of 5–10 μm and then completes the particle separation in the next stage. This device was used for blood cell separation [125].

Microfluidic systems with different characteristics have their own hydrodynamic forces, for instance, the straight channel in a microfluidic geometry is a straightforward design for separating particles depending on inertial forces. However, to order and collect particles with different sizes, multiple equilibrium positions can be employed. Curved spiraling channels rely on the "Dean flow", which results from the curvature of the channel for separating different particles [13].

7.11.2 Protein crystallization

Protein crystallization is the process of obtaining a protein crystal by addition of precipitating agents and controlling the conditions, like temperature, ionic strength, and pH of the solution. This produces a supersaturated solution of the protein in which the natural conformation of the protein molecule is maintained. One of the most important applications of protein crystallization is for X-ray diffraction analysis [126]. The X-ray diffraction patterns of protein crystals are used as raw data to allow the direct visualization of the 3D structure of macromolecules or protein complexes [127]. Testing and examining different chemical conditions, like buffers, salts, and precipitating agents are required for appropriate protein crystallization.

So, in order to optimize crystallization conditions for each protein, a large amount of sample and reagents are needed, and also before protein crystallization, different purification techniques such as chromatography, or ultrafiltration, etc. must be used to obtain highly pure crystals [13]. In this regard, microfluidic technology provides the possibility of evaluating several crystallization conditions simultaneously, with only a small amount of protein sample. Lately, there have been some microfluidic devices designed to perform crystallization experiments using a nano-scale volume. In addition, using a centrifuge-based microfluidic device equipped with vapor-diffusion chambers, a large number of crystallization tests using vapor diffusion are possible. The advantages of this designed microfluidic device for crystallization techniques are, providing the possibility of examination a wider range of crystallization conditions, besides shorter reaction times and lower costs in comparison with conventional crystallization methods [13, 128]. A microfluidic device with a semi-contact dispensing method was designed in which the volume of each droplet was only approximately between 4 and 8 nL and about 100 different crystallization conditions could be tested [129].

7.12 Organ-on-a-chip

Organ-on-a-chip is a term for a microfluidic cell culture system that includes microfluidic channels containing cells. Some of these chips can then be equipped with several different types of cells to investigate the whole-body response to a specific drug and also reduce the requirement for animal testing [130]. Cell culture phases have some drawbacks, for instance, the complexity in harvesting metabolites, the absence of interphase and fluid flow, but the use of organ-on-a-chip devices can overcome these difficulties. The chip can be fabricated by pouring a polymeric liquid onto a silicon substrate to produce the desired patterns on the chip using the soft lithography process. The possibility of exposing the different cells to each other or else keeping them separate is determined via the design of the device. Furthermore, transcellular transport and secretion of various molecules can be monitored using a porous layer for separating the microchannels. This technique provides a degree of control over many parameters, which is impossible with other methods such as 3-D cell cultures. In order to study a single tissue, the simplest organ-on-a-chip system is a single chip with only one kind of cell. More complicated systems can be fabricated to simulate interphases between various kinds of tissues as well as the mechanical stresses that can cause cell signaling. Basically, organ-on-a-chip devices provide an accurate model of in vivo environment by controlling many parameters, for example, mechanical stress, fluid shear stress, and electrochemical gradients. By applying a flexible membrane, mechanical stress can be transferred to adherent cells which induce processes like cell breathing. This successful technology can facilitate drug development and manufacturing processes by modeling the in vivo conditions thus making drug delivery analysis and cytotoxicity assays easier [13].

7.13 The role of microfluidic technology for cancer cell studies

In the case of cancer studies, microfluidic devices are useful for early cancer diagnosis and multiplex screening of cancer cells. Microfluidics have a role in personalized medicine, accurate diagnosis, and prevention of cancer development. Using these devices helps to enhance the efficiency of anti-cancer drug discovery. By analyzing single cells on a multiplexed scale, the identification of heterogeneous subpopulations among cancer cells is possible resulting in a better understanding of the causes and progression of cancer, and the discovery of more efficient treatment strategies. There are several microfluidic devices that have been used to screen multiple markers at the same time in different kinds of cancer [13]. For instance, Fan *et al.* created a device for breast and prostate cancer detection that was able to carry out immuno-detection of 12 different biomarkers simultaneously and the results were validated in 22 patients with known types of cancer [131]. As another example, Wlodkowic *et al.* designed a microarray device with 440 separate traps on which leukemia cancer cells could be immobilized and characterized [132]. The use of microdevices has had a significant impact on improving the efficacy of anti-cancer drugs. Although this technology shows great promise in diagnosis and drug development, more studies must be done to improve the reliability of the analysis in complex environments and clinical samples.

7.14 Autonomous and smart integrated drug delivery microfluidic platforms

Smart drug delivery systems help to maintain drugs at a desired level in the body. By converting implantable microfluidic systems to become autonomous and self-regulating drug delivery platforms, there is a possibility to better treat chronic diseases like rheumatoid arthritis and diabetes using sustained and controlled drug release systems [133, 134]. There are some important parts in such a smart long-term microfluidic drug delivery device; a drug reservoir, a controllable actuator to release desired levels of the drug to the body, a biosensor and a signal processor in order to evaluate a particular analyte, a controlled drug release profile, and a source of energy to power the device [52].

A glucose sensor was fabricated by Tsai *et al.* via immobilizing glucose oxidase onto a hydrogel (Fig. 7.4A). The sensor was protected from surrounding environmental conditions and human body fluids to preserve its sensitivity by being mounted on the lid of a microfabricated vial. By applying a particular electrical potential (800 mV), the lid was opened and the sensor was exposed to the stream of the analyte. Furthermore, it was possible to fix the lid onto a drug reservoir with a sensor to adjust the amount of the released drug [134]. In one interesting study, Son *et al.* produced a wearable patch to treat movement disorders by precise drug delivery (Fig. 7.4B). In this case, they employed a patch with an electroresistive heater/sensor and in order to adsorb and deliver drugs, mesoporous drug-loaded M-silica nanoparticles were employed. A PDMS stamp was employed to print nanoparticles onto

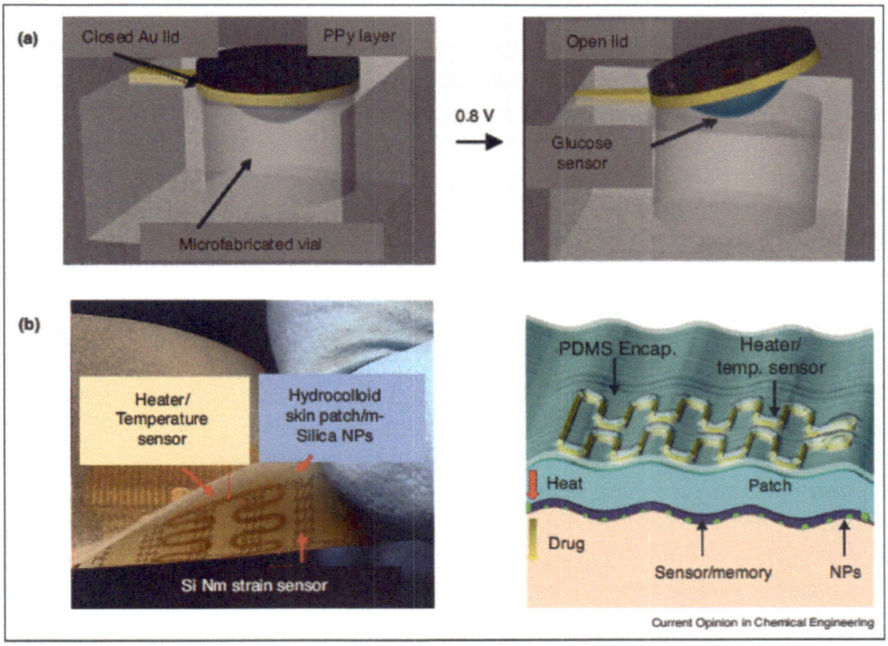

FIG. 7.4

Smart drug delivery microfluidic devices. (A) Schematic of a microfabricated vial and a biosensor which was immobilized on one side of its gold lid, that can be either opened or closed by electroactuation via applying of 800 mV versus Ag/AgCl. (B) Thermal actuation and precise transdermal drug delivery from m-silica nanoparticles (NPs). Wearable electronic patches consisted of the therapeutic actuating elements, diagnostic tools, and data storage modules.

Reprinted with permission from Riahi R, et al. Microfluidics for advanced drug delivery systems. Curr Opin Chem Eng 2015;7:101–12, Elsevier.

one side of the patch. By heating the patch, the loaded drug in the nanoparticles was triggered to release and diffuse across the skin. Also, the temperature sensor could regulate the maximum temperature on the skin for the prevention of skin burns [135].

Fabricating and integrating miniaturized components in a closed-loop design, and producing sensors with selectivity and reliability over the entire implantation period are the main problems for developing smart microfluidic drug delivery systems [52].

7.15 Conclusions and future directions

Microfluidic technology is an outstanding achievement of 21st-century science. Microfluidic systems have made their way into different fields such as drug delivery and other areas of medicine. They are useful for the fabrication of sophisticated drug carriers with specific properties, preprogrammed release profiles, and uniform sizes ranging from hundreds of nanometers to several micrometers. Microfluidic technology has the potential to be used as a platform to investigate interactions between drug carriers and cells, and also the treatment effects of active compounds and drugs. Thus, these platforms can be helpful for filling the gap between animal studies and human clinical trials. Furthermore, direct and localized delivery of drugs to target tissues can be accomplished by using microfluidic systems. Microfluidic systems can deliver the precise dose of drugs to the target sites with many advantages, thus reducing the side effects caused by drug administration at high concentrations. Microfluidic technologies can provide the possibility of analyzing the response of multiple cells, tissues, or organs to a specific drug, thus helping the development of novel therapies. One future direction of microfluidic technologies is to produce very small implantable devices for long-term treatment, with biodegradable properties that allow resorption of the implanted system and avoiding the need for surgical procedures to remove it. So, after the period of the treatment, the implanted system would begin to degrade in the body. For this aim, the components of the device must be made out of biodegradable materials covered by a protective coating layer to avoid degradation during the therapeutic period. When the treatment is finished, the protective layer will be degraded or removed, and rapid degradation of the device can occur by exposure to enzymes in body fluids. However, the development of such a novel field requires advances and collaboration in physics and biological sciences. Another future direction of such systems is the combination of microfluidic devices and sensing platforms for drug delivery. It is expected that, with more research, these devices could be used to measure different biomarkers within the body and tailor appropriate therapies. These systems are expected to revolutionize treatment methods [13, 52].

References

[1] P.S. Dittrich, A. Manz, Lab-on-a-chip: microfluidics in drug discovery, Nat Rev Drug Discov 5 (3) (2006) 210.

[2] B. Ziaie, et al., Hard and soft micromachining for BioMEMS: review of techniques and examples of applications in microfluidics and drug delivery, Adv Drug Deliv Rev 56 (2) (2004) 145–172.

[3] Y.G. Nam, Effect of junction geometry on monodispersed microdroplet generation in microfluidic aqueous two-phase systems, 2014.

[4] G.M. Whitesides, The origins and the future of microfluidics, Nature 442 (7101) (2006) 368.

[5] S. Damiati, et al., Microfluidic devices for drug delivery systems and drug screening, Genes 9 (2) (2018) 103.

[6] F. Ushikubo, et al., Y-and T-junction microfluidic devices: effect of fluids and interface properties and operating conditions, Microfluid Nanofluid 17 (4) (2014) 711–720.

[7] J. Wang, et al., Microfluidics: a new cosset for neurobiology, Lab Chip 9 (5) (2009) 644–652.

[8] K. Jähnisch, et al., Chemistry in microstructured reactors, Angew Chem Int Ed 43 (4) (2004) 406–446.

[9] H. Song, J.D. Tice, R.F. Ismagilov, A microfluidic system for controlling reaction networks in time, Angew Chem Int Ed 42 (7) (2003) 768–772.

[10] J. Pihl, M. Karlsson, D.T. Chiu, Microfluidic technologies in drug discovery, Drug Discov Today 10 (20) (2005) 1377–1383.
[11] Y. Xia, G.M. Whitesides, Soft lithography, Annu Rev Mater Sci 28 (1) (1998) 153–184.
[12] D. Yuan, et al., Recent progress of particle migration in viscoelastic fluids, Lab Chip 18 (4) (2018) 551–567.
[13] E.I. Mancera-Andrade, et al., Microfluidics technology for drug delivery: a review, Front Biosci 10 (2018) 74–91 (Elite Ed.).
[14] T. Fu, et al., Droplet formation and breakup dynamics in microfluidic flow-focusing devices: from dripping to jetting, Chem Eng Sci 84 (2012) 207–217.
[15] N. Filatov, et al., Comparison of step and flow-focusing emulsification methods for water-in-oil monodisperse drops in microfluidic chips, J Phys Conf Ser (2018). IOP Publishing.
[16] C. Kunstmann-Olsen, et al., Uniform droplet splitting and detection using lab-on-chip flow cytometry on a microfluidic PDMS device, Sensors Actuators B Chem 229 (2016) 7–13.
[17] D. Ogończyk, et al., Bonding of microfluidic devices fabricated in polycarbonate, Lab Chip 10 (10) (2010) 1324–1327.
[18] Y. Chen, L. Zhang, G. Chen, Fabrication, modification, and application of poly (methyl methacrylate) microfluidic chips, Electrophoresis 29 (9) (2008) 1801–1814.
[19] A. Muck, et al., Fabrication of poly (methyl methacrylate) microfluidic chips by atmospheric molding, Anal Chem 76 (8) (2004) 2290–2297.
[20] I. Hutter, et al., Polymer-based microfluidic device for measuring membrane protein activities, Microfluid Nanofluid 14 (3–4) (2013) 421–429.
[21] L. El Fissi, D. Vandormael, L.A. Francis, Direct assembly of cyclic olefin copolymer microfluidic devices helped by dry photoresist, Sensors Actuators A Phys 223 (2015) 76–83.
[22] R.K. Jena, C.Y. Yue, Cyclic olefin copolymer based microfluidic devices for biochip applications: ultraviolet surface grafting using 2-methacryloyloxyethyl phosphorylcholine, Biomicrofluidics 6 (1) (2012), 012822.
[23] S. Metz, et al., Polyimide and SU-8 microfluidic devices manufactured by heat-depolymerizable sacrificial material technique, Lab Chip 4 (2) (2004) 114–120.
[24] I. Kobayashi, K. Uemura, M. Nakajima, Formulation of monodisperse emulsions using submicron-channel arrays, Colloids Surf A Physicochem Eng Asp 296 (1–3) (2007) 285–289.
[25] D. Nieto, et al., A laser-based technology for fabricating a soda-lime glass based microfluidic device for circulating tumour cell capture, Colloids Surf B: Biointerfaces 134 (2015) 363–369.
[26] S.A. Nabavi, et al., Dynamics of double emulsion break-up in three phase glass capillary microfluidic devices, J Colloid Interface Sci 450 (2015) 279–287.
[27] A.B. Azouz, et al., Laser processing of quartz for microfluidic device fabrication, Adv Mater Res (2012). Trans Tech Publ.
[28] M.B. Wabuyele, et al., Single molecule detection of double-stranded DNA in poly (methylmethacrylate) and polycarbonate microfluidic devices, Electrophoresis 22 (18) (2001) 3939–3948.
[29] C.-W. Chang, et al., A polydimethylsiloxane–polycarbonate hybrid microfluidic device capable of generating perpendicular chemical and oxygen gradients for cell culture studies, Lab Chip 14 (19) (2014) 3762–3772.
[30] J. Park, J. Li, A. Han, Micro-macro hybrid soft-lithography master (MMHSM) fabrication for lab-on-a-chip applications, Biomed Microdevices 12 (2) (2010) 345–351.

[31] M. Pla-Roca, et al., Micro/nanopatterning of proteins via contact printing using high aspect ratio PMMA stamps and nanoimprint apparatus, Langmuir 23 (16) (2007) 8614–8618.
[32] A. Singh, et al., Nanoengineered particles for enhanced intra-articular retention and delivery of proteins, Adv Healthc Mater 3 (10) (2014) 1562–1567.
[33] P. Couvreur, Nanoparticles in drug delivery: past, present and future, Adv Drug Deliv Rev 65 (1) (2013) 21–23.
[34] Y. Zhang, H.F. Chan, K.W. Leong, Advanced materials and processing for drug delivery: the past and the future, Adv Drug Deliv Rev 65 (1) (2013) 104–120.
[35] J. Puigmartí-Luis, Microfluidic platforms: a mainstream technology for the preparation of crystals, Chem Soc Rev 43 (7) (2014) 2253–2271.
[36] E. Samiei, M. Hoorfar, Systematic analysis of geometrical based unequal droplet splitting in digital microfluidics, J Micromech Microeng 25 (5) (2015), 055008.
[37] N.-T. Nguyen, S.T. Wereley, S.A.M. Shaegh, Fundamentals and applications of microfluidics, Artech House, 2019.
[38] N.S. Bhise, et al., Organ-on-a-chip platforms for studying drug delivery systems, J Control Release 190 (2014) 82–93.
[39] A.M. Bratt-Leal, et al., A microparticle approach to morphogen delivery within pluripotent stem cell aggregates, Biomaterials 34 (30) (2013) 7227–7235.
[40] R. Safavieh, D. Juncker, Capillarics: pre-programmed, self-powered microfluidic circuits built from capillary elements, Lab Chip 13 (21) (2013) 4180–4189.
[41] A. Tamayol, et al., Fiber-based tissue engineering: progress, challenges, and opportunities, Biotechnol Adv 31 (5) (2013) 669–687.
[42] M. Han, et al., Quantum-dot-tagged microbeads for multiplexed optical coding of biomolecules, Nat Biotechnol 19 (7) (2001) 631.
[43] B. Stadler, Preface to special topic: microfluidics in drug delivery, AIP Publishing, 2015.
[44] T. Rossow, et al., Controlled synthesis of cell-laden microgels by radical-free gelation in droplet microfluidics, J Am Chem Soc 134 (10) (2012) 4983–4989.
[45] S. Agnello, et al., Microfluidic production of hyaluronic acid derivative microfibers to control drug release, Mater Lett 182 (2016) 309–313.
[46] V.F. Cardoso, et al., From superhydrophobic-to superhydrophilic-patterned poly (vinylidene fluoride-co-chlorotrifluoroethylene) architectures as a novel platform for biotechnological applications, J Polym Sci B Polym Phys 54 (18) (2016) 1802–1810.
[47] C.A. Serra, Z. Chang, Microfluidic-assisted synthesis of polymer particles, Chem Eng Technol: Ind Chem-Plant Equip-Process Eng-Biotechnol 31 (8) (2008) 1099–1115.
[48] C.-X. Zhao, Multiphase flow microfluidics for the production of single or multiple emulsions for drug delivery, Adv Drug Deliv Rev 65 (11–12) (2013) 1420–1446.
[49] I.U. Khan, et al., Microfluidic conceived pH sensitive core–shell particles for dual drug delivery, Int J Pharm 478 (1) (2015) 78–87.
[50] J. Zhu, R.C. Hayward, Hierarchically structured microparticles formed by interfacial instabilities of emulsion droplets containing amphiphilic block copolymers, Angew Chem Int Ed 47 (11) (2008) 2113–2116.
[51] J.A. Champion, Y.K. Katare, S. Mitragotri, Particle shape: a new design parameter for micro-and nanoscale drug delivery carriers, J Control Release 121 (1–2) (2007) 3–9.
[52] R. Riahi, et al., Microfluidics for advanced drug delivery systems, Curr Opin Chem Eng 7 (2015) 101–112.
[53] C.T. Lo, et al., Controlled self-assembly of monodisperse niosomes by microfluidic hydrodynamic focusing, Langmuir 26 (11) (2010) 8559–8566.

[54] D.E. Owens III, N.A. Peppas, Opsonization, biodistribution, and pharmacokinetics of polymeric nanoparticles, Int J Pharm 307 (1) (2006) 93–102.
[55] T. Kong, et al., Droplet based microfluidic fabrication of designer microparticles for encapsulation applications, Biomicrofluidics 6 (3) (2012), 034104.
[56] J. Wu, et al., Fabrication and characterization of monodisperse PLGA–alginate core–shell microspheres with monodisperse size and homogeneous shells for controlled drug release, Acta Biomater 9 (7) (2013) 7410–7419.
[57] R. Karnik, et al., Microfluidic platform for controlled synthesis of polymeric nanoparticles, Nano Lett 8 (9) (2008) 2906–2912.
[58] C.A. Serra, et al., Microfluidic production of micro-and nanoparticles, Encyclopedia of Polymer Science and Technology, 2002.
[59] N.M. Belliveau, et al., Microfluidic synthesis of highly potent limit-size lipid nanoparticles for in vivo delivery of siRNA, Mol Ther–Nucleic Acids 1 (2012), e37.
[60] C.G. Koh, et al., Delivery of antisense oligodeoxyribonucleotide lipopolyplex nanoparticles assembled by microfluidic hydrodynamic focusing, J Control Release 141 (1) (2010) 62–69.
[61] A. Jahn, et al., Microfluidic directed formation of liposomes of controlled size, Langmuir 23 (11) (2007) 6289–6293.
[62] L. Kang, et al., Microfluidics for drug discovery and development: from target selection to product lifecycle management, Drug Discov Today 13 (1–2) (2008) 1–13.
[63] A.U. Andar, et al., Microfluidic preparation of liposomes to determine particle size influence on cellular uptake mechanisms, Pharm Res 31 (2) (2014) 401–413.
[64] D. Nozdriukhin, et al., The study of monodisperse water-in-oil macroemulsion dynamics in a microfluidic chip, J Phys Conf Ser 917 (4) (2017), 042015.
[65] S.H. Kim, D.A. Weitz, One-step emulsification of multiple concentric shells with capillary microfluidic devices, Angew Chem Int Ed 50 (37) (2011) 8731–8734.
[66] A. Choi, et al., Recent advances in engineering microparticles and their nascent utilization in biomedical delivery and diagnostic applications, Lab Chip 17 (4) (2017) 591–613.
[67] E. Stolovicki, R. Ziblat, D.A. Weitz, Throughput enhancement of parallel step emulsifier devices by shear-free and efficient nozzle clearance, Lab Chip 18 (1) (2018) 132–138.
[68] S. Thatai, et al., Nanoparticles and core–shell nanocomposite based new generation water remediation materials and analytical techniques: a review, Microchem J 116 (2014) 62–76.
[69] O.S. Oluwafemi, et al., A facile completely 'green' size tunable synthesis of maltose-reduced silver nanoparticles without the use of any accelerator, Colloids Surf B: Biointerfaces 102 (2013) 718–723.
[70] A. Ofner, et al., High-throughput step emulsification for the production of functional materials using a glass microfluidic device, Macromol Chem Phys 218 (2) (2017) 1600472.
[71] M.K. Mulligan, J.P. Rothstein, Scale-up and control of droplet production in coupled microfluidic flow-focusing geometries, Microfluid Nanofluid 13 (1) (2012) 65–73.
[72] R. Mathaes, et al., Non-spherical micro-and nanoparticles: fabrication, characterization and drug delivery applications, Expert Opin Drug Deliv 12 (3) (2015) 481–492.
[73] P. Kolhar, et al., Using shape effects to target antibody-coated nanoparticles to lung and brain endothelium, Proc Natl Acad Sci 110 (26) (2013) 10753–10758.
[74] A.R. Studart, H.C. Shum, D.A. Weitz, Arrested coalescence of particle-coated droplets into nonspherical supracolloidal structures, J Phys Chem B 113 (12) (2009) 3914–3919.

[75] H.C. Shum, et al., Droplet microfluidics for fabrication of non-spherical particles, Macromol Rapid Commun 31 (2) (2010) 108–118.
[76] N. Annabi, et al., 25th anniversary article: rational design and applications of hydrogels in regenerative medicine, Adv Mater 26 (1) (2014) 85–124.
[77] D. Dendukuri, et al., Continuous-flow lithography for high-throughput microparticle synthesis, Nat Mater 5 (5) (2006) 365.
[78] J. Kim, et al., Lifting gate polydimethylsiloxane microvalves and pumps for microfluidic control, Anal Chem 84 (4) (2012) 2067–2071.
[79] J.H. Tsui, et al., Microfluidics-assisted in vitro drug screening and carrier production, Adv Drug Deliv Rev 65 (11–12) (2013) 1575–1588.
[80] R. Cheng, et al., Dual and multi-stimuli responsive polymeric nanoparticles for programmed site-specific drug delivery, Biomaterials 34 (14) (2013) 3647–3657.
[81] M. Guo, et al., Multifunctional superparamagnetic nanocarriers with folate-mediated and pH-responsive targeting properties for anticancer drug delivery, Biomaterials 32 (1) (2011) 185–194.
[82] J. Pessi, et al., Microfluidics-assisted engineering of polymeric microcapsules with high encapsulation efficiency for protein drug delivery, Int J Pharm 472 (1–2) (2014) 82–87.
[83] M. de Jesús Rostro-Alanis, et al., Nanobiocatalysis: nanostructured materials–a mini review, Biocatalysis 2 (1) (2016) 1–24.
[84] S. Sharma, et al., An insight into functionalized calcium based inorganic nanomaterials in biomedicine: trends and transitions, Colloids Surf B: Biointerfaces 133 (2015) 120–139.
[85] W.B. Liechty, et al., Polymers for drug delivery systems, Annu Rev Chem Biomol Eng 1 (2010) 149–173.
[86] F. Ito, et al., Preparation and properties of PLGA microspheres containing hydrophilic drugs by the SPG (shirasu porous glass) membrane emulsification technique, Colloids Surf B: Biointerfaces 67 (1) (2008) 20–25.
[87] A. Gañán-Calvo, et al., Building functional materials for health care and pharmacy from microfluidic principles and flow focusing, Adv Drug Deliv Rev 65 (11–12) (2013) 1447–1469.
[88] M.-K. Kim, et al., Capillary microfluidics-derived doxorubicin-containing human serum albumin microbeads for transarterial chemoembolization of hepatic cancer, Mater Sci Eng C 62 (2016) 391–397.
[89] M.A. Kandadai, et al., Microfluidic manufacture of rt-PA-loaded echogenic liposomes, Biomed Microdevices 18 (3) (2016) 48.
[90] H. Xie, et al., One-step fabrication of polymeric Janus nanoparticles for drug delivery, Langmuir 28 (9) (2012) 4459–4463.
[91] J. Wu, et al., Interfacial fast release layer in monodisperse poly (lactic-co-glycolic acid) microspheres accelerates the drug release, Curr Drug Deliv 13 (5) (2016) 720–729.
[92] Q. Xu, et al., Preparation of monodisperse biodegradable polymer microparticles using a microfluidic flow-focusing device for controlled drug delivery, Small 5 (13) (2009) 1575–1581.
[93] S. Dhar, et al., Targeted delivery of cisplatin to prostate cancer cells by aptamer functionalized Pt (IV) prodrug-PLGA–PEG nanoparticles, Proc Natl Acad Sci U S A 105 (45) (2008) 17356–17361.
[94] R.R. Jivani, et al., Biomedical microelectromechanical systems (BioMEMS): revolution in drug delivery and analytical techniques, Saudi Pharmaceut J 24 (1) (2016) 1–20.

[95] N. Nagai, et al., A platform for controlled dual-drug delivery to the retina: protective effects against light-induced retinal damage in rats, Adv Healthc Mater 3 (10) (2014) 1555–1560.

[96] R. Lo, et al., A passive MEMS drug delivery pump for treatment of ocular diseases, Biomed Microdevices 11 (5) (2009) 959.

[97] A.J. Chung, Y.S. Huh, D. Erickson, A robust, electrochemically driven microwell drug delivery system for controlled vasopressin release, Biomed Microdevices 11 (4) (2009) 861–867.

[98] A.J. Chung, et al., Implantable microfluidic and electronic systems for insect flight manipulation, Microfluid Nanofluid 13 (2) (2012) 345–352.

[99] N. Elman, H.H. Duc, M.J. Cima, An implantable MEMS drug delivery device for rapid delivery in ambulatory emergency care, Biomed Microdevices 11 (3) (2009) 625–631.

[100] F.N. Pirmoradi, et al., A magnetically controlled MEMS device for drug delivery: design, fabrication, and testing, Lab Chip 11 (18) (2011) 3072–3080.

[101] R. Langer, Drugs on target, Science 293 (5527) (2001) 58–59.

[102] S.H. Bariya, et al., Microneedles: an emerging transdermal drug delivery system, J Pharm Pharmacol 64 (1) (2012) 11–29.

[103] M.R. Prausnitz, R. Langer, Transdermal drug delivery, Nat Biotechnol 26 (11) (2008) 1261.

[104] P.H. Lambert, P.E. Laurent, Intradermal vaccine delivery: will new delivery systems transform vaccine administration? Vaccine 26 (26) (2008) 3197–3208.

[105] A.L. Teo, et al., Transdermal microneedles for drug delivery applications, Mater Sci Eng B 132 (1–2) (2006) 151–154.

[106] M. Matteucci, et al., A compact and disposable transdermal drug delivery system, Microelectron Eng 85 (5–6) (2008) 1066–1073.

[107] M.A.L. Teo, et al., In vitro and in vivo characterization of MEMS microneedles, Biomed Microdevices 7 (1) (2005) 47–52.

[108] C.Y. Jin, et al., Mass producible and biocompatible microneedle patch and functional verification of its usefulness for transdermal drug delivery, Biomed Microdevices 11 (6) (2009) 1195.

[109] P. Karande, S. Mitragotri, Enhancement of transdermal drug delivery via synergistic action of chemicals, Biochim Biophys Acta Biomembr 1788 (11) (2009) 2362–2373.

[110] M.S. Gerstel, V.A. Place, Drug delivery device, 1976. Google Patents.

[111] R.F. Donnelly, et al., Design, optimization and characterisation of polymeric microneedle arrays prepared by a novel laser-based micromoulding technique, Pharm Res 28 (1) (2011) 41–57.

[112] R.S. Shawgo, et al., BioMEMS for drug delivery, Curr Opinion Solid State Mater Sci 6 (4) (2002) 329–334.

[113] Y. Xie, B. Xu, Y. Gao, Controlled transdermal delivery of model drug compounds by MEMS microneedle array, Nanomedicine 1 (2) (2005) 184–190.

[114] G. Widera, et al., Effect of delivery parameters on immunization to ovalbumin following intracutaneous administration by a coated microneedle array patch system, Vaccine 24 (10) (2006) 1653–1664.

[115] D.V. McAllister, et al., Microfabricated needles for transdermal delivery of macromolecules and nanoparticles: fabrication methods and transport studies, Proc Natl Acad Sci U S A 100 (24) (2003) 13755–13760.

[116] L. Yu, et al., A microfabricated electrode with hollow microneedles for ECG measurement, Sensors Actuators A Phys 151 (1) (2009) 17–22.

[117] A. Caliò, et al., Polymeric microneedles based enzymatic electrodes for electrochemical biosensing of glucose and lactic acid, Sensors Actuators B Chem 236 (2016) 343–349.
[118] K. Siddhapura, H. Harde, S. Jain, Immunostimulatory effect of tetanus toxoid loaded chitosan nanoparticles following microneedles assisted immunization, Nanomedicine 12 (1) (2016) 213–222.
[119] B. Huang, et al., Counting low-copy number proteins in a single cell, Science 315 (5808) (2007) 81–84.
[120] J. Casals-Terré, Y.S. Fung, Q. Chen, F. Du, W. Guo, T. Ma, Z. Nie, H. Sun, R. Wu, W. Zhao, Microfluidic chip-capillary electrophoresis devices, Anal Bioanal Chem 408 (8) (2016) 1989–1991.
[121] V. Chenouard, et al., A rapid and cost-effective method for genotyping genome-edited animals: a heteroduplex mobility assay using microfluidic capillary electrophoresis, J Genet Genomics 43 (5) (2016) 341–348.
[122] L. Zhang, et al., Simultaneous determination of five bioactive constituents in rhizoma chuanxiong by capillary electrophoresis with a carbon nanotube-polydimethylsiloxane composite electrode, J Pharm Biomed Anal 131 (2016) 107–112.
[123] S.W. Ahn, et al., Microfluidic particle separator utilizing sheathless elasto-inertial focusing, Chem Eng Sci 126 (2015) 237–243.
[124] C. Liu, et al., Size-based separation of particles and cells utilizing viscoelastic effects in straight microchannels, Anal Chem 87 (12) (2015) 6041–6048.
[125] J. Nam, et al., Microfluidic device for sheathless particle focusing and separation using a viscoelastic fluid, J Chromatogr A 1406 (2015) 244–250.
[126] A. McPherson, J.A. Gavira, Introduction to protein crystallization, Acta Crystallogr Sect F: Struct Biol Commun 70 (1) (2014) 2–20.
[127] A. McPherson, Introduction to protein crystallization, Methods 34 (3) (2004) 254–265.
[128] L. Wang, et al., A centrifugal microfluidic device for screening protein crystallization conditions by vapor diffusion, Sensors Actuators B Chem 219 (2015) 105–111.
[129] Y. Zhu, et al., Nanoliter-scale protein crystallization and screening with a microfluidic droplet robot, Sci Rep 4 (2014) 5046.
[130] S.N. Bhatia, D.E. Ingber, Microfluidic organs-on-chips, Nat Biotechnol 32 (8) (2014) 760.
[131] Z.H. Fan, W. Tan, DNA nanospheres with microfluidics: a promising platform for cancer diagnosis? Nanomedicine 8 (11) (2013) 1731–1733.
[132] D. Wlodkowic, et al., Microfluidic single-cell array cytometry for the analysis of tumor apoptosis, Anal Chem 81 (13) (2009) 5517–5523.
[133] N.-T. Nguyen, et al., Design, fabrication and characterization of drug delivery systems based on lab-on-a-chip technology, Adv Drug Deliv Rev 65 (11–12) (2013) 1403–1419.
[134] H.K.A. Tsai, et al., Integrating biosensors and drug delivery: a step closer toward scalable responsive drug-delivery systems, Adv Mater 21 (6) (2009) 656–660.
[135] D. Son, et al., Multifunctional wearable devices for diagnosis and therapy of movement disorders, Nat Nanotechnol 9 (5) (2014) 397.

CHAPTER

Microfluidic devices for gene delivery systems

8

Sepideh Ahmadi[a,b], Navid Rabiee[c,*], Mojtaba Bagherzadeh[c], and Mahdi Karimi[d,e,f,g]

[a]*Student Research Committee, Department of Medical Biotechnology, School of Advanced Technologies in Medicine, Shahid Beheshti University of Medical Sciences, Tehran, Iran*

[b]*Cellular and Molecular Biology Research Center, Shahid Beheshti University of Medical Sciences, Tehran, Iran*

[c]*Department of Chemistry, Sharif University of Technology, Tehran, Iran*

[d]*Cellular and Molecular Research Center, Iran University of Medical Sciences, Tehran, Iran*

[e]*Department of Medical Nanotechnology, Faculty of Advanced Technologies in Medicine, Iran University of Medical Sciences, Tehran, Iran*

[f]*Oncopathology Research Center, Iran University of Medical Sciences, Tehran, Iran*

[g]*Research Center for Science and Technology in Medicine, Tehran University of Medical Sciences, Tehran, Iran*

**Corresponding author. E-mail: nrabiee94@gmail.com*

8.1 Introduction

Gene therapy involves the transfer of genetic material in the form of nucleic acids into tissues, cells, or a whole organ, with subsequent expression of the transgene, designed to treat cancer, inherited diseases, or viral infections [1]. In order to carry out effective gene therapy, the discovery of advanced and effective delivery systems capable of transfecting genes into cells in vivo is important.

Transfection means the entry of genetic agents such as DNA or RNA, plasmid DNA, or certain types of RNA such as siRNA or miRNA, into eukaryotic cells, which can modify the gene expression and protein function within the cells. In fact, once the target encoding DNA is inserted into a cell, its protein can be expressed. High amounts of protein can then be extracted by culturing bacterial or eukaryotic cells in the laboratory [2, 3].

Nowadays, the transfer of nucleic acids (low levels of gene transfer and their expression) is considered to be the most important challenge in gene therapy, so that foreign nucleic acids including genes, DNA aptamers or antisense oligonucleotides such as antisense oligonucleotides (ASO) and plasmid DNA (pDNA) can be used. A variety of RNA molecules (siRNA) and microRNA (miRNA) and oligonucleotide (ASO) can be transferred into the cells in order to generate genetically modified

Biomedical Applications of Microfluidic Devices. https://doi.org/10.1016/B978-0-12-818791-3.00010-3

cells [4, 5]. Therefore, it is essential to develop safe and efficient drug delivery systems in order to protect the genetic material from various barriers, including the cell membrane, nuclear membrane, cytosol, and to prevent the destruction of genetic material along the intracellular pathway from endosomes to lysosomes and to escape from endosomes. There are other criteria, such as the particle size and the zeta potential that have a significant effect on the carrier stability in biological environments, such as the tendency of the reticuloendothelial system to trap the carrier. In fact, the use of carriers or other advanced gene transfer methods helps greatly in the transfer of nucleic acids to enable gene therapy [6].

The size of gene delivery carriers is also of the utmost importance in order to transfer large biological entities such as plasmid DNA or CRISPR/cas9. Nowadays, various types of microfluidic systems have been developed, for the production of nanoparticles (NPs) for drug delivery, or for the transfer of genetic material (transfection) which leads to more accurate and efficient gene transfer [7].

Microfluidic systems are devices to produce highly ordered and automated fluid flow that are typically used in controlled biological investigations. The advantages of microfluidic devices are reduced reagent consumption, high surface-to-volume ratio, rapid heat and mass transfer, and also the microenvironment of microfluidic systems permits optimization and good control of multiple procedures used in gene therapy [8, 9].

The production of carriers for genes and nucleic acids using the unique characteristics of microfluidic devices, such as lower reagent volumes and rapidity, has led to the economical development of these devices for gene therapy applications. These devices are able to produce various types of viral and nonviral vectors for gene delivery [10].

Viral vectors such as adenoviruses and adeno-associated viruses (AAVs), rhabdoviruses, retroviruses, and poxviruses, have all been studied for the treatment of diseases such as infections, muscular [11], metabolic [12], ophthalmologic [13], hematologic [14], and different types of cancer [15, 16].

However, despite the ability of viruses to efficiently infect host cells and their high stability, the mutagenic and immunogenic side effects of viruses, as well as the problem to produce viruses in large quantities, remain as limitations hindering their clinical application [17]. The development of a microfluidic system by Vu et al. [18], partially solved the problem of mass production of retroviral vectors. Viral vectors using PT67–GFP packaging cells were produced in a microfluidic system. In this system, the walls of the polydimethylsiloxane (PDMS) channels were coated with bovine serum albumin (BSA) to enhance the virus production.

Nonviral vectors, including NPs, are able to overcome the problem related to the production of an immune response to the viral vectors. Safety is considered as their biggest advantage, but relatively low efficacy is still a limitation [19]. However, a significant increase in nonviral vectors (compared to viral vectors) has been observed in clinical trials from 2000 to 2019 due to their greater safety.

The transfer of naked DNA by physical methods could be a safe and effective strategy in gene delivery applications. In fact, these methods are known as vector-free methods where the transfer of nucleic acids is carried out through the membrane by application of physical force, and the genetic material enters the cell without any carrier [20]. Nowadays, these techniques have not been significantly developed, while viral and nonviral chemical methods are more widely used in experimental research and clinical trials. Damage to cells is considered as one of the major disadvantages of physical methods, but in recent years these problems have been solved by using microfluidic techniques.

In the following chapter, we discuss the use of microfluidics in the production of micro/NPs as nonviral carriers (chemical methods) and their role in the transfer of genetic material, as well as the combination of microfluidic systems with physical methods in the delivery of genetic material, and the role of microfluidic devices in overcoming many of the limitations in gene delivery and gene therapy.

8.2 Microfluidic devices for production of nonviral vectors (micro/NPs)

Nucleic acid transfer into cells can be significantly increased by the use of cationic lipids, such as lipofectamine or other different polymers. These act by compressing the nucleic acids into particles, and forming complexes or lipoplexes with nanometer dimensions. These lipids interact with negatively charged nucleic acids due to them having a positive charge, and can also bind to the cell membrane leading to more efficient endocytosis (for particles less than 100 nm) [21, 22]. Some major limitations include their high toxicity and high price. Conventional synthetic chemistry methods have produced micro/NPs using coprecipitation, emulsion, sol-gel, solvothermal-hydrothermal methods, chemical vapor deposition, or mechanochemical preparation methods such as grinding [23].

The main chemical method for making NPs is the precipitation method. This method is also sometimes called coprecipitation, because it is a process in which a soluble material becomes an insoluble solid structure. The precipitation method has different advantages such as the high quality of the NPs produced, although it can be difficult to produce NPs with the desired size. Some factors can be used for particle growth. Some factors are effective in controlling the particle size, including complexing agents and surfactants [24, 25]. The emulsification method is also considered to be an effective method to produce NPs and ultrafine particles with controlled size and shape [26].

Recently more NPs, including inorganic, organic, liposomes, and polymeric NPs have been developed due to their advantages in order to transfer nucleic acids.

Compared to common batch synthesis methods, microfluidic systems better control the shape and size of the particles, by using liquids, rapid reactions, and mixing, and are more cost-effective [27, 28].

Microfluidic devices are capable of producing a variety of NPs, including semiconductor, metals, and polymeric, which are well controlled and homogeneous [29, 30]. The NP size can be better controlled than those produced by conventional synthetic methods. The addition of reagents during the mixing process and high throughput synthesis make microdevices suitable for NP formulation screening. In Table 8.1, a

Table 8.1 Summary of the advantages and disadvantages of microfluidic techniques in micro/NPs production.

Advantages	Disadvantages
Control over shape and size of particles	Difficult device design
Tunable particle size	Not fully automated
High reproducibility of particle synthesis	Probability of channel clogging
Rapid mixing and reduced in NP synthesis time, high scale-up feasibility	Diffusion of NPs through the PDMS matrix
Less particle size dispersion	Pharmacokinetics cannot be determined
Low reagent consumption	
Label-free	

list of the advantages and disadvantages of microfluidic devices for micro/NP synthesis compared to conventional synthesis methods is presented.

The use of microreactors in microfluidic devices for the synthesis of NPs is important because microreactors lead to improving the control of reaction time, concentration, and temperature of the reagents. Also, they provide heat transfer and better mixing [31, 32]. In order to synthesize NPs, two types of microreactors have been designed: (1) chip-based microreactors; (2) tubing based microreactors [33, 34]. Chip-based microreactors are based on integrating multiple functions into a single chip with channel diameters ranging from tens to hundreds of micrometers. These types of microreactors are usually synthesized from three different types of materials including polymers, silicon, and glass [35]. Silicon and glass can be used to make long-lasting microfluidic devices [36]. Some of their most important benefits include thermal conductivity and thermal stability [37, 38]. Glass substrate microreactors are an alternative to silicon substrate microreactors that are more suitable for high-temperature reactions [39]. However, they are more expensive and it costs a lot to build a microfluidic device.

Polymer-substrate microreactors can be designed using simpler techniques, such as hot embossing or soft lithography compared to other microreactors. They are mostly made of poly(methyl methacrylate) (PMMA) or polydimethyl siloxane (PDMS). These reactors are desirable due to their low cost and ease of fabrication [40, 41]. Polymeric substrate microreactors are easier to prepare and are cheaper than silicon or glass substrates, although they are usually not suitable for high-temperature reactions [42]. Generally, fabricating such a device involves materials including glass capillaries and polymer tubing.

Capillary tubes are also used in the synthesis of NPs. Glass and polytetrafluoroethylene (PTFE, Teflon) tubing are the most common materials in capillary-based microreactors. PTFE has high-temperature compatibility. However, these devices use larger-diameter channels (even at millimeter scale) compared to chip-based microchannels [43, 44]. The synthesis of sub-3 nm citrate-capped gold NPs was performed in a continuous flow PTFE capillary tubing device with an inner diameter of

0.3 mm, using $HAuCl_4$ as a precursor. A mixture of trisodium citrate and gold(III) chloride trihydrate was flowed through capillaries at a high temperature leading to an increased nucleation rate and produced an improved surface-enhanced Raman spectroscopy active surface [45].

Mixing plays an important role in reducing inhomogeneity. In fact, factors such as capillary number (Ca), channel width, and the ratio of viscosities of the dispersed and continuous phases, have effects on the rate of mixing performance. The Reynolds (Re) number is one of the most important parameters in predicting the flow pattern, which is represented by the formula $Re = \rho \nu L/\mu$, ν is the velocity of the fluid, and μ is the viscosity of the fluid, ρ is the density of the fluid, L is the characteristic linear dimension [46, 47].

When the reagents are injected into the microchannels in miscible solvents, a laminar flow is created in which mixing occurs [48]. Mixing occurs within the microchannels more efficiently in batch reactors, due to shorter travel distances and miniaturized fluid dimensions compared to devices with larger channels.

To increase mixing performance, single-phase systems use structures such as herringbone mixer, capillary tube T-junctions, Y-junctions, and hydrodynamic flow focusing [49]. Some of these mixing methods are shown in Fig. 8.1. T-junction, Y-junction, and hydrodynamic flow focusing (HFF) are employed in the preparation of NP suspensions. In a T-junction, one liquid (continuous phase) is injected from the vertical channel, whereas the other liquid (disperse phase) flows through the perpendicular channel [50, 51].

Y-shaped microfluidic devices are used for passive mixing and contain two inlets and one outlet. In the Y-type, the NP solution and nonsolvent flow mix with each other. Fig. 8.1 shows three different types of junctions in microfluidic devices [51, 52].

Based on the flow types in microfluidic devices, the NP synthesis methods can be divided into two types: single-phase and multiple-phase flow synthesis. In continuous flow single phase based microfluidic devices, the mixing of the reagents in microchannels under diffusion laminar flow conditions, mixing efficiency, and temperature and time are the parameters that govern the NP quality [9]. Also, the microfluidic

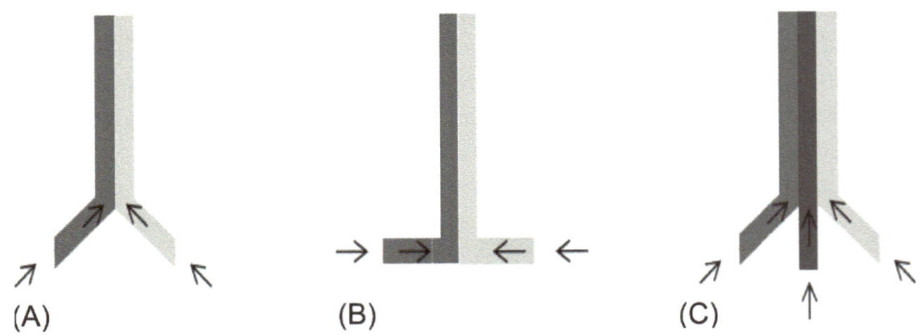

FIG. 8.1

Different types of junctions in microfluidic devices: (A) Y-junction; (B) T-junction; (C) ψ-junction.

production of droplets has been developed. In this system, NP synthesis occurs in droplet reactors to improve the mixing efficiency and decrease the NP size distribution. NP synthesis took place in microdroplet reactors to improve the mixing efficiency in microfluidic channels and further reduces the particle size distribution [53, 54].

In the following section, we discuss continuous flow-based microfluidics and droplet-based microfluidics in more detail and their role in the production of NP for gene delivery.

8.3 Continuous flow systems

A continuous laminar flow streams of single or multiple fluids in a single-phase system, which passes through microchannels and is controlled by external pressure, mechanical pumps, and so on and during that nucleation and growth occurs. This system provided a homogenous environment, fast mixing across the laminar flow and short distances for diffusion and enable of synthesizing several NPs for the gene delivery, including polymer NPs, metallic NPs, and semiconductor quantum dots NPs [55–57]. The microchannel structure is suitable for precisely controlling the reaction time and producing NPs of the preferred size and shape. Continuous modified single-phase systems allow subsequent addition of reagents during the multistep reaction and synthesis process. They can be scaled up to carry out multiple reactions, even on the same chip [58].

In single-phase microfluidic devices there can be a variety of mixing strategies. One common technique for continuous mixing is HFF. Cationic liposomes (CLs) of 100–130 nm diameter with a high yield and good reproducibility were synthesized by Balbino et al. A central flow of lipids dissolved in ethanol was injected into the device, and two lipid flows in ethanol were compressed hydrodynamically by two and three flows of aqueous-based solvents. An increase in the fluid flow rate and a high yield of unilamellar CLs made this method suitable for gene delivery. The factors that govern the NP size and polydispersity include Vf and FRR, including the effect of increasing Vf, which increases the yield. Also, there is a significant relationship between increased FRR and increasing the NP size [59] (Fig. 8.2).

In another study, Balbino et al. [60] reported the assembly of pDNA/CLs composed of stacked bilayers on a laminar-flow-based PMDS/glass microfluidic system. The microchannels were 140 μm wide and 100 μm deep. Compared with common batch processes, these nonviral carriers have been shown to have improved in vitro transfection efficacy with high pDNA loading. Using small-angle X-ray scattering (SAXS) curves, the lipoplexes in the microdevice were established to have stacked bilayers, while larger amounts of pDNA permitted the formation of agglomerates with more stacked bilayers in the batch process. Furthermore, the alignment of shape-anisotropic nanomaterials is of great importance for manufacturing structurally anisotropic products. Nevertheless, rheo-optical studies, which are frequently based on flow-induced approaches, require complex experimental manipulation and are inherently difficult to perform.

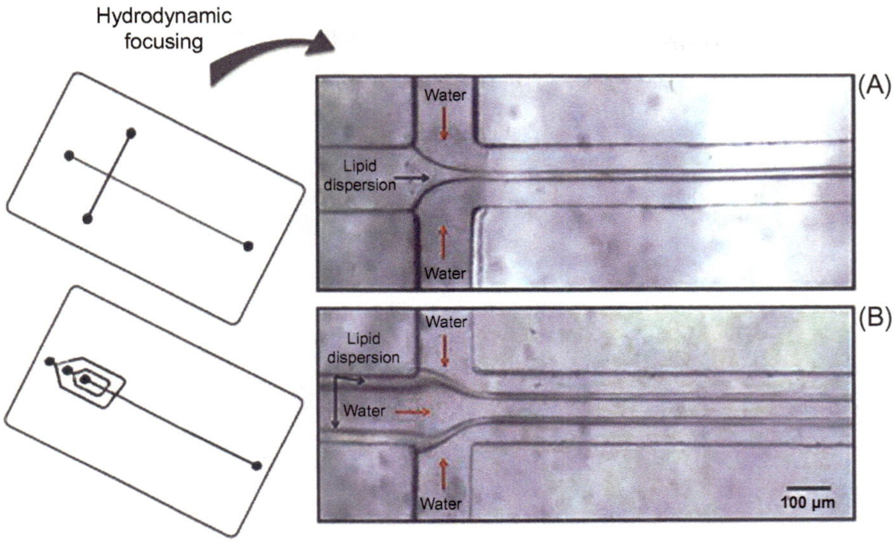

FIG. 8.2

Schematic illustration of two type of (A) single and (B) double hydrodynamic focusing.

Reprinted with permission from Balbino TA, et al., Continuous flow production of cationic liposomes at high lipid concentration in microfluidic devices for gene delivery applications. Chem Eng J. 2013;226:423–33, Elsevier.

Continuous-flow microfluidics was used to produce poly(beta-amino esters)/plasmid DNA NPs with good stability during long-term storage, which exhibited greater in vitro pDNA transfection efficiency in B16, and MDA-MB-231 cancer cells in comparison with conventional transfection reagents such as Lipofectamine^{R} 2000. Fig. 8.3 shows a PDMS/glass chip with two syringe pumps used for mixing DNA and an aqueous polymer [61].

Continuous-flow microfluidic systems can be used in different fields, but optimization and manipulation are needed to arrive at the highest performance. This technique also has some disadvantages compared to the droplet-based microfluidic technique, such as low mixing rate and occurrence of channel clogging [62].

8.4 Droplet-based microfluidic devices

Multiphase flow microfluidics, segmented flow, or droplet microfluidics, include two or more fluids in segmented phases. Droplet-based microfluidics is a nano/microcarrier synthesis technique capable of producing highly homogenous gene-loaded particles [63]. In addition, droplet-microfluidic systems can be used for in vitro/in vivo transfection where genes are encapsulated into separate droplets and it is possible for them to undergo expression in vitro within the droplets using much lower amounts

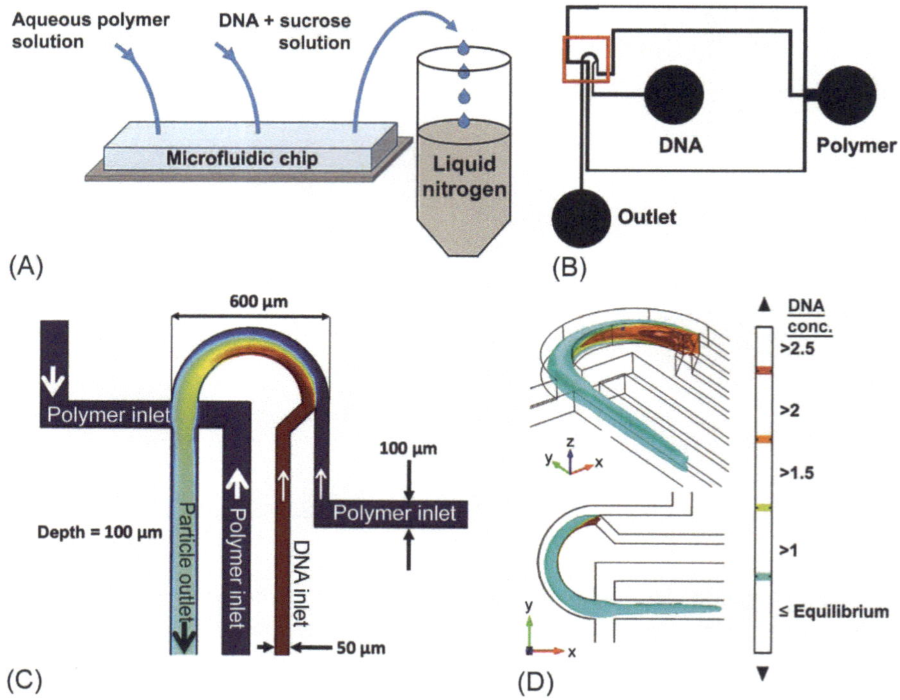

FIG. 8.3

Schematic illustration of 3D-hydrodynamic flow for polyplex formation [61].

Reprinted with permission from Wilson DR, et al., Continuous microfluidic assembly of biodegradable poly(beta-amino ester)/DNA nanoparticles for enhanced gene delivery. J Biomed Mater Res A. 2017;105(6):1813–1825, Wiley.

of reagents. The fabrication of devices for droplet microfluidics can be accomplished by several systems, such as 3D printing [64], optical adhesive bonding [65], or glass etching [66]. The use of laminar flow is another advantage of these systems, which provides heat and mass transfer for transfection [67].

In these systems, the reaction occurs in separate droplets in contrast to continuous flow microreactors. In addition to preventing contamination, each droplet acts independently as a chamber for performing a reaction, and mixing occurs within each individual device section by moving along the channels. The size and number of droplets can be controlled precisely using this method [54]. Like single-phase systems, microchannel structures are designed for optimization of the reaction time and mixing and only a small volume of droplets are needed. Multiphase systems have more flexibility than single-phase systems due to continuous sequential modifications, and because it is more difficult to add reagents to the droplets. Droplet generation mechanisms include optical methods that apply optical forces to form the

NPs; hydrodynamics (T-junction and Y-junction; co-flow and flow-focusing); and electrical method such as dielectrophoresis (DEP) [53].

This method controls the fluid volume in immiscible phases, oil-in-water and liquid-gas phases [68]. Hydrophilic channels are used for oil-in-water emulsions and hydrophobic channels are applied for water-in-oil emulsions [69, 70]. In gas-liquid segmented flow systems, the gaseous phase increases the mixing rate and is used to synthesize polymeric NPs [9]. The gas phase forms a gas-liquid-gas flow and separates the gas and liquid flows. In the liquid-liquid phase, the droplets are encapsulated by a carrier fluid and reactions take place within them, while in the gas-liquid phase, the droplets are separated by gas bubbles and the reactions occur in the continuous phase [54].

Conventional bulk systems can control the droplet size less accurately than other systems. The formation of droplets is based on either active or passive mixing systems. In passive mixing, microchannels are used to produce droplets in the continuous system. [71]. In active mixing, droplets are produced by applying an external force to induce interfacial instability that results in droplet formation [72]. There are various methods for droplet generation geometries in microfluidic devices, including co-flow, flow focusing, and cross-flow [73, 74]. The T-junction is one of the main geometries that can form the basis of other cross-flow geometries and produce highly monodisperse droplets.

Ho et al. established a microfluidic picoliter volume droplet system with a cross-flow type of droplet generator for the fabrication of polyplexes containing pDNA encoding the green fluorescence protein plus a cationic polymer. Cationic and bioreducible block copolymers have previously been shown to possess lower cytotoxicity, high gene delivery efficiency, and the ability to deliver several types of nucleic acids. A comparison of bulk-synthesized and microfluidic droplet methods showed that droplet and bulk-generated carriers resulted in ~60% and ~40% transfection efficiency and ~90% and ~75% cell viability, respectively [75].

In another study, Grigsby et al. established an emulsion-based droplet microfluidic system for the synthesis of polymer-nucleic acid nanocomplexes using the bioreducible linear poly(amidoamine) poly(CBA-ABOL). The polyplexes were more uniform with less aggregation than bulk methods. This nanocomplex increased the transfection efficiency of both pDNA and mRNA in various cell lines, primary cells, and stem cells [76].

Nowadays, the application of microdroplet technology to gene editing is expanding. Microfluidics have a significant effect on reducing any off-target problems, reducing cell death, shortening reaction times, and reducing costs and consumption of culture medium compared to multi-well plates. Gene editing can be carried out by efficient transfection of a plasmid containing sgRNA and Cas9 enzyme into cells to produce DNA double-strand breaks at the specified location [77]. In fact, in recent years, CRISPR-based gene editing has become a fascinating topic in molecular biology and was combined with droplet microfluidics for knockdown of the TP53BP1 gene in K562 cells [78].

In one study, droplet-based microfluidic technology could improve pcDNA3-EGFP plasmid transfection into single cells. Here, a single cell took up a self-assembled lipoplex formed from the plasmid and lipofectamine. This lipoplex was monodisperse and 227 nm in diameter making it suitable for endocytosis. They obtained between 5% and 50% improvements in transfection efficiency for all three cell lines (Jurkat, K562 and THP-1). Application of this technique to CRISPR/Cas9 gene editing allowed the knockout of the *TP53BP1* gene in K562 cells. The results of this study demonstrated a high transfection efficiency and low cell-to-cell variation in hard-to-transfect suspension cells, whether for gene transfer or gene editing, as well as in regenerative medicine using drop microfluidics [78].

High reproducibility and uniform droplet distribution are considered to be the main advantage of droplet-based microfluidics. Other advantages include preventing NPs from contacting the channel walls, and efficient mixing of the reagent streams [33].

In fact, each drop produced by the device is a microreactor on its own, which makes it possible to transport more chemical species due to propagation over shorter distances, and leads to more stable and uniform NP formulations. In addition, the use of droplet manipulation has led to the development of droplet-based microfluidics in different fields. However, one of the disadvantages of this method is that droplet-based chips are mostly used for the synthesis of microparticles, and in general, the synthesis of NPs requires synthesis on more complex chips, including the Herringbone micromixer [53].

Furthermore, droplet-based microfluidic systems are microreactors that decrease the volume employed and are therefore important for molecular analysis. These systems provide a rapid mixing of reagents and higher transfection of cells in vitro, as well as allowing screening of transfection parameters in cell cultures in real time [79]. Table 8.2 summarizes some microfluidic techniques for the production of NPs as nonviral vectors for gene delivery.

8.5 Microfluidic devices based on physical methods for genes transfection

In summary, there are three types of physical methods used for gene transfection. These are used for primary, progenitor, and stem cells, which are considered to be difficult-to-transfect. These approaches can be electrical (such as electroporation), mechanical (such as hydrodynamic force), and direct penetration (such as microinjection) and can lead to permeabilization of the plasma membrane [83]. An important benefit of permeability-based physical delivery is that it is capable of delivering almost any material that can be dispersed in an aqueous solution. Also, these methods are able to overcome many limitations of chemical approaches and do not have the side effects associated with viral carriers. Nevertheless, there are some challenges in using these methods such as cell damage and increased rates of cell death [84].

Table 8.2 Summary of microfluidic techniques for the production of NPs as nonviral vectors.

Microfluidic	Materials	NPs	size	Delivered nucleic acids	Cell type/ mouse model	Efficiency	Ref
Continuous flow microfluidic	PDMS/glass chip	Cationic liposome	88.7 ± 4.7 nm,	pDNA		–	[60]
Continuous flow microfluidic	PDMS/glass chip	Poly(beta-amino-esters) (PBAE)	446 to be 6.2 kDa	pDNA	B16, GB319, and MDA-MB-231	–	[61]
Multi-inlet microfluidic hydrodynamic focusing (MF) devices	poly(methyl methacrylate) (PMMA) plate	Lipopolyplex NPs		Bcl-2 antisense deoxyoligonucleotide (ODN)	K562 human erythroleukemia and G3139 cell	74.8% ± 3.8%	[80]
Microfluidic mixing device	–	Lipid NPs (LNP)	20–100 nm	siRNA	mouse FVII model (in vivo)	excess of 95%	[81]
Emulsion-based droplet microfluidic system	PDMS prepolymer	Bioreducible linear poly(amido amine)	~ 10 nm	pDNA and mRNA encoding GFP	HepG2 and Hmsc cells, HEK293 cells	6%–31%	[76]
Droplet microfluidic	PDMS polymer	Lipoplex (cationic lipid-nucleic acid complex)	277 nm	pcDNA3-EGFP plasmid	three Jurkat, K562 and THP-1 cell lines	≈ 5% to ≈ 50% improved	[78]
Multi-stage microfluidic chip	–	Water core/ PLGA shell/ lipid layer rigid nanovesicles (RNVs) t	140 nm	siRNA/Dox	MCF-7/ADR cells	… ≈ 90%	[82]

Recently, microfluidic systems have been integrated with a variety of physical approaches such as microdroplets, microinjection, electroporation, and hydrodynamic methods, to reduce cell death rates and provide higher efficiency for the transfection of a variety of nucleic acid molecules of different sizes.

8.5.1 Electroporation

Electropermeabilization refers to the creation of reversible pores in the cell membrane using short-pulses of an electric field. DNA and RNA molecules pass through the pores via simple diffusion and can be used for drugs as well as nucleic acids [85]. Electropermeabilization can be divided into different types: electrotransfection, electrogenotherapy, and electroporation [86].

Electroporation is a technique in biology in which electrical pulses are applied to cells to enhance the permeability of the cell membrane to allow chemicals, drugs, or DNA to enter the cells. In fact, electroporation provides high efficiency for the transfer of foreign genes into cells and tissues directly with low toxicity and high efficiency in mammalian cells. These techniques are widely used to treat tumors and different diseases and to produce knockout mice [87].

Some of the most important disadvantages of conventional electroporation methods such as bulk electroporation (BEP) (despite their widespread application) include the need for a high voltage to conduct transfection, which is associated with reduced cell viability and cell damage [88]. Therefore, a possible loss of cell viability must be considered for electroporation systems. Microfluidic systems could partially overcome this drawback of electroporation. For example, a flow-through electroporation method based on the use of syringe pumps, power supplies, and disposable PDMS chips, providing a low voltage and constant voltage can be used to achieve high-efficiency transfection (up to ~75%). Also, this technique is able to transfect large numbers of cells in both in vivo and in vitro conditions using electrotransfection microfluidic devices [89].

Continuous flow systems require high voltages to generate multiple pulses, which can lead to a decrease in cell viability and cause cell damage. Changes in the pulse intensity can be achieved by modifying the system and channel geometry. A continuous-flow multi-pulse electroporation system was designed by Bhattacharjee et al., to generate multiple pulses at a low voltage (~15 to 60V) compared to previously continuous-flow microfluidic designs, leading to increased cell viability (two-fold improvement in cell viability) for pDNA transfection into CHO-K1 cells. In this system, the cells passed through a channel between two poles (cathode and anode) and were much less exposed to the field power and electric pulses. As a result, this system increased the degree of transfection using multiple high electric field pulses and maintained cell viability without damage [90].

Hsi et al. [91] developed a continuous-flow electrotransfection system that automatically switched human primary T cells from the cell culture medium to electroporation medium using acoustophoresis. This technique was used to make changes to the primary cells and to create modified T cells for CAR-T cell therapy.

Transfection of T cells with mRNA encoding mCherry fluorescent protein showed a transfection efficiency of over 60% and a decrease in viability of less than 5%.

The system was constructed from low-cost, polymer-based polystyrene substrate that can be used in cell therapy. But, there is still a need for further research on the development of cost-effective microfluidic systems and large-scale production due to advances being made in cellular therapies.

Droplet microfluidic-based single-cell electroporation has received much attention. This method can target a single cell using droplets containing cells, DNA, and so on [92]. For instance, a PDMS droplet microfluidic-based single-cell electroporation device contained one pair of electrodes, two inlets and one outlet. The cells and DNA were plated in aqueous droplets (in oil) and flowed across a pair of microelectrodes [93]. The improved delivery of EGFP plasmid into Chinese hamster ovary (CHO) cells was demonstrated.

Droplet microfluidics provided high-throughput electroporation to single cells encapsulated in a small volume of water in a continuous nonconductive oil phase [94]. This system was also combined with magnetic tweezers and electroporation by external magnetic fields for high-throughput gene delivery. Chang et al. described a silicon 3D microchannel electroporation (MEP)–magnetic tweezers (MT) system based on photolithography for high throughput transfection of a GATA2 molecular beacon into leukemia cells to investigate GATA2 gene regulation in leukemia. Low voltages and low magnetic fields can be used to control the movement and alignment of cells without damaging them. They developed this system to transfect large numbers of cells (approximately 40,000 cells/cm^2) on a chip with high efficiency and > 90% cell viability [95]. This type of electroporation provides real-time detection, and allows a comprehensive analysis of cells. Also, it provides high efficiency and low voltage transfection.

8.6 Microinjection

Microinjection is a process whereby direct delivery of genetic material is carried out by introducing a glass micropipette into living cells (cells, embryos, eggs, or oocytes of animals) that can be used in many clinical applications, including direct injection of nucleic acids into the nucleus/cytoplasm of animal cells [96]. This technique has many advantages including reduced cost, control of the rate of delivery of genetic material, and reduced immune response due to its virus-free nature, as well as its high efficiency and low cytotoxicity. Compared to electroporation, microinjection requires low amounts of reagents [97]. There are different types of standard microinjection methods based on the moving injection and rotating injection techniques, but their most important disadvantages are cost, low throughput, the need for skilled operators, time-consuming, and low performance. The combination of microfluidic devices with microinjection can be effective in increasing the speed and efficiency [98].

Automated microinjection approaches have been commercialized to enhance the accuracy and speed of microinjection. This system first reported in 1988, with a throughput of 1500 cells/h when carried out on adherent cells [99]. Most automated microinjection approaches are designed to overcome several limitations of manual operation, such as poor reproducibility and operator fatigue.

Microinjection systems have several key parts: cell location adjustment, sensor detection, needle actuator, and dielectrophoresis (DEP) [100].

Azarmanesh et al. [101] developed an automated microinjection device for high-throughput, high speed, and accurate delivery of immiscible liquids/solids into droplets. This system comprised three components: three designs of T-junction (SV2 and SV3), cross-junction microchannels (SV5), and flow-focusing (SV4).

Delivery of cocktail of a plasmid or a synthetic modified mRNA (modRNA) encoding GFP to human foreskin fibroblast (HFF) cells, using automated microinjection showed a high transfection efficiency of 80%. The system consists of a 3-DOF robot manipulator, a cell holder chip, and an objective lens equipped with a CCD camera. This method could perform high transfection (regardless of the cell type) compared to electroporation methods and was especially suitable for hard to transfect cells. This technique also had advantages over DNA delivery systems because of its ability to use modRNA, including allowing it to evaluate single-cell gene expression as well as the number of proteins expressed. Other applications are injecting the Crispr/cas9 system for multiple genome editing [97].

The automated microinjection technique has limitations despite its many advantages, such as the need for a high skill level in order to prevent damage to cells or risk for disrupting the droplets or the cell membrane. This technique still needs to be optimized in order to be used in droplet methods due to the complex injection process of immiscible materials into microdroplets.

8.7 Hydrodynamics-based transfection

Different types of mechanical approaches for membrane permeabilization have been developed using fluid shear forces [102]. These include "cell squeezing" [83], hydrostatic pressure changes, or hydrodynamic delivery [62]. Hydrodynamic delivery means using physical force produced by a sudden increase in hydrostatic pressure that temporarily degrades the cell membrane. This technique is similar to other physical methods, such as microinjection or electroporation, but does not require advanced equipment [62].

In 2019 Jarrell and co-workers [103] described a microfluidic chip with post arrays using hydrodynamic force to induced microfluidic vortex shedding (μVS) to allow intracellular delivery of mRNA into primary T lymphocytes. First, mRNA and cells were mixed together, then by passing the suspension through the ion-etched posts, it created a vortex and disturbed the cell membrane and permitted mRNA to diffuse into the cells. The posts were changeable (10–40 μm) depending on the cell type and size. This method achieved high efficiency (> 60%) and high cell viability

(> 70%) and could be promising for future T cell engineering, gene-modified cell therapy (GMCT) and clinical applications.

A hydroporator is a hydrodynamic cell membrane perforator, which has recently been developed for high-efficiency delivery of macromolecules. This allowed microfluidically controlled cell deformation through a T-junction that caused the cells to collide with the channel walls. Deng et al. presented an internal microfluidic cell hydroporator (iMCH) for delivery of nanomaterials, DNA, RNA, CRISPR-Cas9 or plasmid DNA at efficiencies up to 50% in numerous cell lines. The method focused the cells into a T-junction, where pores formed on the cell membrane as a result of collisions with the spike-like structures on the channel wall. This system had advantages such as low cost, good efficiency, and high controllability. But this system could only deliver materials in vitro and also required cellular internalization of the DNA nanostructures [104].

The same group in 2019 carried out another study using a single-step hydrodynamic microdevice to induce cell deformation in the cells using hydrodynamic shearing, for intracellular delivery of DNA origami (tube- and donut-shaped sequences). They showed that this device was clogging-free, unlike the previous study, which was likely to cause clogging and also used sheath fluids. It showed high efficiency (~90%) without using any vectors and was high-throughput (> 1,600,000 cells per min). In this study, the structural integrity of the nanostructures was maintained up to 1 h after delivery to the cells, so it can be concluded that the inserted DNA would be stable [105]. Table 8.3 summarizes some physical-based microfluidic techniques used in gene delivery.

8.8 Conclusions

The shift from using traditional methods for the delivery of various drugs, proteins, and nucleic acids to using newer microfluidic strategies is continuing. Screening of different parameters due to changes in temperature and reactant concentration and other conditions allow for the synthesis of different types of complex NPs with specific appropriate sizes and shapes. Two mixing strategies of continuous hydrodynamic flow focusing and droplet generation are often used by researchers. Both continuous and droplet flow techniques have been successfully used for the synthesis of NPs. However, continuous synthesis techniques have some limitations due to the strong interaction with the channel walls and possible obstruction. Droplet-based techniques can overcome these limitations and produce higher quality NPs. Also, combining microfluidic systems with physical methods by inducing increases in cell membrane permeability, can increase the efficiency of the transfection of nucleic acids with less damage to the cells. There may be other challenges, including that the NPs produced may not have sufficient efficiency to overcome all the cellular barriers that hinder gene delivery. Some points to be considered are the requirement to be noninvasive, cause less damage to the cells, as well as the cost and ease of use. In fact, it is still challenging to produce nucleic acid transfer systems for clinical

Table 8.3 Summary of physical based microfluidic techniques for gene delivery.

Device type	Materials	Delivered nucleic acids	Cell type	Efficiency	Viability	Ref
Electroporation	Continuous-flow multi-pulse electroporation	Plasmid DNA	CHO-K1 cells	800 V/cm and 900 V/cm were 72% and 78%, respectively	viabilities were 85% and 77%, respectively	[90]
Automated, electrotransfection	Polymer substrate (polystyrene)	mRNA	Primary human T cells	Up to 60%	95%	[91]
Membrane sandwich electroporation (MSE)	poly(methyl methacrylate) (PMMA) substrate	pEGFP and pSEAP plasmids	NIH 3T3 fibroblasts	40%	90%	[106]
Low-voltage dc electroporation	(poly diallyldimethylammonium chloride) (pDADMAC)	EGFP plasmid	K562	60%	80%	[107]
Nanochannel-electroporation (NEP)	Polydimethylsiloxane (PDMS) nanochannels	Chimeric antigen receptor (CAR) encoding plasmids	H9C2 and NK-92 cells	$>70\%$	–	[108]
Microinjection	Polydimethylsiloxane (PDMS, SYLGARD).	Modified mRNA (modRNA)	HFF cells	80%	$97.5\% \pm 2.0\%$ $82.1\% \pm 7.0\%$ (for FITC-dextran injected cells)	[97]
Internal microfluidic cell hydroporter (iMCH)	PDMS/glass	RNA, CRISPR-Cas9 and plasmid DNA	MDA-MB-231 cells	50%	–	[104]
Hydroporator	PDMS-glass	DNA origami	K562 cells	$\sim 90\%$	–	[107]

applications, because nucleic acids are mostly unstable. Even though microfluidics can improve the efficiency of nucleic acid transfer systems, the issue of scaling-up remains a problem with these systems. However, many efforts are underway to accelerate the route from design to commercialization, and the microfluidic synthesis of NPs and microparticles will likely open the door to many new developments in gene therapy in the future.

References

[1] E.L. Scheller, P.H. Krebsbach, Gene therapy: design and prospects for craniofacial regeneration, J Dent Res 88 (7) (2009) 585–596.

[2] K. Pärn, et al., Transfection of infectious RNA and DNA/RNA layered vectors of semliki forest virus by the cell-penetrating peptide based reagent PepFect6, PLoS One 8 (7) (2013), e69659.

[3] T.K. Kim, J.H. Eberwine, Mammalian cell transfection: the present and the future, Anal Bioanal Chem 397 (8) (2010) 3173–3178.

[4] H. Uludag, A. Ubeda, A. Ansari, At the intersection of biomaterials and gene therapy: progress in non-viral delivery of nucleic acids, Front Bioeng Biotechnol 7 (2019) 131.

[5] A.-M. Yu, et al., RNA therapy: are we using the right molecules? Pharmacol Ther 196 (2019) 91–104.

[6] M. Durymanov, J. Reineke, Non-viral delivery of nucleic acids: insight into mechanisms of overcoming intracellular barriers, Front Pharmacol 9 (2018) 971.

[7] N. Hao, Y. Nie, J.X.J. Zhang, Microfluidic synthesis of functional inorganic micro-/nanoparticles and applications in biomedical engineering, Int Mater Rev 63 (8) (2018) 461–487.

[8] H. Jayamohan, et al., Advances in microfluidics and lab-on-a-chip technologies, in: G.P. Patrinos (Ed.), Molecular diagnostics, third ed., Academic Press, 2017, pp. 197–217 (Chapter 11).

[9] J. Ma, et al., Controllable synthesis of functional nanoparticles by microfluidic platforms for biomedical applications – a review, Lab Chip 17 (2) (2017) 209–226.

[10] J. Kim, et al., Microfluidic approaches for gene delivery and gene therapy, Lab Chip 11 (23) (2011) 3941–3948.

[11] J.T. Seto, et al., Gene replacement therapies for duchenne muscular dystrophy using adeno-associated viral vectors, Curr Gene Ther 12 (3) (2012) 139–151.

[12] R.J. Chandler, C.P. Venditti, Gene therapy for metabolic diseases, Transl Sci Rare Dis 1 (1) (2016) 73–89.

[13] M.M. Liu, J. Tuo, C.-C. Chan, Gene therapy for ocular diseases, Br J Ophthalmol 95 (5) (2011) 604–612.

[14] D.W. Russell, M.A. Kay, Adeno-associated virus vectors and hematology, Blood 94 (3) (1999) 864–874.

[15] K. Lundstrom, Viral vectors in gene therapy, Diseases (Basel, Switzerland) 6 (2) (2018) 42.

[16] S.A. Collins, et al., Viral vectors in cancer immunotherapy: which vector for which strategy? Curr Gene Ther 8 (2) (2008) 66–78.

[17] C.S. Lee, et al., Adenovirus-mediated gene delivery: potential applications for gene and cell-based therapies in the new era of personalized medicine, Genes Dis 4 (2) (2017) 43–63.
[18] H.N. Vu, et al., A microfluidic bioreactor for increased active retrovirus output, Lab Chip 8 (1) (2008) 75–80.
[19] F.C. Pérez-Martínez, et al., Barriers to non-viral vector-mediated gene delivery in the nervous system, Pharm Res 28 (8) (2011) 1843–1858.
[20] J. Villemejane, L.M. Mir, Physical methods of nucleic acid transfer: general concepts and applications, Br J Pharmacol 157 (2) (2009) 207–219.
[21] A. Schroeder, et al., Lipid-based nanotherapeutics for siRNA delivery, J Intern Med 267 (1) (2010) 9–21.
[22] K.K. Ewert, et al., Cationic liposome-nucleic acid complexes for gene delivery and silencing: pathways and mechanisms for plasmid DNA and siRNA, Top Curr Chem 296 (2010) 191–226.
[23] T. Iqbal, S. Tufail, S. Ghazal, Synthesis of silver, chromium, manganese, tin and iron nano particles by different techniques, Int J Nanosci Nanotechnol 13 (1) (2017) 19–52.
[24] S. Majidi, et al., Current methods for synthesis of magnetic nanoparticles, Artif Cells Nanomed Biotechnol 44 (2) (2016) 722–734.
[25] H.F. Lu, R.Y. Hong, H.Z. Li, Influence of surfactants on co-precipitation synthesis of strontium ferrite, J Alloys Compd 509 (41) (2011) 10127–10131.
[26] M.A. López-Quintela, et al., Synthesis of nanoparticles in microemulsions, in: L.M. Liz-Marzán, P.V. Kamat (Eds.), Nanoscale materials, Springer US, Boston, MA, 2003, pp. 135–155.
[27] L.-H. Hung, A.P. Lee, Microfluidic devices for the synthesis of nanoparticles and biomaterials, J Med Biol Eng 27 (1) (2006) 1–6.
[28] X. Wang, et al., Synthesis of biomaterials utilizing microfluidic technology, Genes 9 (6) (2018) 283.
[29] R. Karnik, et al., Microfluidic platform for controlled synthesis of polymeric nanoparticles, Nano Lett 8 (9) (2008) 2906–2912.
[30] J. Boken, S.K. Soni, D. Kumar, Microfluidic synthesis of nanoparticles and their biosensing applications, Crit Rev Anal Chem 46 (6) (2016) 538–561.
[31] T.W. Phillips, et al., Nanocrystal synthesis in microfluidic reactors: where next? Lab Chip 14 (17) (2014) 3172–3180.
[32] C.-X. Zhao, et al., Nanoparticle synthesis in microreactors, Chem Eng Sci 66 (7) (2011) 1463–1479.
[33] L.-J. Pan, et al., Controllable synthesis of nanocrystals in droplet reactors, Lab Chip 18 (1) (2018) 41–56.
[34] J. Yue, Multiphase flow processing in microreactors combined with heterogeneous catalysis for efficient and sustainable chemical synthesis, Catal Today 308 (2018) 3–19.
[35] R.L. Hartman, K.F. Jensen, Microchemical systems for continuous-flow synthesis, Lab Chip 9 (17) (2009) 2495–2507.
[36] S. Rashmi Pradhan, F.R. Colmenares-Quintero, C.J. Colmenares Quintero, Designing microflowreactors for photocatalysis using sonochemistry: a systematic review article, Molecules 24 (18) (2019).
[37] C. Iliescu, et al., A practical guide for the fabrication of microfluidic devices using glass and silicon, Biomicrofluidics 6 (1) (2012), 16505.
[38] F. Trachsel, C. Hutter, P.R. von Rohr, Transparent silicon/glass microreactor for high-pressure and high-temperature reactions, Chem Eng J 135 (2008) S309–S316.

[39] S. Marre, et al., Design and packaging of microreactors for high pressure and high temperature applications, Ind Eng Chem Res 49 (22) (2010) 11310–11320.
[40] A. Alrifaiy, O.A. Lindahl, K. Ramser, Polymer-based microfluidic devices for pharmacy, biology and tissue engineering, Polymers 4 (3) (2012).
[41] S. Das, V.C. Srivastava, Microfluidic-based photocatalytic microreactor for environmental application: a review of fabrication substrates and techniques, and operating parameters, Photochem Photobiol Sci 15 (6) (2016) 714–730.
[42] E.Y. Erdem, Microfluidic reactors for the controlled synthesis of monodisperse nanoparticles, Spring, 2013.
[43] J.F. Greene, et al., PTFE-membrane flow reactor for aerobic oxidation reactions and its application to alcohol oxidation, Org Process Res Dev 19 (7) (2015) 858–864.
[44] K. Ren, et al., Whole-Teflon microfluidic chips, Proc Natl Acad Sci U S A 108 (20) (2011) 8162–8166.
[45] H. Huang, et al., Continuous flow synthesis of ultrasmall gold nanoparticles in a microreactor using trisodium citrate and their SERS performance, Chem Eng Sci 189 (2018) 422–430.
[46] J.K. Nunes, et al., Dripping and jetting in microfluidic multiphase flows applied to particle and fiber synthesis, J Phys D Appl Phys 46 (11) (2013), 114002.
[47] H. Liu, Y. Zhang, Droplet formation in microfluidic cross-junctions, Phys Fluids 23 (8) (2011), 082101.
[48] K. Ward, Z.H. Fan, Mixing in microfluidic devices and enhancement methods, J Micromech Microeng 25 (9) (2015) 0960–1317.
[49] N.-T. Nguyen, Z. Wu, Micromixers—a review, J Micromech Microeng 15 (2) (2004) R1–R16.
[50] M.Y.A. Jamalabadi, et al., Effect of injection angle, density ratio, and viscosity on droplet formation in a microfluidic T-junction, Theor Appl Mech Lett 7 (4) (2017) 243–251.
[51] P. Fernandes, Miniaturization in biocatalysis, Int J Mol Sci 11 (3) (2010) 858–879.
[52] Z.Z. Chen, et al., A Y-shaped microfluidic device to study the combined effect of wall shear stress and ATP signals on intracellular calcium dynamics in vascular endothelial cells, Micromachines 7 (11) (2016).
[53] S. Damiati, et al., Microfluidic devices for drug delivery systems and drug screening, Genes 9 (2) (2018).
[54] H. Song, D.L. Chen, R.F. Ismagilov, Reactions in droplets in microfluidic channels, Angew Chem Int Ed Engl 45 (44) (2006) 7336–7356.
[55] M.V. Bandulasena, et al., Continuous synthesis of PVP stabilized biocompatible gold nanoparticles with a controlled size using a 3D glass capillary microfluidic device, Chem Eng Sci 171 (2017) 233–243.
[56] A. Jahn, et al., Preparation of nanoparticles by continuous-flow microfluidics, J Nanopart Res 10 (6) (2008) 925–934.
[57] B. Amoyav, O. Benny, Controlled and tunable polymer particles' production using a single microfluidic device, Appl Nanosci 8 (4) (2018) 905–914.
[58] E. Chiesa, et al., The microfluidic technique and the manufacturing of polysaccharide nanoparticles, Pharmaceutics 10 (4) (2018) 267.
[59] T.A. Balbino, et al., Continuous flow production of cationic liposomes at high lipid concentration in microfluidic devices for gene delivery applications, Chem Eng J 226 (2013) 423–433.
[60] T.A. Balbino, et al., Microfluidic assembly of pDNA/cationic liposome lipoplexes with high pDNA loading for gene delivery, Langmuir 32 (7) (2016) 1799–1807.

[61] D.R. Wilson, et al., Continuous microfluidic assembly of biodegradable poly(beta-amino ester)/DNA nanoparticles for enhanced gene delivery, J Biomed Mater Res A 105 (6) (2017) 1813–1825.
[62] B. Bonamassa, L. Hai, D. Liu, Hydrodynamic gene delivery and its applications in pharmaceutical research, Pharm Res 28 (4) (2011) 694–701.
[63] S.-Y. Teh, et al., Droplet microfluidics, Lab Chip 8 (2) (2008) 198–220.
[64] A.J. Morgan, et al., Simple and versatile 3D printed microfluidics using fused filament fabrication, PLoS One 11 (4) (2016).
[65] P. Wagli, et al., Microfluidic droplet-based liquid-liquid extraction and on-chip IR spectroscopy detection of cocaine in human saliva, Anal Chem 85 (15) (2013) 7558–7565.
[66] S.A. Nabavi, et al., Double emulsion production in glass capillary microfluidic device: parametric investigation of droplet generation behaviour, Chem Eng Sci 130 (2015) 183–196.
[67] E.Y. Basova, F. Foret, Droplet microfluidics in (bio)chemical analysis, Analyst 140 (1) (2015) 22–38.
[68] H. Bazyar, N. van de Beek, R.G.H. Lammertink, Liquid-infused membranes with oil-in-water emulsions, Langmuir 35 (29) (2019) 9513–9520.
[69] L. Derzsi, et al., Hydrophilic polycarbonate for generation of oil in water emulsions in microfluidic devices, Lab Chip 11 (6) (2011) 1151–1156.
[70] L. Shui, A. van den Berg, J.C.T. Eijkel, Interfacial tension controlled W/O and O/W 2-phase flows in microchannel, Lab Chip 9 (6) (2009) 795–801.
[71] S. Liu, et al., Zinc coordination substitute amine: a noncationic platform for efficient and safe gene delivery, ACS Macro Lett 7 (7) (2018) 868–874.
[72] P. Zhu, L. Wang, Passive and active droplet generation with microfluidics: a review, Lab Chip 17 (1) (2016) 34–75.
[73] T. Glawdel, C. Elbuken, C.L. Ren, Droplet generation in microfluidics, in: D. Li (Ed.), Encyclopedia of microfluidics and nanofluidics, Springer US, Boston, MA, 2013, pp. 1–12.
[74] T. Trantidou, et al., Droplet microfluidics for the construction of compartmentalised model membranes, Lab Chip 18 (17) (2018) 2488–2509.
[75] Y.-P. Ho, et al., Tuning physical properties of nanocomplexes through microfluidics-assisted confinement, Nano Lett 11 (5) (2011) 2178–2182.
[76] C.L. Grigsby, et al., Microfluidic preparation of polymer-nucleic acid nanocomplexes improves nonviral gene transfer, Sci Rep 3 (2013), 3155.
[77] X. Han, et al., Cas9 ribonucleoprotein delivery via microfluidic cell-deformation chip for human T-cell genome editing and immunotherapy, Adv Biosyst 1 (1-2) (2017), 1600007.
[78] X. Li, et al., Lipoplex-mediated single-cell transfection via droplet microfluidics, Small 14 (40) (2018) 10.
[79] M.T. Vitor, et al., Droplet-based microfluidic systems for production and transfection invitro of non-viral vectors for gene delivery, J Pharm Pharm Sci 4 (4) (2015) 1–17.
[80] C.G. Koh, et al., Delivery of antisense oligodeoxyribonucleotide lipopolyplex nanoparticles assembled by microfluidic hydrodynamic focusing, J Control Release 141 (1) (2010) 62–69.
[81] N.M. Belliveau, et al., Microfluidic synthesis of highly potent limit-size lipid nanoparticles for in vivo delivery of siRNA, Mol Ther–Nucleic Acids 1 (2012), e37.
[82] L. Zhang, et al., Microfluidic synthesis of rigid nanovesicles for hydrophilic reagents delivery, Angew Chem 127 (13) (2015).

[83] M.P. Stewart, R. Langer, K.F. Jensen, Intracellular delivery by membrane disruption: mechanisms, strategies, and concepts, Chem Rev 118 (16) (2018) 7409–7531.
[84] J.M. Meacham, et al., Physical methods for intracellular delivery: practical aspects from laboratory use to industrial-scale processing, J Lab Autom 19 (1) (2014) 1–18.
[85] M.-P. Rols, Electropermeabilization, a physical method for the delivery of therapeutic molecules into cells, Biochim Biophys Acta Biomembr 1758 (3) (2006) 423–428.
[86] L.D. Cervia, et al., Enhancing electrotransfection efficiency through improvement in nuclear entry of plasmid DNA, Mol Ther–Nucleic Acids 11 (2018) 263–271.
[87] S. Somiari, et al., Theory and in vivo application of electroporative gene delivery, Mol Ther 2 (3) (2000) 178–187.
[88] L. Chang, et al., 3D nanochannel electroporation for high-throughput cell transfection with high uniformity and dosage control, Nanoscale 8 (1) (2016) 243–252.
[89] T. Geng, et al., Flow-through electroporation based on constant voltage for large-volume transfection of cells, J Control Release 144 (1) (2010) 91–100.
[90] N. Bhattacharjee, L.F. Horowitz, A. Folch, Continuous-flow multi-pulse electroporation at low DC voltages by microfluidic flipping of the voltage space topology, Appl Phys Lett 109 (16) (2016), 163702.
[91] P. Hsi, et al., Acoustophoretic rapid media exchange and continuous-flow electrotransfection of primary human T cells for applications in automated cellular therapy manufacturing, Lab Chip 19 (18) (2019) 2978–2992.
[92] M. He, et al., Selective encapsulation of single cells and subcellular organelles into picoliter- and femtoliter-volume droplets, Anal Chem 77 (6) (2005) 1539–1544.
[93] Y. Zhan, et al., Electroporation of cells in microfluidic droplets, Anal Chem 81 (5) (2009) 2027–2031.
[94] S. Le Gac, I. van Uitert, Electroporation in microfluidic devices, in: D. Miklavcic (Ed.), Handbook of electroporation, Springer International Publishing, Cham, 2016, pp. 1–20.
[95] L. Chang, et al., Magnetic tweezers-based 3D microchannel electroporation for high-throughput gene transfection in living cells, Small (Weinheim an der Bergstrasse, Germany) 11 (15) (2015) 1818–1828.
[96] Y. Kikuchi, A. Kimura, Microinjection into the Caenorhabditis elegans embryo using an uncoated glass needle enables cell lineage visualization and reveals cell-non-autonomous adhesion control, bioRxiv (2018) 406991.
[97] Y.T. Chow, et al., Single cell transfection through precise microinjection with quantitatively controlled injection volumes, Sci Rep 6 (2016), 24127.
[98] A. Noori, P.R. Selvaganapathy, J. Wilson, Microinjection in a microfluidic format using flexible and compliant channels and electroosmotic dosage control, Lab Chip 9 (22) (2009) 3202–3211.
[99] W. Ansorge, R. Pepperkok, Performance of an automated system for capillary microinjection into living cells, J Biochem Biophys Methods 16 (4) (1988) 283–292.
[100] Y. Zhao, et al., A review of automated microinjection of zebrafish embryos, Micromachines 10 (1) (2018) 7.
[101] M. Azarmanesh, et al., Passive microinjection within high-throughput microfluidics for controlled actuation of droplets and cells, Sci Rep 9 (1) (2019), 6723.
[102] S. Cooper, et al., Permeabilization of adhered cells using an inert gas jet, J Vis Exp 79 (2013), 50612.
[103] J.A. Jarrell, et al., Intracellular delivery of mRNA to human primary T cells with microfluidic vortex shedding, Sci Rep 9 (1) (2019) 3214.

[104] Y. Deng, et al., Intracellular delivery of nanomaterials via an inertial microfluidic cell hydroporator, Nano Lett 18 (4) (2018) 2705–2710.
[105] M.E. Kizer, et al., Hydroporator: a hydrodynamic cell membrane perforator for high-throughput vector-free nanomaterial intracellular delivery and DNA origami biostability evaluation, Lab Chip 19 (10) (2019) 1747–1754.
[106] Z. Fei, et al., Gene transfection of mammalian cells using membrane sandwich electroporation, Anal Chem 79 (15) (2007) 5719–5722.
[107] S.K. Kim, et al., Continuous low-voltage dc electroporation on a microfluidic chip with polyelectrolytic salt bridges, Anal Chem 79 (20) (2007) 7761–7766.
[108] L. Chang, et al., Dielectrophoresis-assisted 3D nanoelectroporation for non-viral cell transfection in adoptive immunotherapy, Lab Chip 15 (15) (2015) 3147–3153.

CHAPTER

Microfluidic devices in tissue engineering

9

Sajad Bahrami[a], Nafiseh Baheiraei[b,*], Mohammed Najafi-Ashtiani[c], Shirin Nour[d], and Mehdi Razavi[e],

[a]Department of Medical Nanotechnology, Faculty of Advanced Technologies in Medicine, Iran University of Medical Sciences, Tehran, Iran

[b]Tissue Engineering and Applied Cell Sciences Division, Department of Hematology, Faculty of Medical Sciences, Tarbiat Modares University, Tehran, Iran

[c]Department of Physical Therapy, Faculty of Medical Sciences, Tarbiat Modares University, Tehran, Iran

[d]Tissue Engineering Group, Biomedical Engineering Department, Amirkabir University of Technology (Tehran Polytechnic), Tehran, Iran

[e]Biionix^{TM} (Bionic Materials, Implants & Interfaces) Cluster, Department of Internal Medicine, College of Medicine, University of Central Florida, Orlando, FL, United States

**Corresponding author. E-mail: n.baheiraei@modares.ac.ir*

9.1 Introduction

Microfluidics is the recent science of manipulating small volumes of fluids, whether simple or complex, monophase or multiphase, circulating through the networks of microchannels or confined within microchambers [1, 2]. Since the 1990s, microfluidics has advanced exponentially in various fields of modern biomedical and engineering science. Microfluidics first emerged from a miniaturization approach in the 1980s that led to the invention of microelectromechanical systems (MEMS). MEMS involve several branches of science and technology including mechanical, electrical, chemical, thermal, etc. [2].

The main rationale behind microfluidics was to enable better manipulation and control of small volumes of fluids. The small volume of fluids (which now ranges from microliter (10^{-6}) to femtoliter (10^{-15})) can be flowed, pumped, reserved, deviated, or separated within a small laboratory device named lab-on-a-chip (LOC) [3, 4]. There is a similarity between the LOC functions and some natural processes that occur in biology, which highlights the use of microfluidics in mimicking nature. Many biological processes like cellular activity, reactions, and transport, oxygen diffusion through the lung alveoli, blood flow through the capillaries, particle filtering in the kidney, etc. are all microscale phenomena [2].

Working with such a small volume of fluid leads to considerable reductions in the consumption of materials, the time expended, and overall costs of the experiments.

Biomedical Applications of Microfluidic Devices. https://doi.org/10.1016/B978-0-12-818791-3.00008-5

From a physical point-of-view, the low volume of fluids has advantages like laminar regime flow and rapid diffusion time, assuring better control of the fluid behavior [5–8]. Due to the high level of control in a LOC, the precision of the tests will increase and detection can be achieved with lower separation thresholds. Besides, creatively designed LOCs allow multiple simultaneous manipulations and modeling of more complex biological processes [9, 10]. The increasing progress of on-chip technologies has encouraged microfluidic concepts to be used today in a wide range of applications, specifically in health, biotechnology, and pharmacology, e.g., point-of-care detection, drug screening, cell separation, and tissue engineering [11, 12].

Tissue engineering deals with the repair or replacement of damaged tissues within the body that have lost their viability or functionality. Tissue engineering employs the natural biology of a system to allow the development of strategies to replace, repair, maintain or enhance the function of an existing tissue using new viable cells, or engineered tissues and organs [13]. However, cell culture is the most important prerequisite for tissue and organ culture. The need for cellular manipulations in a miniaturized device suggests that the advantages of microfluidics and tissue engineering could be synergistically integrated.

Conventional methods for tissue engineering have been generally limited to two-dimensional (2D) monolayer cell cultures, mainly in conventional Petri dishes whose success is often limited by the key elements of the biological and physiologic characteristics of the environment. However, when using a 2D tissue culture, the distinct phenotype, normal tissue architecture, and tissue-related functions are often lost because of differences between the in vitro and in vivo conditions [14]. The use of 3D cell culture with scaffolds or hydrogels has overcome some obstacles but still suffers from a lack of vascularization leading to insufficient oxygen and nutrient supply [15]. Consequently, researchers have been faced with considerable problems regarding the culture of complex tissues that have a natural thickness greater than the maximum depth of oxygen diffusion, i.e., 200 mm [16]. The scaffolds also have low diffusion properties that restrict the access of cell progenitors or growth factors, which reduces the chance of proper cellular differentiation and growth [17, 18].

This chapter will first discuss some of the prevalent techniques used in the fabrication of microfluidic devices aimed at tissue culture. Also, recent progress in microfluidic-based tissue engineering and some successful examples of LOC-based tissue-engineered organs will be discussed. The final part of this chapter will deal with applications of microfluidics in cancer tissue research.

9.2 Fabrication techniques in microfluidic devices

Microdevices can be fabricated using four classes of techniques, including etching, thermoforming, micromachining, and polymer casting.

9.2.1 Etching

The etching technique is based on protecting a part of the substrate and selectively removing another part to reach a particular depth of material. The removal of material from the substrate, conventionally made from silicon or glass, can be done by using a corrosive fluid (wet etching) or a gas (dry etching) that exert physical or chemical processes, or a combination of them such as reactive ion etching to increase the resolution of microchannels. This technique is rapid, precise, and economical, but is dependent on other techniques to produce protective masks, and also requires a clean room for the fabrication stages [19, 20].

9.2.2 Thermoforming

The thermoforming method includes a variety of techniques to form a thermoplastic material near its transition temperature. For instance, in hot embossing, the polymer materials undergo heating and shaping by the pressure of a stamp to fabricate microchannels or chambers within a microdevice. Hot embossing is rapid and cost-effective but relies on a pressure apparatus and other techniques for the stamps. Injection molding is another technique in this family that injects a molten material into a mold cavity using high pressure. Although injection molding is a high throughput method which can produce high quality on-chip devices, it is costly, intricate and only works on a medium-size scale [21, 22].

9.2.3 Micromachining

Micromachining is the direct use of mechanical tools like lathing, ablation, milling, laser, etc. on plastic or metal substrates to create a microdevice. These techniques allow the creation of patterns with sharp edges but contamination by the debris is hard to remove. The use of micromachining techniques may be economical and rapid, but it is strongly dependent on the quality and precision of the devices and cutting tools [23].

9.2.4 Polymer casting

Polymer casting includes a wide range of techniques that work based on creating a negative image of the desired pattern from a hard material and then pouring a polymer onto it that can be cured by heat or light. The microfluidic device can be finally obtained by peeling the mold off. Among the various techniques used in polymer casting, lithography is the most popular technique for the creation of microdevices. The main principle is the fabrication of a master mold containing patterned surfaces within a microfluidic chip using different techniques such as soft lithography, photolithography, X-ray lithography, etc. Soft lithography is a routine technique that utilizes a patterned elastomer such as polydimethylsiloxane (PDMS) as a mold/stamp to transfer the pattern onto the substrate (Fig. 9.1). Lower costs of tools and materials, high throughput, good resolution, and easy-to-use setup are some benefits of soft lithography, but the preparation of the pattern is still dependent on other lithography or micromachining techniques [24, 25].

Photolithography is another common technique in the fabrication of the devices in microfluidics. Application of this method needs a light source, a photomask, and a photoresist material. The pattern of interest in the chip is transferred from the

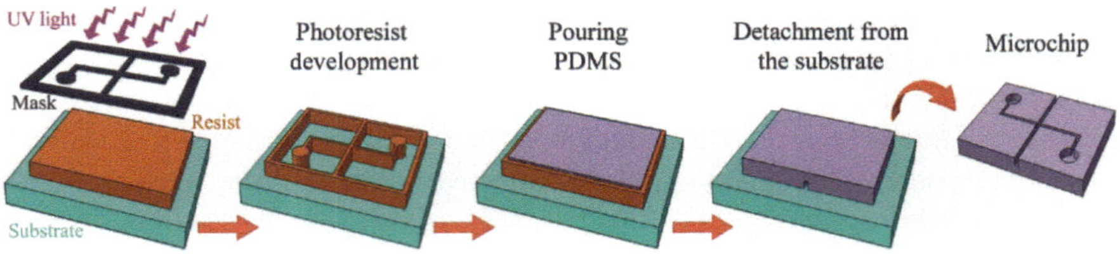

FIG. 9.1

Schematic representation of soft lithography stages (from left to right): exposure of the UV light through the mask to the photoresist material, development of the photoresist pattern to be poured with the PDMS, removing the PDMS cast and detachment of the final microchip from the substrate.

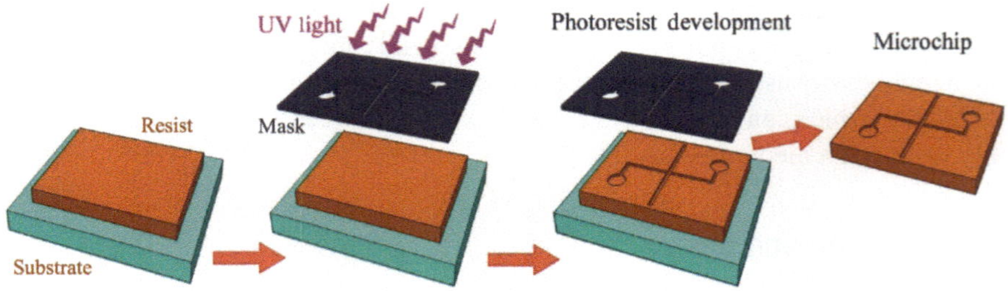

FIG. 9.2

Schematic illustration of the photolithography process including (from left to right) exposure of the UV light to the photoresist material through the photomask, development of the pattern of interest in the photoresist and chemical removal of the substrate to achieve the final microchip.

photomask to the photoresist material by exposure of the light source. The photoresist is a light-sensitive material, which can either become dissolved (positive photoresist) or be cross-linked (negative photoresist) after exposure to the light source. After coating a thin film of the photoresist onto the substrate using a spin coater or dry film lamination, exposure to ultraviolet (UV) light or to an electron beam (with a photomask or even without it) creates specific designed channel shapes. Having solubilized the exposed substrate in a developer solution, the patterned regions can be selectively removed. After baking the remaining structure, the resulting substrate with the resist layer undergoes selective etching so that the removal of the resist layer produces the designed topographies (Fig. 9.2).

9.3 Materials used in microfluidic devices

Numerous materials have been used in the fabrication of microdevices, which depend on the technique chosen technique. These materials can be roughly categorized into four groups, including polymers, hydrogels, inorganic materials, or composites.

9.3.1 Polymers

Polymers are the most commonly used materials in the fabrication of microdevices, because of their availability and economic benefits. Elastomers are often utilized in microfluidics fabrication mainly due to their mechanical properties such as flexibility. Since elastomers tolerate more tension before undergoing rupture and have a low Young's modulus, they are appropriate materials for the complex design of a microfluidic chip [26, 27]. The best example of this category is PDMS, which is widely used in microdevices. PDMS is a transparent, cost-effective material, with low stiffness but a high failure strain, and is permeable to oxygen and carbon dioxide, which are all desirable properties for a microfluidic material. Nevertheless, studies have shown that PDMS can form bubbles in contact with passing gas and also absorbs some hydrophobic molecules [27]. When using thermoforming and micromachining methods, thermoplastic materials like PDMS, polystyrene (PS), polyethylene terephthalate (PET), polyvinyl chloride (PVC), polymethylmethacrylate (PMMA), polyetherimide (PEI) are preferable. In comparison with elastomers, these materials are stiffer, less permeable to molecules and gas, and it is difficult to create an appropriate surface contact with other materials [21].

9.3.2 Hydrogels

Unlike more common polymers like PDMS that are suitable for tissue level microfluidics, hydrogels are used as substrates for cell culture in tissue engineering. Hydrogels are constructed from 3D hydrophilic polymers immersed in an aqueous medium, with easily controllable pore sizes [27] that can realistically mimic the extracellular matrix (ECM); therefore, a microfluidic device can be equipped with hydrogels to support the cultured cells.

9.3.3 Inorganic materials

Inorganic materials are often used in microdevices [28]. The most common examples are glass and silicon that are widely used in etching and micromachining. Silicon is opaque to visible light, too stiff for microvalves or pumps, and difficult to be fabricated as well as being costly. Glass, however, is more available, cheaper, and compatible with the biological materials. However, it is nonpermeable to gases which makes it unsuitable for long term cell culture due to poor oxygen/CO_2 exchange [27].

9.4 Research progress in microfluidics-based tissue engineering

9.4.1 Scaffold fabrication using microfluidics

One of the main problems with the use of scaffolds in tissue engineering (in its conventional framework) is the lack of proper vascularization leading to insufficient oxygen and nutrient supply, which causes the creation of necrotic cores. To address this problem, studies have introduced vascular progenitor cells and growth factors which can induce angiogenesis into the scaffolds. However, the poor diffusion properties of the scaffolds are usually restrictive [29, 30] so that researchers in the field of tissue engineering have used microfluidic technologies to fabricate a porous scaffold consisting of vascular networks resembling the actual vessel diameters in vivo.

The precise design of the microchannels and porosities within the scaffold can enhance the efficiency of microfluidic devices in tissue engineering. One strategy to achieve this goal is to add the hydrogel precursor solution inside a PDMS mold, which contains patterning agents such as microneedles, glass, or polymer fibers. Removal of the needles or dissolving the fibers by special solvents leads to the formation of microchannels or other architectures. As one example, microneedles were used to mold gelatin methacrylate (GelMA) hydrogel as reported by Nichol et al. whereby fabrication of endothelialized tubes within the hydrogel in the presence of fibroblasts led to the production of a microvascularized structure [31]. However, this method has some obstacles, including only limited and simple patterns, difficulty in the creation of interconnectivity between the channels, and being inappropriate for cell-culture applications due to the use of toxic solvents for removal of the patterning agents.

The modification of scaffold properties such as surface patterning and surface functionalization with adhesive substances can also increase the efficiency of microfluidic scaffolds in tissue engineering [32]. For instance, Sarkar et al. fabricated a porous micropatterned polycaprolactone (PCL) scaffold by leaching polylactic-*co*-glycolic acid (PLGA) particles after lithography, and then molding the structure. The culture of vascular smooth muscle cells on this scaffold produced highly aligned and organized cells, compared with nonporous scaffolds without micropatterning [33]. Sheikhi et al. also synthesized beaded-GelMA to decrease the stiffness of a hydrogel and increase the porosity. Their results showed remarkable enhancement in cell viability, adhesion, and proliferation [34]. Recent publications have focused on the use of hydrogels in microfluidic devices in different forms such as microfibers, microparticles, etc. for the engineering of ganglion cells [35], cornea [36], heart [37], and liver [38] tissues, which will be discussed in the following sections.

9.4.1.1 Microfluidic-based microfibrous structures

Fibrous scaffolds have been traditionally fabricated using a spinning technique mainly magneto/electrospinning. In addition, various studies have worked on encapsulation of cells within the inner core of hydrogel-based microfibers that were prepared by a co-axial or multinozzle spinneret. The fiber diameter can be manipulated by adjusting parameters such as the flow rate. However, some properties such as morphology, pore size, mechanical strength and more importantly, the cellular viability or the loading capacity of active agents are poorly controllable [30, 39]. The use of microfluidic devices facilitates the creation of microfibers with different structures and properties that can be readily loaded with cells or therapeutic agents. Shin et al. fabricated alginate microfibers using a co-axial flow microfluidic device with an alginate solution as the core flow and a sheath of $CaCl_2$ solution. The rapid core flow directly caused the larger fiber diameter. These microfibers can be used for encapsulation of drugs, proteins or cells [40]. Another study fabricated hollow cell-laden alginate fibers using a triple flow microfluidic device and co-cultured endothelial cells with smooth muscle cells to mimic vascular morphogenesis more accurately using the fibrous microstructure [41]. In fact, porogen leaching and diffusion mass exchange between the polymer and solvent solutions can improve the porosity of microfibrous scaffolds, which is an important factor in mass transport, cellular viability and also affects the drug release rate, especially in microfluidic-based methods [29, 42].

9.4.1.2 Microfluidic-based microparticles

Microfluidics have been recently used to synthesize hydrogel microparticles with precisely controlled size and shape in order to be used in cell encapsulation or drug delivery applications. Micromolding, emulsions, and lithography-based methods could be used to synthesize particles whereby the hydrogel is cross-linked by photochemical, chemical, or ionic reactions. The regulation of size and shape of microparticles depends on the flow rate, topography, and dimension of the microdevice, concentration of hydrogel and crosslinking agent. These parameters, in fact, govern the gelling time, controlled release of biomolecules, mechanical properties, and thus the cellular viability. For example, a higher flow rate inside the channels leads to smaller particles [37, 43]. Tan et al. used a T-shaped microfluidic device to fabricate alginate microparticles. In this study, sodium alginate solution was chemically cross-linked by $CaCO_3$ solution which resulted in microparticles with a range of 100–140 μm in diameter [44].

Micromolding is also another method for the creation of specific shaped hydrogel microparticles. Briefly, after preparation of the PDMS micromold/stamp, the hydrogel solution (usually a photocurable hydrogel) is added to the mold where the cross-linking step is carried out, and the hydrated particles are collected. One example of this procedure is encapsulated hydrogel microparticles based on polyethylene glycol diacrylate (PEGDA) and methacrylated hyaluronic acid solution, which were shaped after UV exposure in the PDMS microstamp [29].

9.4.2 Stem cell-based microfluidics systems

Generally, the use of primary cells is limited because of their batch-to-batch variation and limited life span. Stem cells are known for their self-renewal ability and high potency to differentiate into various specialized cell types (e.g., neurons, cardiomyocytes, vascular cells, and osteoblasts). In this field, microfluidic devices have also been found to be effective since they can provide multiple environmental cues for the stem cells in a controllable and reproducible manner [45]. For example, Hesari et al. used a hybrid scaffold made by a microfluidic chip to differentiate human induced pluripotent stem cells (iPSCs) into neurons. The results suggested that iPSCs cultured on aligned PLGA nanofibers within a microfluidic chip showed significant differentiation, which was confirmed by increased expression of neural marker genes compared to more common 2D scaffolds [46]. Notably, the combination of microfluidic systems with iPSC-derived vascular cells can play an important role in the formation of vascular structures either within the scaffold or merely as a laboratory research model. Kurokawa et al. created a 3D capillary network by culturing human iPSC-derived endothelial cells in a hydrogel-based microfluidic device, which was stable over 14 days in a human vascular disease model [42]. With the benefit of providing controlled stimulus gradients in stem-cell-based microfluidic systems, they can act as a cellular model for diseases (e.g., cancer, Alzheimer's, Parkinson's), to investigate different biological processes (such as angiogenesis) and also to determine the optimum ratio of parenchymal cells to stem cells ratio for tissue regeneration [39, 42].

It should be noted that the differentiation of various cell types inside microdevices relies on physical, mechanical, and biochemical stimuli, and also the device parameters (e.g., flow rate, culture time, and topography). From a chemical point of view, the optimal composition of culture media, type, and concentration of soluble factors, cell type and culture method (single and co-culture), as well as the culture time all affect the stem cell differentiation [37]. Chung et al. employed a microfluidic device with a tree-like generator in order to culture human neural stem cells under a nonlinear concentration gradient of growth factors (i.e., epidermal growth factor (EGF), fibroblast growth factor-2 (FGF2), and platelet-derived growth factor (PDGF)) and studied their differentiation into astrocytes. For better cell adhesion, all parts of the device (i.e. PDMS channels and glass slide) were coated with poly-L-lysine and mouse laminin. After 7 days, although the stem cells in the control group (i.e., microfluidic chamber without growth factors) were elongated and differentiated into astrocytes, cells in the growth factor containing media showed a significant increase in cell number due to the mitogenic effects of the growth factors while having a lower percentage of differentiated cells. Therefore, they concluded that the optimum growth factor concentration should be adjusted in order to attain a proper cell density as well as for astrocyte differentiation [47]. Another study used a PDMS microfluidic substrate containing 6000 individual cell culture wells seeded with mouse hematopoietic stem cells (HSCs) to investigate the role of medium composition in the cellular fate. Results indicated that changing the composition played an important role in the survival of HSCs from different sources. In fact, some HSCs could tolerate only low perfusion and highly concentrated medium up to 16h (which was the average doubling time of cells) and then they lost their ability to proliferate. Thus, culturing the cells in a microfluidic chip plate could increase cellular viability and functionality due to the controlled and constant replacement of medium without disturbing the cells [48].

Regarding physical and structural factors, it was reported that human mesenchymal stem cells (MSCs) were likely to differentiate into osteoblasts on the rigid microposts of micromolded PDMS substrates. Nevertheless, the expression of adipogenic genes was more pronounced on soft surfaces [31]. One of the major mechanical forces applied to cells in microfluidic devices is fluid shear stress, whereby cellular functionality (especially in vascular cells), viability, migration, and differentiation can be affected. The shear rate can be regulated by either changing the dimensions of the channels or the flow rate of the medium [49]. Toh et al. examined a wide range of fluid shear rates (up to 0.31 dyn/cm^2) by varying the flow rates to identify the effects of shear stress on the proliferation of mouse ESCs. The results of the study by Kim et al. was almost similar to that of Toh et al., which confirmed that higher flow rate (higher shear rates) enabled precise control over the transportation of soluble molecules and maintaining the cellular microenvironment, which can eventually lead to increased proliferation of ESCs and also other cell lines (such as 3T3 fibroblasts) [50, 51]. It is worth mentioning that shear stress is crucial in vascular cell differentiation where a higher shear stress condition exhibits higher levels of differentiation. Using microvalves in the microdevices can easily control the shear force generated by fluid flow and subsequently the degree of cellular activation [52].

On the other hand, induction of cardiogenic and neural differentiation in stem cells and thus better functionality could be affected by electrical stimulation [53]. In this regard, types of electrical fields such as alternative current (AC) or direct current (DC), voltage and frequencies are the determinative factors. Sauer et al. evaluated the degree of differentiation of mouse embryonic fibroblasts incubated in a conductive buffer (called a pulsing buffer) under an electrical current. It was shown that during stimulation of embryoid bodies with the DC pulses (from 100 to 500 V/m) for 90 s, a significant number of embryoid bodies differentiated into cardiomyocytes in the highest electrical field, compared with nonstimulated control samples [54]. Another study indicated the effect of electrical stimulation on the generation of reactive oxygen species (ROS), which plays an important role in cardiac differentiation of human embryonic stem cells (hESCs). After investigation of different electrode materials in an electrical stimulation bioreactor, length of stimulus and age of embryoid bodies, it was suggested that the application of an electric field produced by stainless steel electrodes with an amplitude of 1 V/mm, for 90 s on 4-day embryoid bodies could generate a high amount of ROS, significantly increased cardiogenesis and expression of troponin T [55].

9.5 Organomimetic prospects in microfluidics

9.5.1 Liver-on-a-chip

One of the important human organs for microfluidic research is the liver, which performs numerous functions such as, metabolism, detoxification, and protein synthesis. Lack of sufficient organ donors and an essential need for testing drug hepatotoxicity have caused an advance in the liver tissue engineering field. However, due to the fact that the in vitro 2D culture of hepatocytes leads to the loss of their specific phenotype and activity [29, 30] and also the structural complexity of the liver, simulation of a functional 3D liver tissue could be challenging. With the benefit of microfluidic technology allowing the design of microdevices with an assortment of sizes and shapes, researchers are now able to make 3D like liver models (in either cylindrical or spheroid hepatic cluster shapes) for tissue engineering and drug delivery applications [31, 32].

In 2010, Lee et al. reported the successful creation of a bioartificial liver by using a pure chitosan microfiber chip. After the fabrication of microfibers, they were attached to a PDMS frame and then a PDMS chip whereby the inlet and outlet pores were connected. Noticeably, cultured HepG2 cells on the chip were able to synthesize urea as well as secrete albumin which are specific functions of liver tissue [33]. Another example of a liver-on-a-chip for the study of tissue regeneration was carried out by Powers et al. who reported a successful morphological replication of 3D liver tissue using a microfluidic bioreactor. First, in order to create a 3D scaffold, a silicon chip consisting of arrays of channels with the ability for cellular adhesion was fabricated. Primary rat hepatocytes were then cultured in each channel with a cell-retaining filter where they remained under continuous perfusion. This system provided a controlled oxygen supply and shear stress in the required physiological range leading to the creation of viable cellular spheroids, as well as 3D tissue-like structures for up to 2 weeks [34]. Skardal et al. employed a simple microfluidic method for toxicity screening. The in situ formed scaffold consisted of UV-cross-linkable hyaluronic acid hydrogel combined with hepatic cells prepared in parallel channels of a microfluidic device. The results showed the formation of stable and viable 3D liver tissue which carried out the main hepatic cell functions such as secretion of urea and albumin during 7 days of culture [35].

Liver-on-chip devices with metabolically active liver organoids can be used as a disease model as well as in the field of drug screening and toxicology. In a study by Nakao et al., striking mimicking of liver tissue structure with the creation of bile canaliculi near the hepatic cords was carried out by using a microfluidic device to align the culture of hepatocytes under perfusion. Physiological bile secretion and excretion of other metabolites into the bile canaliculi, which are major metabolic processes of the liver, were observed. Results suggested that the formation of aligned rat primary hepatocytes resembled the actual hepatic canaliculi and could be used for drug screening instead of using animal models [36, 37].

Moreover, combining different organ-on-chip devices can pave the way for the study of the role of different organs in a specific pathological or normal biological phenomenon. As one example, nonalcoholic fatty liver disease (NAFLD) involves both liver and intestines whereby the barrier functions of the intestinal epithelium as well as its bacterial flora are disrupted, which then leads to the release of bacterial pathogens into the liver via the portal vein. Connecting gut-on-chip and liver-on-chip devices can mimic the liver-to-gut axis and could be used to investigate the mechanism and possible cure of this prevalent disease [38, 39].

One of the attractive approaches to the problems of constructing 3D liver tissue and overcoming the limited lifetime of cell cultures is the induction of vascularization within engineered liver tissue, which can produce sinusoid-like models. Co-culture of hepatocytes with vessel forming cells [e.g., human umbilical vein endothelial cells (HUVEC), etc.] has been studied in the fabrication of vascularized hepatic structures. It should be noted that layer-by-layer scaffold fabrication and sequential culture of cell types is crucial to construct functional and perfusable prevascularized 3D liver tissue which could even be transplanted into a mouse model [30, 40, 41].

9.5.2 Gut-on-a-chip

The gut plays a key role in many physiological functions including digestion, absorption, and secretion, as well as metabolism where it cooperates with the liver and pancreas. Moreover, the gut acts as an epithelial barrier against orally consumed substances (toxins in foods or drugs). It should be noted that the regulation of immune response, intestinal homeostasis, and overall health depend on the maintenance of gut microbiome homeostasis [29, 42]. The 2D culture of intestinal cells using Transwell insert culture devices is used for the study of the simple barrier function of cell layers, while 3D tissue structure is required for accurate investigation of the more complex properties of the gut. Despite having several advantages such as excellent availability (easily can be harvested from biopsy samples), a wide range of isolated stem cells, native tissue similarity, and ability to provide personalized medicine, organoid culture lacks the formation of a complete functional 3D intestinal construct, consisting of blood vessels, native peristaltic deformation, natural microbial flora, and also immune cells. For this reason, microfluidic gut-on-chip models have been investigated [37, 43].

To successfully mimic intestinal tissue, it is necessary to provide the desired flow rate and shear stress using fluid pumps, and also to separate hollow channels through a cell adhesive coated porous membrane, which can then be cultured with intestinal epithelial cells [29, 44]. For example, Kim et al. reported the fabrication of a human gut-on-a-chip device, which could replace animal testing due to the comprehensive mimicking of mechanical, structural, functional, microbial, and pathophysiological aspects of the intestine. In this two-channel chip with a separate membrane coated with human intestinal epithelial (Caco-2) cells, the native intestinal microenvironment was simulated by a low flow rate and shear stress with cyclic strain, which then led to the formation of columnar polarized epithelium similar to normal intestinal villi. Moreover, it allowed the co-culture of *Lactobacillus rhamnosus* GG (a gut microbe) for almost 1 week without loss of other cell viability and made this device ideal for studying drug metabolism and toxicity, as well as molecular transportation and intestinal absorption phenomenon within a 3D structure [45]. In another study, the successful co-culture of intestinal microbial cells with intestinal epithelial cells was created in a gut-on-a-chip device, whereby the role of the gut microbiome in intestinal diseases (such as inflammatory bowel disease) could be evaluated. It was shown that a decrease in peristaltic motion could lead to bacterial overgrowth. Thereafter, the release of bacterial endotoxin stimulated the epithelial cells to secrete proinflammatory cytokines, which reduced the barrier function of the injured epithelial layer [46].

Several studies have reported the positive effects of culturing intestinal cells on villus-shaped polymeric scaffolds [39, 42]. Although, the use of intestinal cell lines or stem cells can increase the culture time compared with primary cells (which is less than 24 h), but it is still limited to about 5 days. To address this problem, a combination of organoid and microfluidic devices could be used to form miniaturized organ bioreactors [37, 42]. As one example, Kasendra et al. developed a primary human gut-on-a-chip device using 3D organoids expanded from cells, which were extracted from healthy intestinal biopsy samples. The contact of the parallel channels containing cultured cells, intestinal microvascular endothelium, and also the epithelial cell layer enhanced cell viability and function over a longer period. In addition, continuous flow within the microchannels could differentiate the epithelial cell layer into lineages similar to the normal intestine. Significantly, this microdevice could be used to quantitatively analyze digestion, secretion, and barrier function of the human duodenum over a prolonged period (multiple days) [47].

Thus, organoid culture in gut-on-a-chip devices can be employed as a platform with many applications including the study of metabolism, drug mechanisms of action, tissue morphogenesis, and disease mechanisms, which can be even patient-specific. The ability to control the cellular complexity and also genetic and molecular aspects of a specific disease are other unique properties of this type of intestinal chip disease model [31, 48].

9.5.3 Brain-on-a-chip

Microfluidic devices can promote neural tissue engineering aimed at in vitro mimicking of nerve cells and the brain-on-a-chip in a 3D controllable manner. In fact, microfluidics could be promising for mimicking some neurodegenerative diseases like Alzheimer's and Parkinson's. This system provides variability in the physiochemical, mechanical, and biomaterial properties inside a chip. Different properties of microfluidics can imitate the ECM microenvironment and cell interactions to monitor the development of neural structures [56]. As one example, hESCs were co-cultured with PA6 stromal cells. Neurite outgrowth and axon guidance of the neural cells derived from hESCs were studied using microfluidics technology [57]. Aiming to use a microfluidic device as a gradient generator, a gradient of CXCL12 (stromal cell-derived factor 1-α) was created, which increased neural cell differentiation and the directionality of migration [58]. To study human neurodevelopment in vitro, brain organoids could be used. 3D tissue culture lacks sufficient nutrient exchange at the center of the tissue and does not allow the imaging of the entire mass of the organoids. Therefore, a microfabricated chamber was successfully developed to investigate the dynamics of organoid growth, cell differentiation, and the cell cycle [59]. This device limited tissue growth in the z-direction, but growth in the lateral directions was unlimited, which helped the organoid to reach a diameter of more than 1.5 mm with efficient nutrient exchange and high-magnification microscopic imaging [59].

Microfluidic platforms have also been investigated to study stem cell differentiation behavior. In one study by Cheng et al., chemical and physical-chemical stimulation were used to culture human placenta-derived multipotent stem cells (PDMCs) inside a microfluidic device. The device provided a precise in vitro microenvironment in which PDMCs could be effectively differentiated into neuronal cells [60]. Also, 3D neural tissues were derived from embryonic stem cells using a microfluidic biochip [61].

The blood-brain barrier (BBB) is the highly selective physiological barrier to protect the nervous system, composed of microvascular endothelial cells, ECM, pericytes, and astrocytes. The complex nature of the BBB and necessity for all three mentioned cell types makes the BBB challenging to simulate [62, 63]. Due to the limitation of single-cell cultures and the nonhuman physiology of animal models, providing more effective microfluidic BBB models could be useful for investigating the BBB function and possible treatment of related neurological diseases. A microfluidic model of the neurovascular unit (NVU) was developed with a brain parenchymal compartment and influx/efflux across the BBB. This device contained three chips: one brain chip in the middle and two BBB chips (influx and efflux) on either side. The BBB chips contained primary human brain microvascular endothelial cells (hBMVECs) and primary brain microvascular pericytes dispersed among astrocytes that were cultured on the lower and upper surfaces of the chip, respectively, to mimic the brain microvessel external wall. The brain chip contained neural cells that had been differentiated from hippocampus derived neural stem cells. Different medium (artificial cerebral spinal fluid) flowed through the device and the efflux was analyzed. In vivo physiological functions of the NVU were investigated through the expression of metabolic enzymes and reversible effects of a neuroactive drug (methamphetamine) [64]. This device revealed details of metabolic activities that were unachievable using previous approaches. Traditional models are limited in the spatiotemporal control of the NVU and neuron/BBB interactions and use static mono- and co-cultures of human cells. Control over the structural properties of microchips and applying a dynamic flow with various cells and different polymers as a scaffold could be useful in imitation of BBB related diseases to replace in vivo approaches.

9.5.4 Kidney-on-a-chip

The main function of the kidneys is to purify the blood by removal of waste materials like urea, salts, and creatinine by urine formation in the renal tubules. In addition to natural waste filtration, the kidneys are also responsible to balance the amount of chemicals and salts within the body. The main goal of the microfluidic tissue engineering of the kidney is to create a kidney-on-a-chip comprising renal microstructures in order to imitate the absorption and reabsorption of natural substances, or drugs in the case of nephrotoxicity studies. Assessment of the degree of toxicity of a certain drug to the human kidney is a crucial stage of pharmaceutical testing [65] that have conventionally been performed in animal models, that are faced with inaccuracy or ethical issues [66]. Nevertheless, organ-on-a-chip technologies offer an alternative nephrotoxicity testing method in vitro [67].

Although some efforts have been made to construct an on-chip nephron as the functional unit of the kidney [67], mimicking the entire renal function, requires the culture of more than one cell type since kidney microstructures contain many blood vessels, renal ducts, and many different cell types. Therefore, the first attempts to fabricate a kidney-on-a-chip were limited to merely considering one part of the kidney, e.g., proximal tubules, glomerulus, collecting ducts, etc.

The majority of the kidney-on-a-chip models use molds (mostly PDMS) including the microchannels or chambers separated by an ECM-coated porous membrane (mostly polyester) to allow molecular transportation. Recent designs have employed hollow fiber microtubes or tubular hydrogels to contain the cultured cells within a tubule.

Baudoin et al. fabricated one of the first microfluidic devices based on replica molding with PDMS plasma bonding, in order to culture canine kidney cells in a kidney-on-a-chip model. Their model was aimed at assessment of the effects of model parameters like flow rate and number of cultured cells [68]. Jang and Suh used a PDMS mold and polyester porous membrane to culture rat inner medullary collecting duct cells and found that the fluidic shear stress roughly equal to 1 dyn/cm^2 for 5 h was optimal for cell-cell interactions, polarization, and cytoskeletal reorganization [69]. By culturing human proximal tubular cells inside the hollow fibers, Sanechika et al. formed a bioartificial renal tubule able to reabsorb water, sodium, and glucose [70].

Jang et al. also used PDMS microfabrication techniques and polyester porous membrane to prepare a surface coated with ECM for the culture of primary human kidney epithelial cells. They controlled all the fluidic parameters like shear stress and flow rates to better imitate the actual kidney conditions. Then, cisplatin was injected into the interstitial medium to assess its nephrotoxicity [71]. By using a fibrin-coated 0.3 μm hollow fiber microfluidic device, Ng et al. cultured proximal tubular epithelial cells and found that the cells were correctly polarized for reabsorbing suitable substances [72]. Kim et al. used the photolithography technique for the fabrication of a microfluidic device to host canine kidney cells cultured in a kidney-on-a-chip model. Then, the effects of two different gentamicin dosage regimens on the kidney cell toxicity over 24 h were examined with control of fluid conditions like the shear stress [73].

9.5.5 Heart-on-a-chip

The heart is the main organ of the human cardiovascular system that pumps blood through the vessels and capillaries that feed the body tissues. The heart muscle itself requires a blood supply via the coronary capillaries, which when blocked can cause myocardial infarction, the most prevalent worldwide heart disorder. Treatments of heart attack and failure rely on the prescription of drugs, but again the optimum dosage should be tested. In spite of the prevalent use of animals in studies, recent findings showed inaccurate results besides the ethical dilemmas involved [74–76].

The use of organ-on-a-chip technology can benefit cardiac researchers. Nevertheless, constructing a heart-on-a-chip is not as easy as other organs since mimicking its natural environment is difficult. The cardiomyocytes (CMs) undergo cyclic contractions due to heartbeat. The consequence is the existence of sinusoidal uniaxial strains in the CMs along the direction of the fibers embedded in the ECM. Therefore, a heart-on-a-chip microdevice should at least include the ECM in a 3D environment allowing cell-cell and cell-ECM interactions and also the simulation of the heartbeat stimulation [77]. Furthermore, the microdevice should be able to control chemical and mechanical conditions during the cell culture which are not available using conventional culture methods due to poor vascularization and the absence of anisotropy and 3D nature of the cell assembly [78].

The general procedure for the fabrication of a heart-on-a-chip is to first provide a substrate for MC culture in direct contact with the beating tissue. The majority of the studies have used PDMS bonded on thin glass sheets. Also, the CMs are commonly derived from the rat or human iPSC-derived CMs. The stimulation can be applied either electrically or mechanically [74]. The electrical stimuli often utilize the insertion of microelectrodes to conduct AC currents with certain frequencies, e.g., 2 Hz in the study of Agarwal et al. [79]. The CMs subjected to this electrical current are aligned along the direction of the electrical field [80, 81]. The mechanical stimulation has included a variety of actuating systems to induce uniaxial strain in the CMs. Some studies have used pneumatic actuation to imitate contraction/relaxation in the biphasic behavior of the real heart environment [77, 82]. Other studies have used thin film stretching to mimic the heartbeat deformation [83, 84]. A novel heart-on-a-chip design was developed by Schneider et al. who applied centrifugal forces on the CMs to avoid manual injection of excess cells and allow proper alignment of the CMs, with viability and functionality [78].

Since the main application of the heart-on-a-chip is to perform preclinical tests on cardiotoxicity, many studies that used a microfluidic model of the heart examined the effect of different drugs on the CMs. For instance, the toxicity of isoproterenol was assessed using a microfluidic heart-on-a-chip model made from polycarbonate with an aluminum substrate to culture human iPSC-derived CMs under electrical stimulations (~15 V, 2 Hz, 10 ms pulse duration AC current) of a deformable cantilever thin film [79]. Qian et al. also evaluated the toxicity of norepinephrine as a neurotransmitter in CMs cultured in polystyrene chambers, which were electrically stimulated [85]. The degree of toxicity of isoproterenol (mainly used for the treatment of bradycardia and heart block) in the iPSC-derived CMs was also analyzed by Maoz et al. who fabricated an electrically-stimulated microfluidic heart-on-a-chip model from the PDMS bonded onto glass [86].

9.6 Microfluidic models of cancer tissue

Cancer is difficult to treat due to the complex and heterogeneous composition of cells, molecules, and microenvironments, as well as the alteration of tumor structure in different growth stages [87, 88]. Many cancerous tumors secrete growth factors that stimulate the growth of blood vessels. This process directs nutrients and oxygen from healthy tissues to cancerous cells to support their abnormal and rapid growth. In addition, cancer can spread via the blood vessels or lymphatics to other areas of the body. Since patients can benefit from treatments that stop the growth of these blood vessels [89], researchers are interested in finding new technologies for studying tumor blood vessels. Furthermore, cell cultures in 2D or 3D or application of liquid flow can facilitate the investigation of other key factors affecting cancer initiation and progression [90, 91]. Applications of microfluidics for modeling cancer tissue in vitro can be categorized into three main groups: (1) cancer cells 2D and 3D culture and co-culture; (2) in vitro models of tumor spheroids and tumor tissue modeling; and (3) in vitro models of tumors that include multiorgan structures.

9.6.1 Cancer cells 2D and 3D culture and co-culture

Application of microfluidics in cancer research and cancer mimicking in vitro has been explored by a simple culture of one or two types of cells [92, 93]. This application continued over the years to study the basic process of cancer cell behavior including attachment, proliferation, and migration. For example, improvements in cell trapping, attachment/detachment, and migration behavior were shown using MDA-MB-231 human breast cancer cells in a vertically integrated array (VIA) microdevice [94]. The real-time monitoring of basic cancer mechanisms has been investigated by designing a two-layer microfluidic system able to supply oxygen-containing CaSki cervical cancer cells allowing the monitoring of migration and online biomarkers [95].

More cancer characteristics such as invasion, angiogenesis, and metastasis have also been investigated using microdevices [96, 97]. In cancer therapy, targeting the different stages of cancer progression is important. Each stage of cancer progression has own complex properties; for example, circulating tumor aggregates have the significant metastatic potential [96]. In another study, a microfluidic device was fabricated to imitate the transendothelial invasion of tumor aggregates [96]. Analysis of extravasation in salivary gland adenoid cystic carcinoma (ACC) cell aggregates and the effects of chemical stimulation on transendothelial invasion were performed using this device. Suppression of invasion across a HUVEC layer by the drug AMD3100 was shown; however, invasion of the aggregates into the ECM was stimulated by CXCL12 (CXC chemokine ligand 12).

Interactions and communications of cancer cells with other cells and tissues play an important role in cancer behavior such as angiogenesis [98, 99]. Investigation into tumor-stromal interactions using microdevices can provide opportunities for improvements over common co-culture approaches, particularly regarding the static condition and limited numbers of compartments [100, 101]. In this regard, microfluidics can provide a more realistic 3D environment with better control over the microenvironmental factors, external biochemical and biomechanical factors, and improved levels of compartmentalization [100, 102]. For example, co-culture patterns using hemichannels were more drug-responsive compared to monocultures and flat surfaces [103], and the influence of macrophages and myofibroblasts on the migration rate of lung cancer cells co-cultured in a microchip were studied [104]. Different shapes and geometries of microdevices, and various microscale physical properties have been successfully used for the culture and/or co-culture of different cancer cells.

9.6.2 In vitro models of tumor spheroids and tumor tissue

Tumor spheroids are important in cancer research as tumor models. However there are difficulties in traditional spheroid generation (e.g., rotating cultures, spinner flasks, and 96-well plates), meaning that new approaches are needed for uniform-sized spheroid generation for use in drug screening [90, 100, 105]. Advantageous properties of microfluidics, include developing different shapes and/or geometries, cost-effectiveness of high-throughput screening, 3D environment, and precise control of microscale phenomena [106]. A hemispherical SpheroChip model was designed for HT-29 colon carcinoma and Hep-G2 liver carcinoma culture to form spheroids [106]. The spatiotemporal controllability and media exchange of such devices can provide more precise setups for long-term metabolic monitoring and drug screening.

Different microfluidic approaches have been explored for the recapitulation of tumor tissue in vitro. Traditional microdevices suffer from limitations for in situ and real-time tumor analysis and monitoring the effects of external stimuli on tumor behavior [107]. Extensive studies have been reported in the last decade that use synergistic combinations of biological engineering methods with microfluidics to overcome these restrictions. However, the fabrication of more practical devices and better translation to clinical laboratories are required. For example, it was shown that the integration of a microfluidic system with pneumatic microstructures (PμSs) to produce 3D tumor spheroids was possible using PDMS with subsequent control over the localization of U251, HepG2, and MCF-7 cancer cells [95]. Furthermore, gradient distribution, high density, and local accumulation of U251 cells could be achieved, as well as three different types of 3D tumor using off-switch PμSs.

9.6.3 In vitro models of tumor including multiorgans

Further investigations of the critical processes in cancer progression (such as metastasis) require the development of advanced dual-organ and multi organ-on-a-chip technologies. Due to the relationship between invasive and metastatic cancer and poor patient prognosis, single tumor organ studies will be insufficient. For instance, cancer metastasis to distant organs leads to treatment resistance and also causes more than 90% of cancer-related mortality [108, 109]. This underlines the importance of investigations into cancer cell/tissue/organs and cancer interactions with other healthy tissues. In this context, organ-on-a-chip and body-on-a-chip devices were introduced for mimicking the structural properties and physiological functions of an organ or multiple organs within a microdevice in vitro. Conventional 3D tumor modeling lacks the effects of physiological processes in the recapitulation and is not fully integrated with the whole human body [90, 100]. A microdevice with three channels for culture media and four independent gel channels was developed and consisted of collagen channels loaded with human osteo-differentiated bone marrow-derived mesenchymal stem cells (hBM-MSCs) as a bone-like microenvironment with seeded HUVECs in the central channel to produce an endothelial covering. The process of extravasation and migration of MDA-MB-231 human breast cancer cells was investigated using this micrometastatic system, showing specific metastatic behavior of breast cancer to bone (Fig. 9.3) [110].

Examination of the effects of therapeutic moieties like pharmaceutical substance or nanoparticles in the human body requires modeling of multiorgan-on-a-chip systems [111, 112]. Recent technologies have facilitated the design and fabrication of separate chambers in microdevices for culturing different cell types from different organs, and including the physicomechanical properties of vessels and other structures.

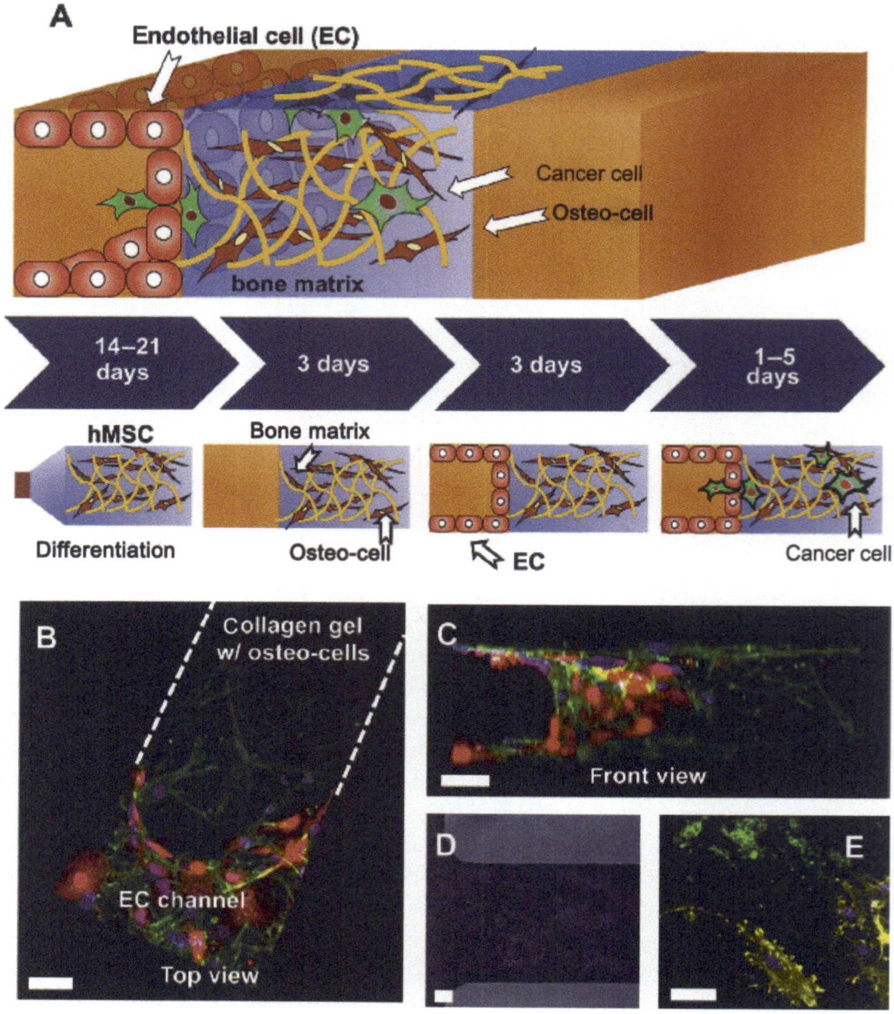

FIG. 9.3

Breast cancer micrometastasis to bone. (A) hBM-MSCs *(brown)* seeding within microdevices and deposition in ECM *(yellow filaments)*; Seeding of endothelial cells (ECs) *(red)* and in result generation of a monolayer; addition of cancer cells *(green)* and analysis of their micrometastasis generation. (B and C) Top (B) and a front view (C) of the 3D region between 2 PDMS walls. HUVECs (RFP) complete covering the channel walls and osteo-differentiated hBM-MSCs distribution within the collagen. (D) Optical microscopy of calcium deposits Alizarin Red staining within a gel channel. (E) Osteocalcin *(green)* secretion ability of osteo-differentiated hBM-MSCs by staining of 2D projection of a confocal stack highlights the ability of osteo-differentiated hBM-MSCs.
Scale bars: 50 μm [110].

Reprinted with permission from Elsevier.

One example is a multiorgan device investigated the cytotoxicity of anticancer drugs in a microcell culture analog (μCCA) with multiple cell types embedded in 3D hydrogels within the interconnected chambers [113]. The 3D hydrogel, interconnections, and the microdevice mimicked the 3D ECM, blood flow, and pharmaceutical profile, respectively. Hepatoma cells (HepG2/C3A) and colon cancer cells (HCT-116) were encapsulated in Matrigel, and myeloblasts (Kasumi-1) were encapsulated in alginate. These were cultured in the liver, tumor, and marrow chambers, respectively. This device was used for investigation of hepatotoxicity and hematological toxicity showing the prodrug-drug metabolism in the liver and the subsequent cancer cell death. Another microfluidic chip was designed with two parallel compartments connected via fluidic channels. The multiorgan chip contained two separate chambers for HepG2 and HeLa cells, representing the liver and the tumor model, respectively [114].

Overall, microsystems offer many advantages over traditional 2D and 3D systems for tumor tissue engineering [90, 91, 100] including (1) advanced physiological mimicry of the tumor microenvironment; (2) providing spatiotemporal controllability and functionality; (3) diffusion-based molecular transport for gradient formation; (4) applying polymers with different diameters and shapes; (5) investigating cancer behavior with co-culture systems and application of multi-ECM components; (6) providing high-throughput screening systems using a smaller sample size.

9.7 Conclusions and challenges

Despite the numerous advances in microfluidic-based tissue engineering, there are still some challenges associated with cell culture, controlling cellular microenvironment, and cellular analysis. Considering the dramatic difference between cellular behavior in 2D and 3D microenvironments, developing techniques using 3D bioprinting are required for the creation of 3D moieties (e.g., microgels) inside microfluidic devices. It is also necessary for future studies to investigate methods for longer-term cell culture, more uniform cell loading and microtopographies, continuous cellular hydration and nutrient delivery, and accurate and simultaneous analysis of the total protein content of cell lysates or biological samples. By meeting these requirements, microfluidic devices can be upgraded to become robust and rapid diagnostic and therapeutic tools.

References

[1] K. Schwab, E. Henriksen, J. Worlock, M.L. Roukes, Measurement of the quantum of thermal conductance, Nature 404 (2000) 974.

[2] P. Tabeling, Introduction to microfluidics, Oxford University Press, Oxford, England, 2005.

[3] M. Leman, F. Abouakil, A.D. Griffiths, P. Tabeling, Droplet-based microfluidics at the femtolitre scale, Lab Chip 15 (2015) 753–765.

[4] J.-u. Shim, R.T. Ranasinghe, C.A. Smith, S.M. Ibrahim, F. Hollfelder, W.T. Huck, D. Klenerman, C. Abell, Ultrarapid generation of femtoliter microfluidic droplets for single-molecule-counting immunoassays, ACS Nano 7 (2013) 5955–5964.

[5] S. Takayama, E. Ostuni, P. LeDuc, K. Naruse, D.E. Ingber, G.M. Whitesides, Laminar flows: subcellular positioning of small molecules, Nature 411 (2001) 1016.

[6] C.L. Hansen, E. Skordalakes, J.M. Berger, S.R. Quake, A robust and scalable microfluidic metering method that allows protein crystal growth by free interface diffusion, Proc Natl Acad Sci U S A 99 (2002) 16531–16536.

[7] A. Bange, H.B. Halsall, W.R. Heineman, Microfluidic immunosensor systems, Biosens Bioelectron 20 (2005) 2488–2503.

[8] B. Gale, A. Jafek, C. Lambert, B. Goenner, H. Moghimifam, U. Nze, S. Kamarapu, A review of current methods in microfluidic device fabrication and future commercialization prospects, Inventions 3 (2018) 60.

[9] D. Caballero, S.M. Blackburn, M. De Pablo, J. Samitier, L. Albertazzi, Tumour-vessel-on-a-chip models for drug delivery, Lab Chip 17 (2017) 3760–3771.

[10] D. Huh, B.D. Matthews, A. Mammoto, M. Montoya-Zavala, H.Y. Hsin, D.E. Ingber, Reconstituting organ-level lung functions on a chip, Science 328 (2010) 1662–1668.

[11] Š. Selimović, H. Kaji, H. Bae, A. Khademhosseini, Microfluidic systems for controlling stem cell microenvironments, in: Microfluidic cell culture systems, Elsevier, 2019, pp. 31–63.

[12] S.A.P. Rajan, P. Hambright, R.C. Burke, A.R. Hall, Microfluidics in cell and tissue studies, in: Tumor organoids, Springer, 2018, pp. 149–170.

[13] R. Langer, J.P. Vacanti, Tissue engineering, Science (1993) 920–926.

[14] S.N. Bhatia, D.E. Ingber, Microfluidic organs-on-chips, Nat Biotechnol 32 (2014) 760.

[15] J.T. Borenstein, H. Terai, K.R. King, E. Weinberg, M. Kaazempur-Mofrad, J. Vacanti, Microfabrication technology for vascularized tissue engineering, Biomed Microdevices 4 (2002) 167–175.

[16] W.-C. Tian, E. Finehout, Microfluidic systems for engineering vascularized tissue constructs, in: Microfluidics for biological applications, Springer, 2008, pp. 223–240.

[17] A. Bein, W. Shin, S. Jalili-Firoozinezhad, M.H. Park, A. Sontheimer-Phelps, A. Tovaglieri, A. Chalkiadaki, H.J. Kim, D.E. Ingber, Microfluidic organ-on-a-chip models of human intestine, Cell Mol Gastroenterol Hepatol 5 (2018) 659–668.

[18] V. van Duinen, S.J. Trietsch, J. Joore, P. Vulto, T. Hankemeier, Microfluidic 3D cell culture: from tools to tissue models, Curr Opin Biotechnol 35 (2015) 118–126.

[19] R.A. Dorey, Ceramic thick films for MEMS and microdevices, William Andrew, 2011.

[20] M. Toofan, J. Toofan, A brief review of the cleaning process for electronic device fabrication, in: Developments in surface contamination and cleaning, Elsevier, 2015, pp. 185–212.

[21] P.N. Nge, C.I. Rogers, A.T. Woolley, Advances in microfluidic materials, functions, integration, and applications, Chem Rev 113 (2013) 2550–2583.

[22] F.C. Huang, Y.F. Chen, G.B. Lee, CE chips fabricated by injection molding and polyethylene/thermoplastic elastomer film packaging methods, Electrophoresis 28 (2007) 1130–1137.

[23] B. Yan, A. Wang, C. Huang, F. Huang, Study of precision micro-holes in borosilicate glass using micro EDM combined with micro ultrasonic vibration machining, Int J Mach Tool Manuf 42 (2002) 1105–1112.

[24] A. Yadegari, F. Fahimipour, M. Rasoulianboroujeni, E. Dashtimoghadarm, M. Omidi, H. Golzar, M. Tahriri, L. Tayebi, Specific considerations in scaffold design for oral tissue engineering, in: Biomaterials for oral and dental tissue engineering, Elsevier, 2017, pp. 157–183.

[25] O. Sahin, M. Ashokkumar, P.M. Ajayan, Micro-and nanopatterning of biomaterial surfaces, in: Fundamental biomaterials: metals, Elsevier, 2018, pp. 67–78.
[26] H. Becker, C. Gärtner, Polymer microfabrication technologies for microfluidic systems, Anal Bioanal Chem 390 (2008) 89–111.
[27] K. Ren, J. Zhou, H. Wu, Materials for microfluidic chip fabrication, Acc Chem Res 46 (2013) 2396–2406.
[28] S.C. Terry, J.H. Jerman, J.B. Angell, A gas chromatographic air analyzer fabricated on a silicon wafer, IEEE Trans Electron Devices 26 (1979) 1880–1886.
[29] H. Kimura, Y. Sakai, T. Fujii, Organ/body-on-a-chip based on microfluidic technology for drug discovery, Drug Metab Pharmacokinet 33 (2018) 43–48.
[30] T. Osaki, V. Sivathanu, R.D. Kamm, Vascularized microfluidic organ-chips for drug screening, disease models and tissue engineering, Curr Opin Biotechnol 52 (2018) 116–123.
[31] A. Skardal, T. Shupe, A. Atala, Organoid-on-a-chip and body-on-a-chip systems for drug screening and disease modeling, Drug Discov Today 21 (2016) 1399–1411.
[32] J.T. Borenstein, G. Vunjak-Novakovic, Engineering tissue with BioMEMS, IEEE Pulse 2 (2011) 28–34.
[33] K.H. Lee, S.J. Shin, C.B. Kim, J.K. Kim, Y.W. Cho, B.G. Chung, S.H. Lee, Microfluidic synthesis of pure chitosan microfibers for bio-artificial liver chip, Lab Chip 10 (2010) 1328–1334.
[34] M.J. Powers, K. Domansky, M.R. Kaazempur-Mofrad, A. Kalezi, A. Capitano, A. Upadhyaya, P. Kurzawski, K.E. Wack, D.B. Stolz, R. Kamm, L.G. Griffith, A microfabricated array bioreactor for perfused 3D liver culture, Biotechnol Bioeng 78 (2002) 257–269.
[35] A. Skardal, M. Devarasetty, S. Soker, A.R. Hall, In situ patterned micro 3D liver constructs for parallel toxicology testing in a fluidic device, Biofabrication 7 (2015), 031001.
[36] Y. Nakao, H. Kimura, Y. Sakai, T. Fujii, Bile canaliculi formation by aligning rat primary hepatocytes in a microfluidic device, Biomicrofluidics 5 (2011) 22212.
[37] A. Fatehullah, S.H. Tan, N. Barker, Organoids as an in vitro model of human development and disease, Nat Cell Biol 18 (2016) 246–254.
[38] S. Ishida, Organs-on-a-chip: current applications and consideration points for in vitro ADME-Tox studies, Drug Metab Pharmacokinet 33 (2018) 49–54.
[39] D. Huh, G.A. Hamilton, D.E. Ingber, From 3D cell culture to organs-on-chips, Trends Cell Biol 21 (2011) 745–754.
[40] A. Skardal, T. Shupe, A. Atala, chip systems for drug screening and disease modeling, Drug Discov Today 21 (2016) 1399–1411.
[41] T. Takebe, R.R. Zhang, H. Koike, M. Kimura, E. Yoshizawa, M. Enomura, N. Koike, K. Sekine, H. Taniguchi, Generation of a vascularized and functional human liver from an iPSC-derived organ bud transplant, Nat Protoc 9 (2014) 396–409.
[42] A. Bein, W. Shin, S. Jalili-firoozinezhad, M.H. Park, A. Sontheimer-phelps, A. Tovaglieri, A. Chalkiadaki, H.J. Kim, D.E. Ingber, Microfluidic organ-on-a-chip models of human intestine, Cell Mol Gastroenterol Hepatol 5 (2018) 659–668.
[43] P. Jung, T. Sato, A. Merlos-Suárez, F.M. Barriga, M. Iglesias, D. Rossell, H. Auer, M. Gallardo, M.A. Blasco, E. Sancho, H. Clevers, E. Batlle, Isolation and in vitro expansion of human colonic stem cells, Nat Med 17 (2011) 1225.
[44] A. Balijepalli, V. Sivaramakrishan, Organs-on-chips: research and commercial perspectives, Drug Discov Today 22 (2017) 397–403.

[45] H.J. Kim, D. Huh, G. Hamilton, D.E. Ingber, Human gut-on-a-chip inhabited by microbial flora that experiences intestinal peristalsis-like motions and flow, Lab Chip 12 (2012) 2165–2174.

[46] H.J. Kim, H. Li, J.J. Collins, D.E. Ingber, Contributions of microbiome and mechanical deformation to intestinal bacterial overgrowth and inflammation in a human gut-on-a-chip, Proc Natl Acad Sci U S A 113 (2016) E7–15.

[47] M. Kasendra, A. Tovaglieri, A. Sontheimer-Phelps, S. Jalili-Firoozinezhad, A. Bein, A. Chalkiadaki, W. Scholl, C. Zhang, H. Rickner, C.A. Richmond, H. Li, D.T. Breault, D.E. Ingber, Development of a primary human small intestine-on-a-chip using biopsy-derived organoids, Sci Rep 8 (2018) 2871.

[48] J.F. Pereira, N.T. Awatade, C.A. Loureiro, P. Matos, M.D. Amaral, P. Jordan, The third dimension: new developments in cell culture models for colorectal research, Cell Mol Life Sci 73 (2016) 3971–3989.

[49] A. Cochrane, H.J. Albers, R. Passier, C.L. Mummery, A.V.D. Berg, V.V. Orlova, A.D.V.D. Meer, Advanced in vitro models of vascular biology: human induced pluripotent stem cells and organ-on-chip technology, Adv Drug Deliv Rev (2018).

[50] Y.C. Toh, J. Voldman, Multiplex microfluidic perfusion identifies shear stress, in: 14th International conference on miniaturized systems for chemistry and life sciences, 2010, pp. 10–12.

[51] L. Kim, M.D. Vahey, H.Y. Lee, J. Voldman, Microfluidic arrays for logarithmically perfused embryonic stem cell culture, Lab Chip 6 (2006) 394–406.

[52] D. Park, J. Lim, J.Y. Park, S.-H. Lee, Concise review: stem cell microenvironment on a chip: current technologies for tissue engineering and stem cell biology, Stem Cells Transl Med 4 (2015) 1352–1368.

[53] Y. Zhao, N. Rafatian, E.Y. Wang, N.T. Feric, B.F.L. Lai, E.J. Knee-Walden, P.H. Backx, M. Radisic, Engineering microenvironment for human cardiac tissue assembly in heart-on-a-chip platform, Matrix Biol (2019).

[54] H. Sauer, G. Rahimi, J. Hescheler, M. Wartenberg, Effects of electrical fields on cardiomyocyte differentiation of embryonic stem cells, J Cell Biochem 75 (1999) 710–723.

[55] E. Serena, E. Figallo, N. Tandon, C. Cannizzaro, S. Gerecht, N. Elvassore, G. Vunjak-Novakovic, Electrical stimulation of human embryonic stem cells: cardiac differentiation and the generation of reactive oxygen species, Exp Cell Res 315 (2009) 3611–3619.

[56] M. Karimi, S. Bahrami, H. Mirshekari, S.M.M. Basri, A.B. Nik, A.R. Aref, M. Akbari, M.R. Hamblin, Microfluidic systems for stem cell-based neural tissue engineering, Lab Chip 16 (2016) 2551–2571.

[57] N. Lee, J.W. Park, H.J. Kim, J.H. Yeon, J. Kwon, J.J. Ko, S.-H. Oh, H.S. Kim, A. Kim, B.S. Han, Monitoring the differentiation and migration patterns of neural cells derived from human embryonic stem cells using a microfluidic culture system, Mol Cells 37 (2014) 497.

[58] H. Xu, S.C. Heilshorn, Microfluidic investigation of BDNF-enhanced neural stem cell chemotaxis in CXCL12 gradients, Small 9 (2013) 585–595.

[59] E. Karzbrun, R.Y. Tshuva, O. Reiner, An on-chip method for long-term growth and real-time imaging of brain organoids, Curr Protoc Cell Biol 81 (2018), e62.

[60] Y.-C. Cheng, C.-W. Tsao, M.-Z. Chiang, C.-A. Chung, C.-C. Chien, W.-W. Hu, R.-C. Ruaan, C. Li, Microfluidic platform for human placenta-derived multipotent stem cells culture and applied for enhanced neuronal differentiation, Microfluid Nanofluid 18 (2015) 587–598.

[61] A. Sandoz, I. Charvet, L. Stoppini, Development of a microfluidic biochip for chronic monitoring of 3D neural tissues derived from human embryonic stem cells, Procedia Eng 59 (2013) 46–50.
[62] T.-E. Park, N. Mustafaoglu, A. Herland, R. Hasselkus, R. Mannix, E.A. FitzGerald, R. Prantil-Baun, A. Watters, O. Henry, M. Benz, Hypoxia-enhanced Blood-Brain Barrier Chip recapitulates human barrier function and shuttling of drugs and antibodies, Nat Commun 10 (2019) 2621.
[63] R. Cecchelli, V. Berezowski, S. Lundquist, M. Culot, M. Renftel, M.-P. Dehouck, L. Fenart, Modelling of the blood–brain barrier in drug discovery and development, Nat Rev Drug Discov 6 (2007) 650.
[64] B.M. Maoz, A. Herland, E.A. FitzGerald, T. Grevesse, C. Vidoudez, A.R. Pacheco, S.P. Sheehy, T.-E. Park, S. Dauth, R. Mannix, A linked organ-on-chip model of the human neurovascular unit reveals the metabolic coupling of endothelial and neuronal cells, Nat Biotechnol 36 (2018) 865.
[65] I. Kola, J. Landis, Can the pharmaceutical industry reduce attrition rates? Nat Rev Drug Discov 3 (2004) 711.
[66] S.W. Paine, K. Ménochet, R. Denton, D.F. McGinnity, R.J. Riley, Prediction of human renal clearance from preclinical species for a diverse set of drugs that exhibit both active secretion and net reabsorption, Drug Metab Dispos 39 (2011) 1008–1013.
[67] E. Weinberg, M. Kaazempur-Mofrad, J. Borenstein, Concept and computational design for a bioartificial nephron-on-a-chip, Int J Artif Organs 31 (2008) 508–514.
[68] R. Baudoin, L. Griscom, M. Monge, C. Legallais, E. Leclerc, Development of a renal microchip for in vitro distal tubule models, Biotechnol Prog 23 (2007) 1245–1253.
[69] K.-J. Jang, K.-Y. Suh, A multi-layer microfluidic device for efficient culture and analysis of renal tubular cells, Lab Chip 10 (2010) 36–42.
[70] N. Sanechika, K. Sawada, Y. Usui, K. Hanai, T. Kakuta, H. Suzuki, G. Kanai, S. Fujimura, T.A. Yokoyama, M. Fukagawa, Development of bioartificial renal tubule devices with lifespan-extended human renal proximal tubular epithelial cells, Nephrol Dial Transplant 26 (2011) 2761–2769.
[71] K.-J. Jang, A.P. Mehr, G.A. Hamilton, L.A. McPartlin, S. Chung, K.-Y. Suh, D.E. Ingber, Human kidney proximal tubule-on-a-chip for drug transport and nephrotoxicity assessment, Integr Biol 5 (2013) 1119–1129.
[72] C.P. Ng, Y. Zhuang, A.W.H. Lin, J.C.M. Teo, A fibrin-based tissue-engineered renal proximal tubule for bioartificial kidney devices: development, characterization and in vitro transport study, Int J Tissue Eng 2013 (2013).
[73] S. Kim, S.C. LesherPerez, C. Yamanishi, J.M. Labuz, B. Leung, S. Takayama, Pharmacokinetic profile that reduces nephrotoxicity of gentamicin in a perfused kidney-on-a-chip, Biofabrication 8 (2016), 015021.
[74] M. Kitsara, D. Kontziampasis, O. Agbulut, Y. Chen, Heart on a chip: micro-nanofabrication and microfluidics steering the future of cardiac tissue engineering, Microelectron Eng (2018).
[75] S. Bahrami, N. Baheiraei, M. Mohseni, M. Razavi, A. Ghaderi, B. Azizi, N. Rabiee, M. Karimi, Three-dimensional graphene foam as a conductive scaffold for cardiac tissue engineering, J Biomater Appl (2019), https://doi.org/10.1177/0885328219839037.
[76] H.B. Van der Worp, D.W. Howells, E.S. Sena, M.J. Porritt, S. Rewell, V. O'Collins, M.R. Macleod, Can animal models of disease reliably inform human studies? PLoS Med 7 (2010), e1000245.

[77] A. Marsano, C. Conficconi, M. Lemme, P. Occhetta, E. Gaudiello, E. Votta, G. Cerino, A. Redaelli, M. Rasponi, Beating heart on a chip: a novel microfluidic platform to generate functional 3D cardiac microtissues, Lab Chip 16 (2016) 599–610.
[78] O. Schneider, L. Zeifang, S. Fuchs, C. Sailer, P. Loskill, User-friendly and parallelized generation of human induced pluripotent stem cell-derived microtissues in a centrifugal heart-on-a-chip, Tissue Eng Part A 25 (2019) 786–798.
[79] A. Agarwal, J.A. Goss, A. Cho, M.L. McCain, K.K. Parker, Microfluidic heart on a chip for higher throughput pharmacological studies, Lab Chip 13 (2013) 3599–3608.
[80] N. Tandon, A. Marsano, R. Maidhof, K. Numata, C. Montouri-Sorrentino, C. Cannizzaro, J. Voldman, G. Vunjak-Novakovic, Surface-patterned electrode bioreactor for electrical stimulation, Lab Chip 10 (2010) 692–700.
[81] M. Yang, X. Zhang, Electrical assisted patterning of cardiac myocytes with controlled macroscopic anisotropy using a microfluidic dielectrophoresis chip, Sens Actuators A: Phys 135 (2007) 73–79.
[82] H. Parsa, B.Z. Wang, G. Vunjak-Novakovic, A microfluidic platform for the high-throughput study of pathological cardiac hypertrophy, Lab Chip 17 (2017) 3264–3271.
[83] J.U. Lind, T.A. Busbee, A.D. Valentine, F.S. Pasqualini, H. Yuan, M. Yadid, S.-J. Park, A. Kotikian, A.P. Nesmith, P.H. Campbell, Instrumented cardiac microphysiological devices via multimaterial three-dimensional printing, Nat Mater 16 (2017) 303.
[84] A. Grosberg, P.W. Alford, M.L. McCain, K.K. Parker, Ensembles of engineered cardiac tissues for physiological and pharmacological study: heart on a chip, Lab Chip 11 (2011) 4165–4173.
[85] F. Qian, C. Huang, Y.-D. Lin, A.N. Ivanovskaya, T.J. O'Hara, R.H. Booth, C.J. Creek, H.A. Enright, D.A. Soscia, A.M. Belle, Simultaneous electrical recording of cardiac electrophysiology and contraction on chip, Lab Chip 17 (2017) 1732–1739.
[86] B.M. Maoz, A. Herland, O.Y. Henry, W.D. Leineweber, M. Yadid, J. Doyle, R. Mannix, V.J. Kujala, E.A. FitzGerald, K.K. Parker, Organs-on-chips with combined multi-electrode array and transepithelial electrical resistance measurement capabilities, Lab Chip 17 (2017) 2294–2302.
[87] G.P. Gupta, J. Massagué, Cancer metastasis: building a framework, Cell 127 (2006) 679–695.
[88] M. Allinen, R. Beroukhim, L. Cai, C. Brennan, J. Lahti-Domenici, H. Huang, D. Porter, M. Hu, L. Chin, A. Richardson, Molecular characterization of the tumor microenvironment in breast cancer, Cancer Cell 6 (2004) 17–32.
[89] F. Pezzella, Cancer and blood vessels: a complex relationship, J Lung Cancer Diagn Treat 1 (2016) 104.
[90] K.E. Sung, D.J. Beebe, Microfluidic 3D models of cancer, Adv Drug Deliv Rev 79 (2014) 68–78.
[91] Z. Zhang, S. Nagrath, Microfluidics and cancer: are we there yet? Biomed Microdevices 15 (2013) 595–609.
[92] D.T. Chiu, N.L. Jeon, S. Huang, R.S. Kane, C.J. Wargo, I.S. Choi, D.E. Ingber, G.M. Whitesides, Patterned deposition of cells and proteins onto surfaces by using three-dimensional microfluidic systems, Proc Natl Acad Sci U S A 97 (2000) 2408–2413.
[93] W. Saadi, S.-J. Wang, F. Lin, N.L. Jeon, A parallel-gradient microfluidic chamber for quantitative analysis of breast cancer cell chemotaxis, Biomed Microdevices 8 (2006) 109–118.
[94] M. Chanasakulniyom, A. Glidle, J.M. Cooper, Cell proliferation and migration inside single cell arrays, Lab Chip 15 (2015) 208–215.
[95] X. Lin, Q. Chen, W. Liu, J. Zhang, S. Wang, Z. Lin, J.-M. Lin, Oxygen-induced cell migration and on-line monitoring biomarkers modulation of cervical cancers on a microfluidic system, Sci Rep 5 (2015).

[96] Q. Zhang, T. Liu, J. Qin, A microfluidic-based device for study of transendothelial invasion of tumor aggregates in realtime, Lab Chip 12 (2012) 2837–2842.
[97] C. Kim, J. Kasuya, J. Jeon, S. Chung, R.D. Kamm, A quantitative microfluidic angiogenesis screen for studying anti-angiogenic therapeutic drugs, Lab Chip 15 (2015) 301–310.
[98] N. Ferrara, R.S. Kerbel, Angiogenesis as a therapeutic target, Nature 438 (2005) 967–974.
[99] J. Folkman, Angiogenesis: an organizing principle for drug discovery? Nat Rev Drug Discov 6 (2007) 273–286.
[100] E.W. Young, Cells, tissues, and organs on chips: challenges and opportunities for the cancer tumor microenvironment, Integr Biol 5 (2013) 1096–1109.
[101] Z. Xu, Y. Gao, Y. Hao, E. Li, Y. Wang, J. Zhang, W. Wang, Z. Gao, Q. Wang, Application of a microfluidic chip-based 3D co-culture to test drug sensitivity for individualized treatment of lung cancer, Biomaterials 34 (2013) 4109–4117.
[102] S. Chung, R. Sudo, P.J. Mack, C.-R. Wan, V. Vickerman, R.D. Kamm, Cell migration into scaffolds under co-culture conditions in a microfluidic platform, Lab Chip 9 (2009) 269–275.
[103] P.-A. Vidi, T. Maleki, M. Ochoa, L. Wang, S.M. Clark, J.F. Leary, S.A. Lelièvre, Disease-on-a-chip: mimicry of tumor growth in mammary ducts, Lab Chip 14 (2014) 172–177.
[104] T.-H. Hsu, Y.-L. Kao, W.-L. Lin, J.-L. Xiao, P.-L. Kuo, C.-W. Wu, W.-Y. Liao, C.-H. Lee, The migration speed of cancer cells influenced by macrophages and myofibroblasts co-cultured in a microfluidic chip, Integr Biol 4 (2012) 177–182.
[105] A.Y. Hsiao, Y.-s. Torisawa, Y.-C. Tung, S. Sud, R.S. Taichman, K.J. Pienta, S. Takayama, Microfluidic system for formation of PC-3 prostate cancer co-culture spheroids, Biomaterials 30 (2009) 3020–3027.
[106] K. Kwapiszewska, A. Michalczuk, M. Rybka, R. Kwapiszewski, Z. Brzózka, A microfluidic-based platform for tumour spheroid culture, monitoring and drug screening, Lab Chip 14 (2014) 2096–2104.
[107] W. Liu, J.-C. Wang, J. Wang, Controllable organization and high throughput production of recoverable 3D tumors using pneumatic microfluidics, Lab Chip 15 (2015) 1195–1204.
[108] C.L. Chaffer, R.A. Weinberg, A perspective on cancer cell metastasis, Science 331 (2011) 1559–1564.
[109] S. Valastyan, R.A. Weinberg, Tumor metastasis: molecular insights and evolving paradigms, Cell 147 (2011) 275–292.
[110] S. Bersini, J.S. Jeon, G. Dubini, C. Arrigoni, S. Chung, J.L. Charest, M. Moretti, R.D. Kamm, A microfluidic 3D in vitro model for specificity of breast cancer metastasis to bone, Biomaterials 35 (2014) 2454–2461.
[111] M.B. Esch, A.S. Smith, J.-M. Prot, C. Oleaga, J.J. Hickman, M.L. Shuler, How multi-organ microdevices can help foster drug development, Adv Drug Deliv Rev 69 (2014) 158–169.
[112] D. Wlodkowic, J.M. Cooper, Tumors on chips: oncology meets microfluidics, Curr Opin Chem Biol 14 (2010) 556–567.
[113] J.H. Sung, M.L. Shuler, A micro cell culture analog (μCCA) with 3-D hydrogel culture of multiple cell lines to assess metabolism-dependent cytotoxicity of anti-cancer drugs, Lab Chip 9 (2009) 1385–1394.
[114] H. Lee, D.S. Kim, S.K. Ha, I. Choi, J.M. Lee, J.H. Sung, A pumpless multi-organ-on-a-chip (MOC) combined with a pharmacokinetic–pharmacodynamics (PK–PD) model, Biotechnol Bioeng 114 (2017) 432–443.

CHAPTER

Microfluidics in organic chemistry

10

Beheshteh Khodadadi Chegeni*

Oncopathology Research Center, Iran University of Medical Sciences, Tehran, Iran

**Corresponding author. E-mail: Beheshteh.khodadadi@gmail.com*

10.1 Introduction

Over the past decades, the study of organic chemistry reactions has allowed the synthesis of molecules such as natural products, drugs, and polymers. The investigation of organic molecules and chemical reactions within microfluidic systems has emerged as an ideal route to solve critical issues in organic chemistry and industry. This novel technology, which has developed via to perform reactions under continuous flow conditions instead of conventional batch chemistry, as a basic tool for chemical synthesis has created new promising horizons and new opportunities in many areas of research and it is growing rapidly, especially in industry. The limitations of conventional chemical synthesis include the requirement for the vigorous stirring of reaction mixtures, the presence of by-products, unstable intermediates, and so on.

The vast majority of efforts in microscale chemical reactions have been performed to address these limitations [1–3]. Macroscale reactions have many restrictions, such as poor control of mass transfer, large quantities of toxic or expensive reagents, low selectivity, producing many by-products, the requirement for high temperatures, and long reaction times that could be precisely controlled in microscale reactions [4–8]. The microreactors avoid waste of reactants and energy by reducing the side reactions. For example, microreactors can be designed for the improvement of gas-liquid-solid reactions relying on the principles of gas-liquid chromatography [9].

Microfluidic reactors can manipulate and control fluids using components with internal dimensions ranging between several micrometers and hundreds of micrometers. The first microfluidic device was described in 1940 [10], after which the technology for microfluidic reactions for the synthesis of chemical materials was expanded by many researchers in different institutes, such as GlaxoSmithKline (United Kingdom) [11], Imperial College London (United Kingdom) [12], and so on. Generally, the size of the microfluidic structure and the properties of the produced materials are very important factors in the applicability of microfluidic reactors.

Biomedical Applications of Microfluidic Devices. https://doi.org/10.1016/B978-0-12-818791-3.00011-5

The range of materials used for fabrication of the different types of microfluidic reactors is extensive, e.g., polymers, ceramics, and so on that are generally selected according to the type of the desired reaction.

Mass transfer is one of the most important advantages of microfluidic reactors, that can be enhanced by increasing the interfacial contact between the phases. Mixing times can come down to several milliseconds and an approximately complete mixture can be obtained within a few seconds in microfluidic reactors. The higher ratio of the surface area to volume in microfluidic reactors can cause higher heat-exchange efficiency compared to bulk reactors. This ultimately causes rapid heating and cooling of reaction mixtures within the microstructures.

Coiled tubing, chip-based, packed-bed, and tube-in-tube reactors and the new microfluidic nebulator are some important types of reactors that have been used for conducting organic reactions.

Besides, better control and simplicity of intermediates and selective reactions can be achieved via microfluidic devices, compared to conventional bulk reactors. The possibility of performing multistep sequences of individual reactions is another benefit of microfluidic technology.

In this chapter, we review the important advantages of microfluidic reactors for the improvement of synthetic methods for organic compounds, materials, and drugs. We begin Section 10.2 with an introduction to the different types of microreactors in organic chemistry. In the following sections, we review several important syntheses that have been optimized by microfluidic reactors over a broad range of organic chemistry.

10.2 Microfluidic devices used in organic chemistry

Today, various types of microfluidic devices have been developed from materials such as polymers [13, 14], ceramics [15], and silicon [16] for organic reactions. Their designs depend on the properties of the constructed materials and the reactions, but can still be considered to be in an early stage. These reactors play an important role in chemical synthesis with improved conditions, so they are promising in expeditious organic synthesis. In this section, some useful and efficient microfluidic reactors are introduced and their features (pros and cons) are analyzed and discussed for organic synthetic procedures.

A nebulator type of microfluidic device that produces amorphous nanoparticles (NPs) with a very small size using a supersonic spray drier was reported. Supersonic airspeeds could be achieved at moderate pressure in this device. The device was constructed from poly(dimethylsiloxane) (PDMS) with six air inlets and could control the flow of air [17]. The microfluidic nebulator had many advantages such as being constructed of an amorphous material that enhanced the bioavailability of hydrophobic drugs [18], lack of crystal structures due to high drying speed [19], increasing the solubility of amorphous materials, enhancing their stability in storage by reducing the particle size, and no requirement for excipients [17, 20]. Hydrophobic organic drugs (e.g., fenofibrate and clotrimazole) were produced by the microfluidic nebulator with a smaller size, excellent stability, well separated, and remained amorphous for several months [20, 21].

A coiled tubing microreactor is another type of microfluidic device used in a broad spectrum of organic syntheses. These microreactors can be constructed of inert material such as thermosetting polymers [e.g., perfluoroalkoxy (PFA), polyetheretherketone (PEEK), Teflon, or stainless steel]. Fluorination [22], nitration [23], halogenation [24, 25], and oxidation [26, 27] are some interesting and important reactions that have been performed in this microreactor.

Nitrile synthesis is one of the prominent reactions in organic chemistry. This reaction has found little application due to the very high temperatures required and generally has low yields. These reactions on a large scale can be dangerous due to the high vapor pressure produced by the solvent evaporation. This problem can be solved using microfluidic technology.

Kappe et al. used the coiled tubing type microreactor for nitrile synthesis (Fig. 10.1). Nitrile synthesis is an acid-nitrile exchange reaction with acetonitrile solvent, without using any catalyst and needs high-temperature conditions. Kappe et al. showed that different types of aromatic and aliphatic carboxylic acids could be converted to the corresponding nitriles (Table 10.1) and applied the same conditions for benzoic acid. They observed that in entries 2–6, despite the conditions such as high temperature, very good compatibility was achieved with halogen, nitro, alcohol, and ester functional groups (Table 10.1). In most instances, nitriles were successfully synthesized in good to excellent yield [25].

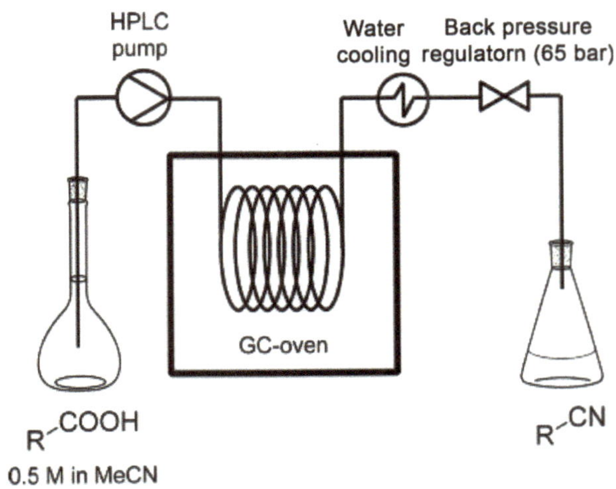

FIG. 10.1

Schematic diagram of the continuous-flow setup used for the preparation of organic nitriles from carboxylic acids.

Reproduced with permission from Cantillo D, Kappe CO. Direct preparation of nitriles from carboxylic acids in continuous flow. J Org Chem 2013;78(20):10567–71. Copyright (2013), The Journal of Organic Chemistry.

Table 10.1 Synthesis of organic nitriles from carboxylic acids and acetonitrile in continuous flow.[a]

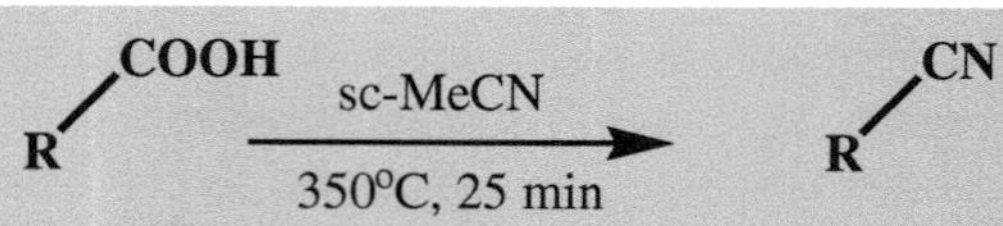

Entry	Substrate	Conversion (%)[b]	Yield[c]
1	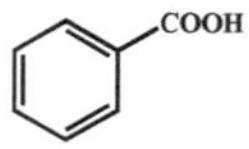	95	**89**
2	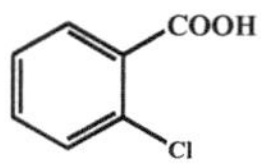	99	**97**
3	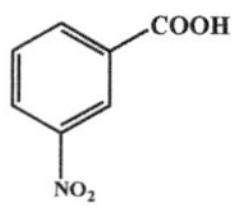	94	**90**
4	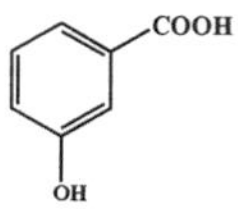	92	**78**
5	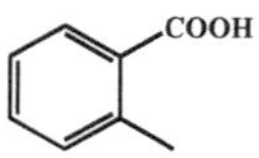	92	**90**
6	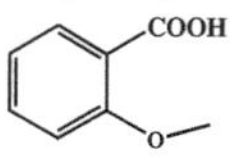	98	**92**
7	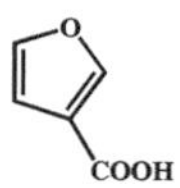	91	**86**
8	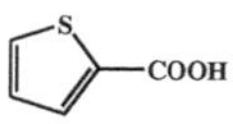	88	**82**
9	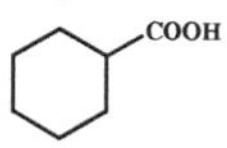	–[d]	**72**
10	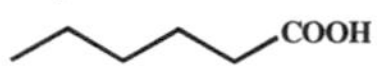	–[d]	**78**
11	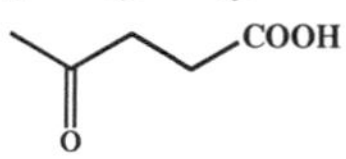	–[d]	**85**

[a] *Conditions: 0.5 M acid in acetonitrile, 350°C, 0.4 mL min^{-1} (25 min residence time).*
[b] *HPLC conversion (215 nm).*
[c] *Isolated yields from 10 mL (5 mmol) of the crude reaction mixture.*
[d] *Not determined.*

Flash vacuum pyrolysis (FVP) is a particular type of gas-phase thermolysis with the advantages of avoiding secondary reactions in the heating zone and produces a series of desired stable materials. In FVP, typically a sublimed substrate is produced in vacuum heated to temperatures of typically 400–1100°C and this is typically performed by a continuous-flow process. Therefore, intramolecular transformation reactions at high-temperature (for instance, eliminations, rearrangements, or cyclization processes) can be performed using this protocol [28, 29]. However, translating the procedure from a small-scale to a large-scale is difficult. Coiled tubing microreactors could resolve these issues, and also decrease the reaction time under the high-T/p conditions. For example, Kappe et al. in 2012 used a high-T/p liquid-phase "flash flow pyrolysis" (FFP) technique for the thermolysis of 2,2-dimethyl-1,3-dioxane-4,6-dione (Meldrum's acid) derivatives, pyrrole-2,3-diones, and pyrrole-2-carboxylic esters and obtained very good selectivity, for example, close to 90% for acylketene-acetone and about 98% for the oxoketene dimer [30].

The diethylaminosulfur trifluoride reagent, used for the synthesis of fluoro derivatives of alcohols and carbonyl compounds has some problems, for instance, volatility and water sensitivity, low conversion efficiency, and forming by-products in traditional batch methods. Ley et al. used a continuous-flow device constructed with flow tubes made from nonreactive plastic (PEEK, PTFE, PFA) to facilitate a class of fluorination syntheses such as nucleophilic, electrophilic fluorination, and trifluoromethylation. In this study, the technique not only overcame the existing challenges but also had a high efficiency of about 94% [22].

Development in microfluidic and lab-on-a-chip technologies have created excellent opportunities due to the miniaturization of the fluidic environment. A network of miniaturized channels enables microfluidic reactors to be embedded within a lab-on-chip [16]. These reactors have been prepared by techniques such as injection molding, hot embossing, or phase-separation-micromolding. Reactions under well-defined conditions can be performed using a lab-on-chip microfluidic reactor that is made of chemically and physically resistant substances with high thermal conductivity.

Another important class of compounds is β-amino alcohols that can be used in the synthesis of pharmaceutical drugs, namely, oxazolidones using β-amino alcohol precursors. Ring-opening of epoxides by reaction with amines is one of the most important and frequently used approaches to prepare β-amino compounds [31]. The addition of several equivalents of propan-2-amine, in a polar protic solvent for about 2 to 5 h are typically the conditions for this reaction in conventional batch synthesis. Studies have shown that the use of microreactors can match or exceed the efficiency in many cases. Jamison et al. used a lab-on-chip microfluidic device to prepare the pharmaceutical drugs, indacaterol and metoprolol (marketed under the trade-name Lopressor) (Fig. 10.2). Metoprolol is a specific drug to treat hypertension (high blood pressure) with β-amino alcohol functional groups. Synthesis of metoprolol by a silicon-chip-based microfluidic process could be performed at 240°C with only 15 s residence time and a yield of metoprolol up to 7 gh^{-1}. Thus, this reaction was improved by utilizing a silicon-chip-based microfluidic device [32].

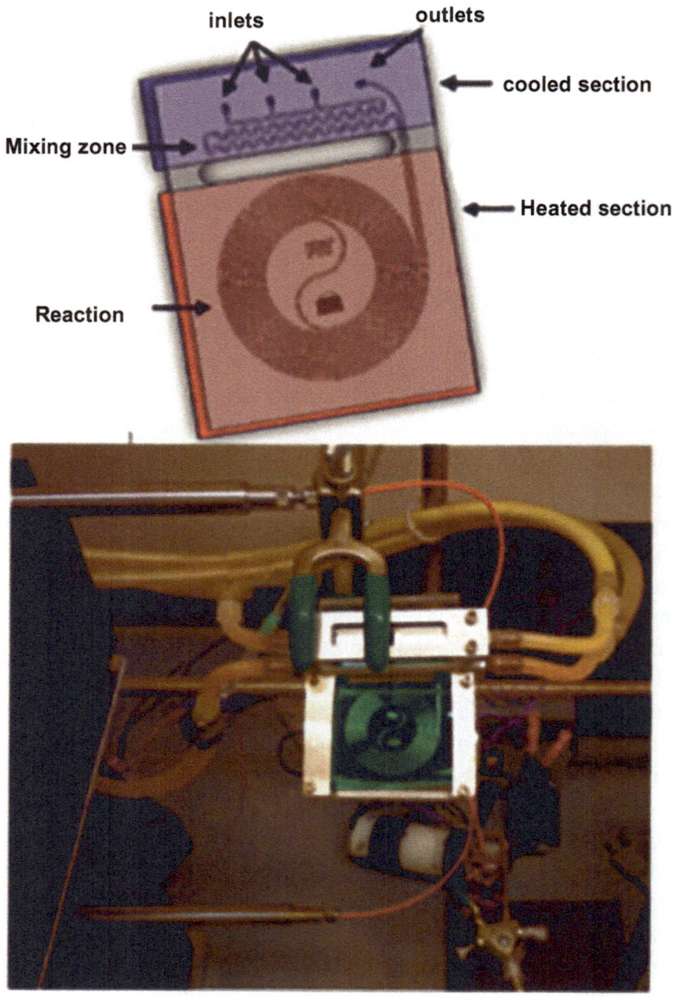

FIG. 10.2

Microreactor layout diagram and setup for preparing epoxide.

Reproduced with permission from Bedore MW, Zaborenko N, Jensen KF, Jamison TF. Aminolysis of epoxides in a microreactor system: a continuous flow approach to β-amino alcohols. Org Process Res Dev 2010;14(2):432–40. Copyright (2010), Organic Process Research & Development.

Another microfluidic reactor used for two-phase liquid-gas reactions was a ring-shaped microfluidic device with the outside being a thick-walled impermeable tube, and an internal PTFE tube constructed of a gas-permeable Teflon AF-2400 membrane as a selective membrane for passing gases and excluding liquids [33, 34]. Teflon AF-2400 is an amorphous commercially available polymer of 1,1,2,2-tetrafluoroethene and perfluoro-dimethyl dioxolane monomers whose permeability to a variety of gases (such as O_3) can be tailored.

This microfluidic reactor with the gas-permeable membrane was studied for improving the safety of both homogeneous and heterogeneous catalytic reactions with only minimal gas content and effectively removing excess unreacted materials.

Ozonolysis is an extremely useful synthetic reaction. Ozonation a highly efficient biphasic exothermic gas/liquid reaction that produces ozonides and/or hydroperoxides in the liquid phase, but explosive mixtures of solvent vapors plus oxygen and ozone gases are present in the gas phase [35]. This reaction has a hazardous nature because of the intermediate ozonides and peroxy materials [36]. Hence, a microstructured reactor could be useful for ozonolysis reactions, for instance, a two-step process for the production of intermediates in the synthesis of vitamin D analogs employs an ozonolysis reaction with the unsaturated bonds of alkenes and a subsequent reduction step [37].

One of the most widely used and important reactions is the catalytic hydrogenation of unsaturated bonds that is the cornerstone of many important synthetic routes [38, 39]. This reaction is popular because hydrogen molecules are very cheap, readily available, nontoxic, and it can be used in excess, and the unreacted gas can be simply removed at the end of the procedure. However, the hydrogenation reaction has serious problems. High concentrations of hydrogen proportional to the pressure (Boyle's law for gas-phase, Henry's law for solutions) that are used in most hydrogenation processes have a significant safety consideration.

Hydrogenations could be carried out using the continuous microfluidic protocol, with a low volume local operating reactor, could be safer compared to the corresponding batch procedure with a large volume. A ring-shaped microfluidic reactor was able to quickly deliver the gas to the liquid reactant flow through a central semipermeable Teflon AF-2400 tubing. Ley et al. used an efficient, economical, and scalable tube-in-tube reactor/injector for both homogeneous and heterogeneous hydrogenation, in which only a small volume of gas needed pressurization. They found that the permeable tubing allowed gas uptake into the solution, by both a burette method and a new computer-assisted "bubble counting" method and the reaction proceeded rapidly [40].

Another achievement of the tube-in-tube microfluidic procedure was a carbonylation reaction with improved safety. Carbon monoxide (CO) is a practical source of carbonyl groups used for the production of a broad range of carbonyl compounds, including aldehydes, ketones, carboxylic acids, etc. CO is problematic using batch techniques owing to the difficulty in handling the odorless, colorless, toxic, tasteless, and inflammable gas, CO. These microfluidic devices consisted of a two-chamber reactor with two novel solid CO precursors that were employed in this novel approach for low-pressure carbonylation reactions with improved simplicity and safety [33].

Another type of microfluidic reactor used for many reactions (hydrogenation, oxidation, acid-catalyzed reactions, etherification) is known as a microfluidic packed-bed reactor [41]. Bourne et al. used a self-optimizing packed-bed continuous flow reactor, coupled with online analysis for the optimization of 1-pentanol methylation in supercritical carbon dioxide (scCO_2) using dimethyl carbonate (DMC) and methanol as alkylating agents with an γ-alumina catalyst [42]. They found higher yields of pentyl methyl ether reacting with DCM under milder conditions using four reaction parameters.

Leitner and coworkers studied the asymmetric catalytic transformation of low-volatility organic substrates by a highly efficient continuous-flow process. The procedure involved a chiral transition-metal complex in a supported ionic liquid phase (SILP) with $scCO_2$ flow. They obtained high enantioselectivity and quantitative conversion in the hydrogenation of dimethyl itaconate, yielding an analytically pure isolated product using an automated high-pressure continuous-flow setup. The optimized system with $0.7\,kg\,L^{-1}\,h^{-1}$ space-time yield and productivity of more than 100 kg product per gram of rhodium, or 14 kg per gram of ligand, produced good selectivity and yield of chemically and optically pure materials making it attractive for larger-scale applications [43].

Similarly, the packed-bed microfluidic reactor can be used for organic synthesis such as hydrogenation of complex a pharmaceutical intermediate, *rac*-sertraline in $scCO_2$. In this study, superior levels of selectivity were attained at 40°C, 175 bar pressure using a palladium/calcium carbonate ($Pd/CaCO_3$) catalyst. Under optimized conditions, lower levels of side reactions such as dechlorination and dehydrogenation were observed. The obtained selectivity could be related to the rapid heat transfer ability of $scCO_2$ in removing the excess heat from the catalyst surface [44]. The packed-bed microfluidic reactor can also be used for carbonylative coupling reactions. By using a microfluidic continuous flow reactor (X-Cube) operating at high pressure and high temperature, halogenated aryl carboxylic acids were effectively transformed into the corresponding dicarboxylic acid monoamides, and the optimal reaction parameters (solvent, base, catalyst, pressure, temperature) were rapidly optimized with a higher overall reaction rate, compared to the batch technique. As a result, the packed-bed microfluidic reactor was able to automate parallel reactions of compound libraries and allowed many optimized syntheses [45].

10.3 Effect of microfluidics on reducing by-products in organic synthesis

The synthesis of complex organic molecules, which are usually multistep reactions, requires the removal of by-products and the isolation and purification of reaction intermediates [46, 47] Since the early 1970s, optimizing synthetic reactions has received significant attention [48, 49]. The multistep substitution of functional groups such as aryl, vinyl, and alkyl halide/pseudohalide can be carried out using a nucleophile in the presence of a metal catalyst. In these reactions, C–C and C–X bonds are formed in three steps including (1) oxidative addition, (2) transmetallation, and (3) reductive elimination [50, 51].

The Suzuki-Miyaura cross-coupling reaction (SMC) is one of the most important metal-catalyzed reactions. In SMC reactions, the coupling of functional groups such as aryl, vinyl, and alkyl halides/pseudo halides with organoboron compounds takes place under basic conditions through carbon-carbon bond-formation [52, 53].

However, multistep reactions have many problems such as the formation of intermediates and by-products. In recent decades, continuous-flow reactors have attracted considerable attention in multistep synthesis due to their advantages of improved heat- and mass-transfer, the safety of operation, strict control of residence time, isolation of sensitive reactions from air and moisture, the facility of scale-up, and operating many devices simultaneously compared to traditional batch reactors [54].

Buchwald et al. in 2011 reported the use of SMC for linking various phenols with different arylboronic acids. They showed that a continuous-flow microfluidic system could be very effective in converting phenols to their corresponding aryl triflates, and subsequently transform the intermediate triflates into biaryls without the formation of any by-products.

The process in which an acyl group is added to a compound is called acylation. This reaction is a very important method in the formation of ferrocene derivative, such as ferrocenyl ketones as valuable intermediates. Di-acetylferrocene is a by-product obtained from the classical Friedel-Crafts acetylation [55–57]. Lei et al. used a microfluidic chip as the reactor for a fast and very selective acylation of ferrocene (Fig. 10.3). Synthesis of acylferrocenes from ferrocene with high yields could be obtained at room temperature without any by-product. Microfluidic chips provide precise control of temperature, and efficient mixing to improve this synthetic route [7].

Despite an abundance of examples, the exact mechanism of acetyl chloride esterification is still unknown. In general, the mechanism suggested for base-catalyzed acetylation includes a base-assisted nucleophilic reaction of the alcohol with acetyl chloride [58]. Intermediates such as the quaternary acetyl ammonium ion [59] or a highly reactive ketene formed via base-assisted alpha-elimination of hydrochloric acid from acetyl chloride [60]. Oosthoek-de Vries et al. studied the acetylation of benzyl alcohol using nuclear magnetic resonance (NMR) spectroscopy to determine the kinetics and mechanism of the reaction. The reaction products were identified by a combination of conventional 2D NMR techniques. According to their study, ketene and acetyl ammonium ion were the intermediates of the acetylation of benzyl alcohol in the presence of DIPEA and a tetrahedral intermediate was proposed for the reaction mechanism. The rate of reaction increased rapidly by replacing DIPEA with TEA [61].

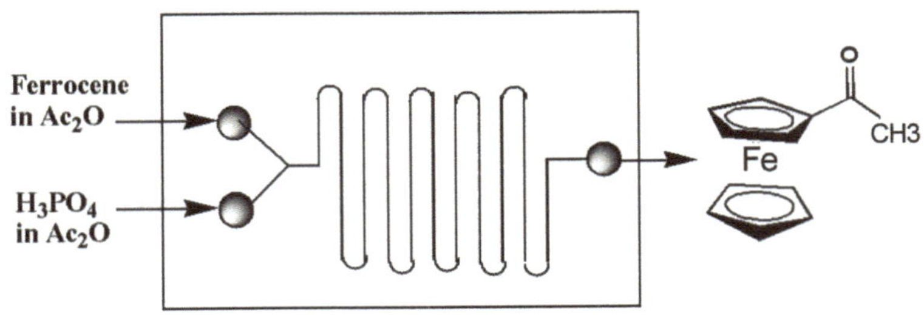

FIG. 10.3

Schematic structure of the microfluidic chip.

10.4 Effect of microfluidics on mass transfer in organic synthesis

Mass transfer is difficult in a multiphase or multistep reaction. Multiphase catalytic reactions including gas-liquid, gas-liquid-liquid, or gas-liquid-solid reactions are one of the most important reactions in both laboratory research and the chemical and pharmaceutical industries [62, 63]. However, these heterogeneous reactions often have a slow rate due to the extremely low efficiency and mass transfer rates compared to homogeneous reactions. In general, these reactions can be accelerated by increasing the contact surface between the two or three reacting phases, for instance, additional equipment or rapid stirring [64]. The use of microchannel devices with a high specific interfacial region per unit of volume from 10,000 to 50,000 $m^2 m^{-3}$, versus only 100 $m^2 m^{-3}$ for conventional reactors, can help to achieve efficient multiphase reactions. In these devices, the solid phase can be immobilized on the microchannel wall and the liquid or gas phase can flow over it. In general, multiphase microfluidic reactors suggest possessing wide and well-defined interfacial areas, rapid mixing, and fewer mass-transfer limitations [64–66].

Absorption of CO_2 into aqueous alkanolamines, the reaction of hydrogen sulfide with aqueous iron (III) sulfate, and ozonolysis, or the hydrogenation, fluorination, and chlorination of organic materials are some examples of gas-liquid reactions [67, 68]. Gas-liquid reactions have a wide variation of rate constants due to mass-transfer limitation and a poor interface between the gas and liquid phases [69, 70].

Chen et al. for the first time reported that CO_2 absorption in a gas-liquid reaction could occur by utilizing aqueous monoethanolamine in a T-type rectangular microchannel reactor with a hydraulic diameter of 408 μm. They found that for the absorption of CO_2 by aqueous monoethanolamine, the improved mass transfer enhanced the chemical reaction [71].

The effective combination of catalytic NPs (which increase the surface area) with microfluidic devices (that decrease the diffusion length) can improve multiphase reactions such as three-phase hydrogenation under mild reaction conditions by increasing mass transfer [72] (Fig. 10.4). Reactions with mass transfer limitation between the gas, liquid, and solid phases, are commonly performed at a high temperature and high hydrogen pressure over long periods, but have disadvantages such side reactions, lack of operator safety, and high consumption of energy [73, 74]. In this method, hydrogen diffusion to the catalytic sites can be increased via the combination of nanocatalysts and microfluidics which can eliminate mass transfer limitations [72].

In recent years, gas-liquid-liquid (G/L/L) multiphase flow has been used in microfluidics [75]. Önal et al. [76] studied the selective hydrogenation of α,β-unsaturated aldehydes with aqueous multiphase catalysis in a capillary microreactor, with two connected mixers in one line that can improve the surface to volume ratio. After that, Zhang et al. [77] used these parameters for their kinetic model of multiphase reaction. They studied the Beckmann rearrangement of cyclohexanone oxime in a multiphase microreactor. The addition of gas-phase while avoiding coalescence was considered an advantage to increase the mass-transfer rate in this system.

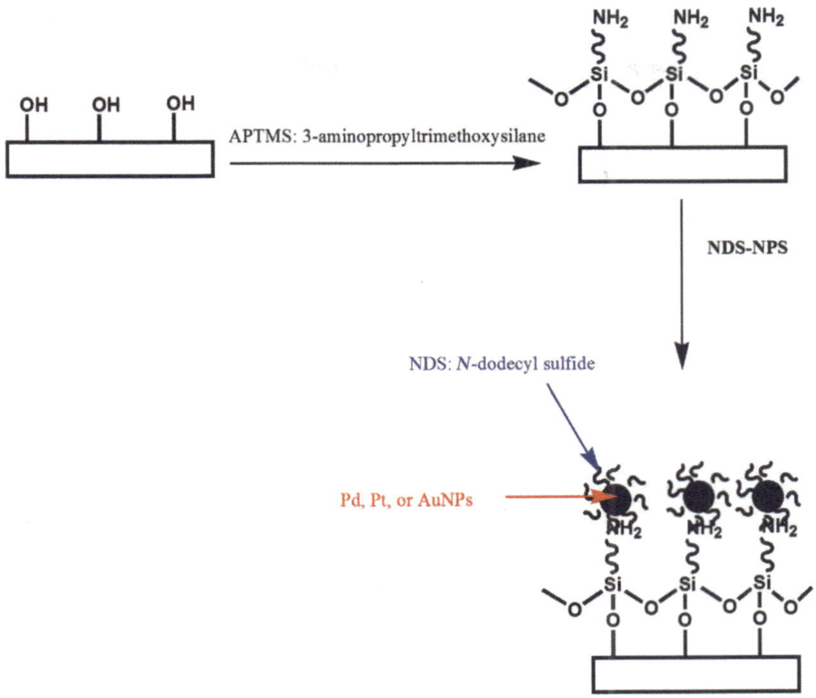

FIG. 10.4

Scheme for immobilization of NDS-stabilized NPs in a microfluidic reactor. The reactor surfaces were first treated with oxygen plasma to introduce hydroxyl groups, then aminosilanized by APTMS to form primary amine groups to which Pd, Pt, or AuNPs can attach through their stabilizing ligands to complete the immobilization [72].

10.5 Microreactors for the high-temperature synthesis

Microchannels with a high surface/volume ratio enable efficient heat transfer and can control the reaction temperature through better utilization or elimination of heat [78, 79]. As a consequence, reactions at high-temperature conditions can be performed in microreactors [80, 81] (and related continuous-flow reactors [82, 83]). A stainless steel microreactor can operate at high temperatures and pressures. In this microreactor, the reaction mixture is introduced into the steel coils and a heat exchanger using one (or more) standard high-performance liquid chromatography (HPLC) pumps. The pressure is controlled within a range of 50–200 bar of pressure, and the temperature is controlled at the outside of the coil, which controls the reaction temperature inside the coil [84].

Organic nitriles have a wide range of application as intermediates in the synthesis of different functional groups [85] or heterocycle compounds [86] and can be prepared from carboxylic acids. Although the reaction is easy for nitrile synthesis, this reaction generally should be heated above 300°C to attain sufficient rates, and still can have low yields. Moreover, this reaction has found little application, especially on a large scale due to the high vapor pressure produced from solvent evaporation. Microfluidic technology allowed a controllable procedure to be carried out at high-temperature high pressure (HTPT) conditions [87–90]. For example, the synthesis of benzonitrile from benzoic acid via a batch process produced by-products of benzamide and *N*-acetylbenzamide, which is not suitable for practical applications. Benzonitrile can be synthesized from benzoic acid in a 25 min residence time at high temperature and pressure (350°C and 65 bar) and about 94% yield. The microreactor is compatible with many functional groups, for instance, nitro, halogen, ester, etc. at high temperatures [91].

Kappe and coworkers investigated Diels-Alder reactions. They synthesized the cyclohexene adduct from 2,3-dimethyl butadiene and acrylonitrile in a microreactor with stainless steel coils. The Diels-Alder reaction is an important chemical reaction between a conjugated diene and an alkene. This cycloaddition generally can be performed within 20 min at 240°C (or 10 min at 250°C) in toluene as well as a sealed-vessel batch microwave. They showed full conversion was attained at 250°C (60 bar set pressure) at 0.8 mL min^{-1}flow rate [92].

The synthesis of tetrahydrocarbazole is another example of a reaction performed by stainless-steel coiled tubing microreactors. Conversion of 3-bromoanisole into 3-anisaldehyde in two-steps is difficult to scale up due to its very exothermic nature, and the yield is generally reduced with increasing the size of the reactor. Conversion of 3-bromoanisole into 3-anisaldehyde was successfully performed in a microreactor, and the heat-exchange capabilities were improved [93].

10.6 Effect of microfluidics on control of conversion and selectivity in organic synthesis

Conventional reactions use convection and turbulence for mixing the reactants. Microfluidic systems operating in the laminar flow regime with low Reynold numbers, where diffusion causes mass transfer for mixing and can be reduced using split-and-recombine mixing elements in this microreactor. Turbulent mixing in conventional reactions can produce high concentration gradients, while more homogeneous diffusion and reproducible reactions can be achieved in microfluidic reactors, which increases selectivity and remarkably decreases the formation of side products [94].

Synthesis of benzaldehyde by oxidation of benzyl alcohol is an important reaction in organic chemistry and the chemical industry [95]. In the traditional method, environmentally harmful organic solvents such as toluene [96], acetonitrile [97], and so on were used for oxidation of benzyl alcohol and the use of water as a safe solvent for oxidation also have low conversion and selectivity problems [98]. Rao et al. synthesized benzaldehyde using a microreactor with high conversion and selectivity in an aqueous solution. The system was constructed by immobilizing a gold-based catalyst on the surface of cyclic olefin copolymer (COC) microreactors. The AuNPs had high selectivity (94%) for benzaldehyde over at least 9 h of catalytic activity but the yield was only 20%, indicating relatively low productivity. In comparison, AuNP@ zeolite immobilized microreactors had high selectivity for benzaldehyde (>99%) with 42.4% conversion of benzyl alcohol that could be related to the synergistic interaction between the dual active sites of zeolite and AuNPs [99].

The selective alkylation of phenyl acetonitrile was used for monoalkylation in a microchannel reactor. In this reaction, by increasing the volumetric aqueous-to-organic phase flow ratio, the rate of reaction was increased, but the selectivity of the reaction was decreased due to the formation of side products by deprotonation reactions. The main goal of the research reported by Schouten and his colleagues in 2010 was the microfluidic control of the conversion and selectivity of this reaction. The conversion and selectivity of the synthesis in a microchannel reactor with 250-μm internal diameter were increased compared to a stirred batch reactor.

10.7 Multiphase microfluidic strategies for the synthesis of microparticles

Over the last decade, a large range of microparticles and microcapsules including hydrogels and microgels have been synthesized using multiphase microfluidic systems [100–102]. These can be used in a wide range of organic material syntheses [102, 103]. Microgels are typically polymerized in two separate steps, including droplet production, followed by cross-linking initiation via a temperature gradient, irradiation with UV, or a chemical reaction that performed by a catalyst [104–106]. Palladium (Pd)-loaded poly-hydromethylsiloxane (PHMS) gel could generate catalytically active Pd^0 by reducing the Pd^{2+} and could be used as the catalyst for reactions such as cross-coupling. These gels have advantages, such as avoiding the energy-intensive separation step, using less harsh solvents, and incorporating the catalyst into a porous scaffold [103, 107].

The synthesis of microparticles using conventional microfluidic procedures is difficult due to problems with PHMS, such as PHMS cross-linking by the hydrosilylation chemical method that has fast reaction kinetics, is poorly water-soluble, and forms the microparticles in a single step that which could eventually lead to clogging of the microchannels. Moreover, PHMS is incompatible with conventional PDMS-based microfluidic devices. Hence, Abolhasani and coworkers in 2018 prepared microparticles from an elastic silicone elastomer, with good loading capacity, and a tunable size by a multiphase microfluidic strategy. Off-the-shelf components were used to construct the capillary-based coaxial flow-focusing microfluidic device. They synthesized monodisperse PHMS microparticles in a single step. They built a microparticle-packed bed reactor (μPBR) by loading the microparticles into a tubular Teflon reactor (Fig. 10.5) and used them as microreaction vessels [103]. The award of the Nobel Prize in Chemistry for 2010 to Akira Suzuki and two other researchers is testimony to their valuable contribution to this cross-coupling reaction [108]. The μ-PBR reactor has many advantages such as enhancing the catalytic surface area and mass transport while maintaining catalytic activity and the advantages of a flow process [109–111].

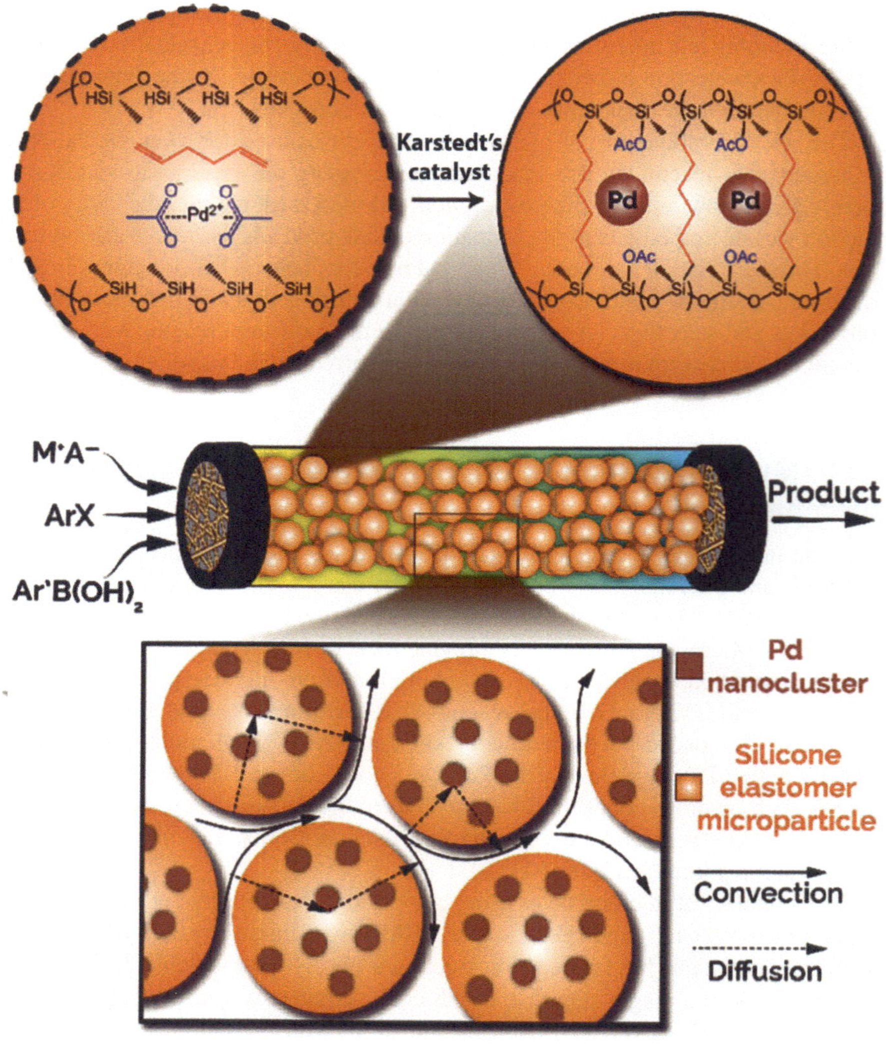

FIG. 10.5

Schematic of Pd-loaded PHMS microparticle synthesis by hydrosilylation cross-coupling and construction of the μ-PBR.

Reproduced with permission from Bennett JA, Kristof AJ, Vasudevan V, Genzer J, Srogl J, Abolhasani M. Microfluidic synthesis of elastomeric microparticles: a case study in catalysis of palladium-mediated cross-coupling. AIChE J 2018;64(8):3188–97. Copyright (2018), American Institute of Chemical Engineers Journals.

10.8 Summary

In this chapter, the important advantages of microfluidic reactors for the improvement of the synthesis of organic compounds and drugs have been reviewed. We began Section 10.2 with an introduction to different types of useful and efficient reactors in organic synthesis. These microfluidic devices owing to the improved mass and heat transfer are suitable for rapid and exothermic reactions. In the following section, we reviewed the advantages of the microfluidic reactor for the improvement of some selected important organic reactions.

We finished the chapter with two illustrative multiphase microfluidic strategies that use microfluidics for the synthesis of microparticles.

References

[1] M.M. Singh, Z. Szafran, R.M. Pike, Microscale chemistry and green chemistry: complementary pedagogies, J Chem Educ 76 (12) (1999) 1684.

[2] J.G. Ibanez, M.M. Singh, R.M. Pike, Z. Szafran, Laboratory experiments on electrochemical remediation of the environment part 3: microscale electrokinetic processing of soils, J Chem Educ 75 (5) (1998) 634.

[3] N. Kockmann, M. Gottsponer, B. Zimmermann, D.M. Roberge, Enabling continuous-flow chemistry in microstructured devices for pharmaceutical and fine-chemical production, Chemistry 14 (25) (2008) 7470–7477.

[4] K.S. Elvira, X. Casadevall i Solvas, R.C. Wootton, A.J. de Mello, The past, present and potential for microfluidic reactor technology in chemical synthesis, Nat Chem 5 (11) (2013) 905–915. 24153367. (Epub 2013/10/25. eng).

[5] S.H. DeWitt, Micro reactors for chemical synthesis, Curr Opin Chem Biol 3 (3) (1999) 350–356.

[6] P.L. Mills, D.J. Quiram, J.F. Ryley, Microreactor technology and process miniaturization for catalytic reactions—a perspective on recent developments and emerging technologies, Chem Eng Sci 62 (24) (2007) 6992–7010.

[7] R.-J. Hu, M. Lei, H.-S. Xiong, X. Mu, Y.-G. Wang, X.-F. Yin, Highly selective acylation of ferrocene using microfluidic chip reactor, Tetrahedron Lett 49 (2) (2008) 387–389.

[8] S.-Y. Teh, R. Lin, L.-H. Hung, A.P. Lee, Droplet microfluidics, Lab Chip 8 (2) (2008) 198–220.

[9] V. Hessel, P. Angeli, A. Gavriilidis, H. Löwe, Gas – liquid and gas – liquid – solid microstructured reactors: contacting principles and applications, Ind Eng Chem Res 44 (25) (2005) 9750–9769.

[10] J.S.L. Philpot, The use of thin layers in electrophoretic separation, Trans Faraday Soc 35 (1940) 38–46.

[11] E. Garcia-Egido, S.Y.F. Wong, B.H. Warrington, A Hantzsch synthesis of 2-aminothiazoles performed in a heated microreactor system, Lab Chip 2 (1) (2002) 31–33.

[12] R. Srinivasan, S.L. Firebaugh, I. Hsing, J. Ryley, M.P. Harold, K.F. Jensen, et al. (Eds.), Chemical performance and high temperature characterization of micromachined chemical reactors, Proceedings of international solid state sensors and actuators conference (transducers '97), 19 June 1997, 1997.

[13] A. Guber, M. Heckele, D. Herrmann, A. Muslija, V. Saile, L. Eichhorn, et al., Microfluidic lab-on-a-chip systems based on polymers—fabrication and application, Chem Eng J 101 (2004) 447–453.
[14] J.P. Rolland, R.M. Van Dam, D.A. Schorzman, S.R. Quake, J.M. DeSimone, Solvent-resistant photocurable "Liquid Teflon" for microfluidic device fabrication, J Am Chem Soc 126 (8) (2004) 2322–2323.
[15] R. Knitter, D. Göhring, P. Risthaus, J. Haußelt, Microfabrication of ceramic microreactors, Microsyst Technol 7 (3) (2001) 85–90.
[16] K. Geyer, J.D.C. Codée, P.H. Seeberger, Microreactors as tools for synthetic chemists—the chemists' round-bottomed flask of the 21st century? Chemistry 12 (33) (2006) 8434–8442.
[17] E. Amstad, M. Gopinadhan, C. Holtze, C.O. Osuji, M.P. Brenner, F. Spaepen, et al., Nanoparticles. Production of amorphous nanoparticles by supersonic spray-drying with a microfluidic nebulator, Science 349 (6251) (2015) 956–960. 26315432. (Epub 2015/09/01. eng).
[18] R. Laitinen, K. Lobmann, C.J. Strachan, H. Grohganz, T. Rades, Emerging trends in the stabilization of amorphous drugs, Int J Pharm 453 (1) (2013) 65–79. 22569230. (Epub 2012/05/10. eng).
[19] Y. Kawabata, K. Wada, M. Nakatani, S. Yamada, S. Onoue, Formulation design for poorly water-soluble drugs based on biopharmaceutics classification system: basic approaches and practical applications, Int J Pharm 420 (1) (2011) 1–10. 21884771. (Epub 2011/09/03. eng).
[20] E. Amstad, F. Spaepen, D.A. Weitz, Crystallization of undercooled liquid fenofibrate, Phys Chem Chem Phys 17 (44) (2015) 30158–30161.
[21] E. Amstad, F. Spaepen, D.A. Weitz, Stabilization of the amorphous structure of spray-dried drug nanoparticles, J Phys Chem B 120 (34) (2016) 9161–9165. 27441485. (Epub 2016/07/22. eng).
[22] M. Baumann, I.R. Baxendale, L.J. Martin, S.V. Ley, Development of fluorination methods using continuous-flow microreactors, Tetrahedron 65 (33) (2009) 6611–6625.
[23] D. Cantillo, M. Damm, D. Dallinger, M. Bauser, M. Berger, C.O. Kappe, Sequential nitration/hydrogenation protocol for the synthesis of triaminophloroglucinol: safe generation and use of an explosive intermediate under continuous-flow conditions, Org Process Res Dev 18 (11) (2014) 1360–1366.
[24] J.R. Breen, G. Sandford, D.S. Yufit, J.A.K. Howard, J. Fray, B. Patel, Continuous gas/liquid-liquid/liquid flow synthesis of 4-fluoropyrazole derivatives by selective direct fluorination, Beilstein J Org Chem 7 (2011) 1048–1054. 21915207. (Epub 2011/08/02. eng).
[25] D. Šterk, M. Jukič, Z. Časar, Application of flow photochemical bromination in the synthesis of a 5-bromomethylpyrimidine precursor of rosuvastatin: improvement of productivity and product purity, Org Process Res Dev 17 (1) (2013) 145–151.
[26] P.J. Nieuwland, K. Koch, N. van Harskamp, R. Wehrens, J.C. van Hest, F.P. Rutjes, Flash chemistry extensively optimized: high-temperature Swern-Moffatt oxidation in an automated microreactor platform, Chem Asian J 5 (4) (2010) 799–805. 20166118. (Epub 2010/02/19. eng).
[27] Z. He, T.F. Jamison, Continuous-flow synthesis of functionalized phenols by aerobic oxidation of Grignard reagents, Angew Chem Int Ed Eng 53 (13) (2014) 3353–3357. 24554581. (Epub 2014/02/21. eng).

[28] R.F.C. Brown, Pyrolytic methods in organic chemistry. Application of flow and flash vacuum pyrolytic techniques, Academic Press, New York, 1980 (XII, 347 S., geb. $ 38.50. 1981;93(6–7):625).

[29] M. Karpf, Organic synthesis at high temperatures. Gas-phase flow thermolysis [new synthetic methods (57)], Angew Chem Int Ed Eng 25 (5) (1986) 414–430.

[30] D. Cantillo, H. Sheibani, C.O. Kappe, Flash flow pyrolysis: mimicking flash vacuum pyrolysis in a high-temperature/high-pressure liquid-phase microreactor environment, J Org Chem 77 (5) (2012) 2463–2473.

[31] T.-X. Métro, J. Appenzeller, D. Gomez Pardo, J. Cossy, Highly enantioselective synthesis of β-amino alcohols, Org Lett 8 (16) (2006) 3509–3512.

[32] M.W. Bedore, N. Zaborenko, K.F. Jensen, T.F. Jamison, Aminolysis of epoxides in a microreactor system: a continuous flow approach to β-amino alcohols, Org Process Res Dev 14 (2) (2010) 432–440.

[33] C. Brancour, T. Fukuyama, Y. Mukai, T. Skrydstrup, I. Ryu, Modernized low pressure carbonylation methods in batch and flow employing common acids as a CO source, Org Lett 15 (11) (2013) 2794–2797.

[34] M. O'Brien, I.R. Baxendale, S.V. Ley, Flow ozonolysis using a semipermeable teflon AF-2400 membrane to effect gas – liquid contact, Org Lett 12 (7) (2010) 1596–1598.

[35] V. Tyagi, A.K. Gupta, Efficient and convenient method for workup of ozonolysis reaction using sodium hydrosulfite, Synth Commun 42 (6) (2012) 843–848.

[36] D. Noller, S. Mazurowski, G. Linden, F. De Leeuw, O. Mageli, Correction—a relative hazard classification of organic peroxides, Ind Eng Chem 57 (6) (1965) 17.

[37] S. Hübner, U. Bentrup, U. Budde, K. Lovis, T. Dietrich, A. Freitag, et al., An ozonolysis–reduction sequence for the synthesis of pharmaceutical intermediates in microstructured devices, Org Process Res Dev 13 (2009) 952–960.

[38] R. Noyori, T. Ohkuma, M. Kitamura, H. Takaya, N. Sayo, H. Kumobayashi, et al., Asymmetric hydrogenation of .beta.-keto carboxylic esters. A practical, purely chemical access to .beta.-hydroxy esters in high enantiomeric purity, J Am Chem Soc 109 (19) (1987) 5856–5858.

[39] S. Nishimura, Handbook of heterogeneous catalytic hydrogenation for organic synthesis, Wiley-VCH, New York, 2001. 700 pp. $175.00. ISBN:0-471-39698-2. Org Process Res Dev. 2001 ;5(6):669–70.

[40] M. O'Brien, N. Taylor, A. Polyzos, I.R. Baxendale, S.V. Ley, Hydrogenation in flow: homogeneous and heterogeneous catalysis using Teflon AF-2400 to effect gas–liquid contact at elevated pressure, Chem Sci 2 (7) (2011) 1250–1257.

[41] X. Han, M. Poliakoff, Continuous reactions in supercritical carbon dioxide: problems, solutions and possible ways forward, Chem Soc Rev 41 (4) (2012) 1428–1436.

[42] R.A. Bourne, R.A. Skilton, A.J. Parrott, D.J. Irvine, M. Poliakoff, Adaptive process optimization for continuous methylation of alcohols in supercritical carbon dioxide, Org Process Res Dev 15 (4) (2011) 932–938.

[43] U. Hintermair, G. Franciò, W. Leitner, A fully integrated continuous-flow system for asymmetric catalysis: enantioselective hydrogenation with supported ionic liquid phase catalysts using supercritical CO2 as the mobile phase, Chem Eur J 19 (14) (2013) 4538–4547.

[44] P. Clark, M. Poliakoff, A. Wells, Continuous flow hydrogenation of a pharmaceutical intermediate, [4-(3,4-dichlorophenyl)-3,4-dihydro-2H-naphthalenyidene]methylamine, in supercritical carbon dioxide, Adv Synth Catal 349 (17–18) (2007) 2655–2659.

[45] R. Jones, L. Gödörházy, D. Szalay, J. Gerencsér, G. Dormán, L. Ürge, et al., A novel method for high-throughput reduction of compounds through automated sequential injection into a continuous-flow microfluidic reactor, QSAR Comb Sci 24 (6) (2005) 722–727.
[46] K. Tamao, K. Sumitani, M. Kumada, Selective carbon-carbon bond formation by cross-coupling of Grignard reagents with organic halides. Catalysis by nickel-phosphine complexes, J Am Chem Soc 94 (12) (1972) 4374–4376.
[47] R.J.P. Corriu, J.P. Masse, Activation of Grignard reagents by transition-metal complexes. A new and simple synthesis of trans-stilbenes and polyphenyls, J Chem Soc Chem Commun (3) (1972) 144.
[48] J. Antilla, in: A. de Meijere (Ed.), Metal-catalyzed cross-coupling reactions, Second Completely Revised and Enlarged Edition: Volumes 1 and 2, Wiley-VCH Verlag GmbH & Co. KGaA, Weinheim, Germany, 2004. (George-August-Universität, Göttingen) and Francois Diederich (ETH, Zürich). xxii + xxii + 916 pp. $450.00. ISBN:3-527-30518-1. J Am Chem Soc 2005;127:10121–2.
[49] B.E. de Pedro, J. Priego, A. Gironda-Martínez, F. González, J. Benavides, J. Blas, et al., Mild and efficient palladium-mediated C–N cross-coupling reaction between DNA-conjugated aryl bromides and aromatic amines, ACS Comb Sci 21 (2) (2019) 69–74.
[50] D. Roy, Y. Uozumi, Recent advances in palladium-catalyzed cross-coupling reactions at ppm to ppb molar catalyst loadings, Adv Synth Catal 360 (4) (2018) 602–625.
[51] D. Shen, Y. Xu, S.-L. Shi, A bulky chiral N-heterocyclic carbene palladium catalyst enables highly enantioselective Suzuki–Miyaura cross-coupling reactions for the synthesis of biaryl atropisomers, J Am Chem Soc 141 (37) (2019) 14938–14945.
[52] R. Martin, S.L. Buchwald, Palladium-catalyzed Suzuki-Miyaura cross-coupling reactions employing dialkylbiaryl phosphine ligands, Acc Chem Res 41 (11) (2008) 1461–1473. 18620434. PMC2645945. [Epub 2008/07/16. eng].
[53] F. Bellina, A. Carpita, R. Rossi, Palladium catalysts for the Suzuki cross-coupling reaction: an overview of recent advances, Synthesis-Stuttgart 15 (2004) 2419–2440.
[54] T. Wirth, Microreactors in organic chemistry and catalysis, John Wiley & Sons, 2013.
[55] P.L. Pauson, Ferrocene and related compounds, Q Rev Chem Soc 9 (4) (1955) 391–414.
[56] V. Weinmayr, Hydrogen fluoride as a condensing agent. V. Reactions of dicyclopentadienyliron in anhydrous hydrogen fluoride, J Am Chem Soc 77 (11) (1955) 3009–3011.
[57] L.-L. Lai, T.-Y. Dong, A novel method to synthesize unsymmetrical disubstituted ferrocenes, J Chem Soc Chem Commun (20) (1994) 2347–2348.
[58] K. Ishihara, H. Kurihara, H. Yamamoto, An extremely simple, convenient, and selective method for acetylating primary alcohols in the presence of secondary alcohols, J Org Chem 58 (15) (1993) 3791–3793.
[59] P. Hubbard, W.J. Brittain, Mechanism of amine-catalyzed ester formation from an acid chloride and alcohol, J Org Chem 63 (3) (1998) 677–683. 11672060. (Epub 2001/10/24. eng).
[60] D.H. Paull, A. Weatherwax, T. Lectka, Catalytic, asymmetric reactions of ketenes and ketene enolates, Tetrahedron 65 (34) (2009) 3771–6803. 21494417. PMC3074489. [Epub 2009/08/22. eng].
[61] A.J. Oosthoek-de Vries, P.J. Nieuwland, J. Bart, K. Koch, J.W.G. Janssen, P.J.M. van Bentum, et al., Inline reaction monitoring of amine-catalyzed acetylation of benzyl alcohol using a microfluidic stripline nuclear magnetic resonance setup, J Am Chem Soc 141 (13) (2019) 5369–5380.

[62] P.L. Mills, R.V. Chaudhari, Multiphase catalytic reactor engineering and design for pharmaceuticals and fine chemicals, Catal Today 37 (4) (1997) 367–404.
[63] J. Yue, Multiphase flow processing in microreactors combined with heterogeneous catalysis for efficient and sustainable chemical synthesis, Catal Today 308 (2018) 3–19.
[64] J. Kobayashi, Y. Mori, K. Okamoto, R. Akiyama, M. Ueno, T. Kitamori, et al., A microfluidic device for conducting gas-liquid-solid hydrogenation reactions, Science 304 (5675) (2004) 1305–1308.
[65] F.C. MacKintosh, J. Käs, P.A. Janmey, Elasticity of semiflexible biopolymer networks, Phys Rev Lett 75 (24) (1995) 4425–4428.
[66] W. Xu, Y. Su, Y. Song, M. Shang, L. Zha, Q. Lu, Process analysis on preparation of cyclobutanetetracarboxylic dianhydride in a photomicroreactor within gas–liquid taylor flow, Ind Eng Chem Res 57 (7) (2018) 2476–2485.
[67] G.T. Rochelle, Amine scrubbing for CO_2 capture, Science 325 (5948) (2009) 1652–1654.
[68] M. Brzozowski, M. O'Brien, S.V. Ley, A. Polyzos, Flow chemistry: intelligent processing of gas–liquid transformations using a tube-in-tube reactor, Acc Chem Res 48 (2) (2015) 349–362.
[69] A. Aboudheir, P. Tontiwachwuthikul, A. Chakma, R. Idem, Kinetics of the reactive absorption of carbon dioxide in high CO2-loaded, concentrated aqueous monoethanolamine solutions, Chem Eng Sci 58 (2003) 5195–5210.
[70] P.D. Vaidya, E.Y. Kenig, Gas–liquid reaction kinetics: a review of determination methods, Chem Eng Commun 194 (12) (2007) 1543–1565.
[71] C. Ye, G. Chen, Q. Yuan, Process characteristics of CO2 absorption by aqueous monoethanolamine in a microchannel reactor, Chin J Chem Eng 20 (1) (2012) 111–119.
[72] R. Lin, X. Ma, T. Fielitz, S. Obare, R. Ofoli, Facile hydrogenation of carbon-carbon double bonds using catalytic noble nanoparticles immobilized in microfluidic reactors, Catal Commun 18 (2012) 168–175.
[73] J. Kobayashi, Y. Mori, S. Kobayashi, Multiphase organic synthesis in microchannel reactors, Chem Asian J 1 (1–2) (2006) 22–35. 17441035. (Epub 2007/04/19. eng).
[74] M. Irfan, T.N. Glasnov, C.O. Kappe, Heterogeneous catalytic hydrogenation reactions in continuous-flow reactors, ChemSusChem 4 (3) (2011) 300–316.
[75] Z. Chen, J. Xu, Y. Wang, Gas-liquid-liquid multiphase flow in microfluidic systems—a review, Chem Eng Sci 202 (2019) 1–14.
[76] Y. Önal, M. Lucas, P. Claus, Application of a capillary microreactor for selective hydrogenation of α,β-unsaturated aldehydes in aqueous multiphase catalysis, Chem Eng Technol 28 (2005) 972–978.
[77] J. Zhang, K. Wang, X. Lin, Y. Lu, G. Luo, Intensification of fast exothermic reaction by gas agitation in a microchemical system, AIChE J 60 (7) (2014) 2724–2730.
[78] C. Wiles, P. Watts, Continuous flow reactors, a tool for the modern synthetic chemist, Eur J Org Chem 2008 (10) (2008) 1655–1671.
[79] K. Diao, Y. Zhao, Heat transfer performance of sintered Cu microchannels produced by a novel method, Int J Heat Mass Transf 139 (2019) 537–547.
[80] P.W. Miller, N.J. Long, A.J. de Mello, R. Vilar, H. Audrain, D. Bender, et al., Rapid multiphase carbonylation reactions by using a microtube reactor: applications in positron emission tomography 11C-radiolabeling, Angew Chem Int Ed Eng 46 (16) (2007) 2875–2878. 17348061. (Epub 2007/03/10. eng).
[81] B.C. Hamper, E. Tesfu, Direct uncatalyzed amination of 2-chloropyridine using a flow reactor, Synlett 2007 (14) (2007) 2257–2261 (Epub 13.08.2007. Eng.).

[82] E. Comer, M.G. Organ, A microreactor for microwave-assisted capillary (continuous flow) organic synthesis, J Am Chem Soc 127 (22) (2005) 8160–8167. 15926844. (Epub 2005/06/02. eng).
[83] M. Baumann, I.R. Baxendale, S.V. Ley, N. Nikbin, C.D. Smith, J.P. Tierney, A modular flow reactor for performing Curtius rearrangements as a continuous flow process, Org Biomol Chem 6 (9) (2008) 1577–1586.
[84] T. Iwasaki, J.-I. Yoshida, Free radical polymerization in microreactors. Significant improvement in molecular weight distribution control, Macromolecules 38 (4) (2005) 1159–1163.
[85] Applications of nitriles as reagents for organic synthesis with loss of the nitrile functionality (including cycloaddition reactions), in: Category 3, compounds with four and three carbon heteroatom bonds, Georg Thieme Verlag, Stuttgart, 2004. Science of synrthesis. Available from: http://www.thieme-connect.de/products/ebooks/lookinside/10.1055/sos-SD-019-00272.
[86] J. Roh, K. Vávrová, A. Hrabálek, Synthesis and functionalization of 5-substituted tetrazoles, Eur J Org Chem 2012 (31) (2012) 6101–6118.
[87] V. Hessel, D. Kralisch, N. Kockmann, T. Noel, Q. Wang, Novel process windows for enabling, accelerating, and uplifting flow chemistry, ChemSusChem 6 (5) (2013) 746–789. 23606410. (Epub 2013/04/23. eng).
[88] T. Noël, S.L. Buchwald, Cross-coupling in flow, Chem Soc Rev 40 (10) (2011) 5010–5029.
[89] C. Wiles, P. Watts, Continuous flow reactors: a perspective, Green Chem 14 (1) (2012) 38–54.
[90] M. Baumann, I.R. Baxendale, S.V. Ley, The flow synthesis of heterocycles for natural product and medicinal chemistry applications, Mol Divers 15 (3) (2011) 613–630.
[91] D. Cantillo, C.O. Kappe, Direct preparation of nitriles from carboxylic acids in continuous flow, J Org Chem 78 (20) (2013) 10567–10571.
[92] T. Razzaq, T.N. Glasnov, C.O. Kappe, Continuous-flow microreactor chemistry under high-temperature/pressure conditions, Eur J Org Chem 2009 (9) (2009) 1321–1325.
[93] D. Kralisch, G. Kreisel, Assessment of the ecological potential of microreaction technology, Chem Eng Sci 62 (2007) 1094–1100.
[94] J. Yoshida, A. Nagaki, T. Iwasaki, S. Suga, Enhancement of chemical selectivity by microreactors, Chem Eng Technol 28 (3) (2005) 259–266.
[95] R. Ali, K. Nour, A. Al-Warthan, M.R.H. Siddiqui, Selective oxidation of benzylic alcohols using copper-manganese mixed oxide nanoparticles as catalyst, Arab J Chem 8 (4) (2015) 512–517.
[96] X. Zhang, X. Ke, H. Zhu, Zeolite-supported gold nanoparticles for selective photooxidation of aromatic alcohols under visible-light irradiation, Chem Eur J 18 (26) (2012) 8048–8056.
[97] M. Sharma, B. Das, M. Sharma, B.K. Deka, Y.B. Park, S.K. Bhargava, et al., Pd/Cu-oxide nanoconjugate at zeolite-Y crystallite crafting the mesoporous channels for selective oxidation of benzyl-alcohols, ACS Appl Mater Interfaces 9 (40) (2017) 35453–35462. 28933824. (Epub 2017/09/22. eng).
[98] J. Ftouni, M. Penhoat, J.-S. Girardon, A. Addad, E. Payen, C. Rolando, Immobilization of gold nanoparticles on fused silica capillary surface for the development of catalytic microreactors, Chem Eng J 227 (2013) 103–110.
[99] X. Rao, A. Abou Hassan, C. Guyon, E.O. Martinez Ruiz, M. Tatoulian, S. Ognier, Synthesis of benzaldehyde with high selectivity using immobilized AuNPs and AuNPs@zeolite in a catalytic microfluidic system, Lab Chip 19 (17) (2019) 2866–2873.

[100] C. Martino, T.Y. Lee, S.H. Kim, A.J. de Mello, Microfluidic generation of PEG-b-PLA polymersomes containing alginate-based core hydrogel, Biomicrofluidics 9 (2) (2015) 024101. 25825616. PMC4352166. [Epub 2015/04/01. eng].

[101] S. Cho, Y. Li, M. Seo, E. Kumacheva, Nanofibrillar stimulus-responsive cholesteric microgels with catalytic properties, Angew Chem Int Engl 55 (45) (2016) 14014–14018. 27735118. (Epub 2016/10/30. eng).

[102] M. Khanmohammadi, S. Sakai, T. Ashida, M. Taya, Production of hyaluronic-acid-based cell-enclosing microparticles and microcapsules via enzymatic reaction using a microfluidic system, J Appl Polym Sci 133 (16) (2016) 1–8, https://doi.org/10.1002/app.43107.

[103] J.A. Bennett, A.J. Kristof, V. Vasudevan, J. Genzer, J. Srogl, M. Abolhasani, Microfluidic synthesis of elastomeric microparticles: a case study in catalysis of palladium-mediated cross-coupling, AIChE J 64 (8) (2018) 3188–3197.

[104] R.K. Shah, J.-W. Kim, J.J. Agresti, D.A. Weitz, L.-Y. Chu, Fabrication of monodisperse thermosensitive microgels and gel capsules in microfluidic devices, Soft Matter 4 (12) (2008) 2303–2309.

[105] T. Rossow, J.A. Heyman, A.J. Ehrlicher, A. Langhoff, D.A. Weitz, R. Haag, et al., Controlled synthesis of cell-laden microgels by radical-free gelation in droplet microfluidics, J Am Chem Soc 134 (10) (2012) 4983–4989. 22356466. (Epub 2012/02/24. eng).

[106] D. Baah, T. Floyd-Smith, Microfluidics for particle synthesis from photocrosslinkable materials, Microfluid Nanofluid 17 (3) (2014) 431–455.

[107] I. Stibingerova, S. Voltrova, S. Kocova, M. Lindale, J. Srogl, Modular approach to heterogenous catalysis. Manipulation of cross-coupling catalyst activity, Org Lett 18 (2) (2016) 312–315.

[108] S.E. Hooshmand, B. Heidari, R. Sedghi, R. Varma, Recent advances in the Suzuki-Miyaura cross-coupling reaction using efficient catalysts in eco-friendly media, Green Chem 21 (2018) 381–405.

[109] J. Zhang, A.R. Teixeira, L.T. Kögl, L. Yang, K.F. Jensen, Hydrodynamics of gas–liquid flow in micropacked beds: pressure drop, liquid holdup, and two-phase model, AIChE J 63 (10) (2017) 4694–4704.

[110] J. Zhang, A.R. Teixeira, K.F. Jensen, Automated measurements of gas-liquid mass transfer in micropacked bed reactors, AIChE J 64 (2) (2018) 564–570.

[111] C. Hu, R.L. Hartman, High-throughput packed-bed microreactors with in-line analytics for the discovery of asphaltene deposition mechanisms, AIChE J 60 (10) (2014) 3534–3546.

CHAPTER

Microfluidic paper-based devices 11

Akbar Hasanzadeh[a,b,*] and Iman Hashemzadeh[a,b]

[a]Department of Medical Nanotechnology, Faculty of Advanced Technologies in Medicine, Iran University of Medical Sciences, Tehran, Iran

[b]Advances Nanobiotechnology and Nanomedicine Research Group (ANNRG), Iran University of Medical Sciences, Tehran, Iran

**Corresponding author. E-mail: akbarhasanzadeh16@gmail.com*

11.1 Introduction

Microfluidic paper-based analytical devices, so-called μPADs, were described for the first time by Whitesides and colleagues in 2007 [1]. For the fabrication of μPADs, either hydrophobic or hydrophilic microstructures have been patterned onto paper substrates using a range of methods. The advantages of μPADs, such as low-cost, minimal sample consumption, portability, disposability, and ease of construction have led to the use of μPADs as a good alternative for polymer and glass-based conventional microfluidic systems in the fields of food safety [2], environmental monitoring [3], and clinical diagnosis [4–7] as well as bioterrorism prevention [8, 9]. Besides, the use of miniaturized equipment allowing laboratory operations on microstructured devices donate has suggested that μPADs can be promising platforms to use for applications in field testing, and point of care (POC) diagnosis [10, 11]. A broad range of chemical and physical techniques have been applied for μPADs fabrication including, wax printing [12, 13], photolithography [14, 15], flexography [16, 17], laser treatment [18, 19], screen-printing [20], plasma treatment [21], plotting [22], ink stamping [23], inkjet etching [24], paper cutting and shaping, inkjet printing [25], lacquer spraying, chemical vapor phase deposition [26], hand-held corona treatment [27], and wet etching [28]. These techniques will be explained in the following section.

11.2 Fabrication techniques

Inkjet printing, wax patterning, laser treatment, and photolithography are categories of fabrication techniques for μPADs, but we have classified the fabrication methods based on chemical and physical processes in this chapter.

Biomedical Applications of Microfluidic Devices. https://doi.org/10.1016/B978-0-12-818791-3.00007-3

11.2.1 Physical techniques

11.2.1.1 Wax printing

Wax printing was one of the first approaches for the fabrication of hydrophobic microstructures on naturally hydrophilic paper substrates in μPADs. In this method, hydrophobic boundaries are created by an inexpensive wax pattern.

For the construction of μPADs, a printer device, which was able to print wax onto paper substrates with predesigned patterns, was introduced by Lu et al. in 2009 [29]. After porous filter paper was printed by the wax, it was heated in an oven to melt the wax, which penetrated the paper substrate to shape clear microscale channels upon the substrate surface. Although this easy and simple fabrication method does not need expensive or complicated equipment, but only requires a wax printer and an oven; the resolution of this device constructed using wax pattering was restricted to millimeters.

Songjaroen and colleagues described a novel wax dipping technique to fabricate wax μPADs. Briefly, a laser cutting technique was used to design the iron template. The paper substrate was then positioned on the glass slide and the patterned mold was placed upon the paper. A permanent magnet was affixed to the back of the glass slide to temporarily maintain the template in contact. In the next step, to print the pattern on the paper, the filter paper and glass slide assembly were dipped into the melted wax with a temperature approximately 120–130°C for 1 s. After the temperature of the assembly reached the ambient temperature, the glass slide was detached from the paper and the iron mold was also separated as well. In the last step, the hydrophilic and hydrophobic zones of the μPADs were generated. The total time for construction of μPADs without using complicated instruments was only about 1 min as an advantage of this method [30].

11.2.1.2 Plotting

This method was called plotting because a plotter device was used for the creation of patterns on paper. In this method, a repurposed *x*-*y*-plotter was utilized by Whitesides and colleagues to manufacture μPADs [22]. Firstly, polydimethylsiloxane (PDMS), a hydrophobic polymer, was dissolved in hexane and applied as ink for the modified *x*-*y*-plotter to print the desired pattern onto filter paper. The solution of PDMS then penetrated the deep parts of the paper and finally formed a sealed hydrophobic wall, which prevented the passage of aqueous solutions. The minimum width of the channels and space between channels was about 1 mm. The use of PDMS as an elastomer allowed users to fold and bend patterned papers without destroying the integrity of the channels. Notwithstanding the cost-effectiveness and flexibility of μPADs fabricated by this plotting technique, the maintenance and control of the hydrophobic barriers with a defined size is difficult using this method, which is a limitation for the design of complex patterns.

11.2.1.3 Inkjet etching

The etching is a procedure generally used for semiconductor fabrication, but etching employs solutions and reactive ions as well as other mechanical procedures more suitable for electronic components. The etching of holes and trenches into polymers film was the first time that the inkjet etching concept was used [31]. Abe and coworkers utilized an inkjet etching method to construct μPADs [24]. In the first step, the hydrophobic filter paper was soaked in 1.8 wt% polystyrene dissolved in toluene for about 2 h and then removed from the solution. After evaporation of the extra solvent from the filter paper, the patterning of polystyrene in the desired pattern was created by an inkjet printer device. The patterns and channels required 10–20 repeated applications to eliminate the polystyrene sediment within the zones. Using this procedure, the hydrophobic boundaries and hydrophilic channels were formed. In this approach, the peeling of the polystyrene from the desired zones on the surface of the paper using a solution (toluene) can be considered as etching. A high resolution in the μPADs fabricated by the previously mentioned technique is an advantage, but the construction process is relatively complicated.

11.2.1.4 Flexographic printing

The flexographic printing method is a direct and simple printing method using polystyrene to form fluid conducting barriers and layers on the filter paper. Subsequently, polystyrene penetrates to the depth of the paper substrate and builds hydrophobic walls. In this method, polystyrene plays the role of ink for printing. The penetration of polystyrene into the paper substrate helps to form very thin hydrophobic channels, which leads to the lower consumption of samples. The consumption of materials is modest and the instruments are fairly simple; therefore, this method can be considered to be suitable for the production of large-scale paper-based fluidic devices. However, this technique maybe not appropriate for laboratory prototype construction [17].

11.2.1.5 Laser treatment

Laser-based fabrication techniques of various kinds have been used for the construction of μPADs. In one example, hydrophobic channels were manufactured using light-activated polymerization of a photopolymer. In this technique, the fabricated hydrophobic barriers had a width of about 120 μm [32]. Besides, the use of a CO_2 laser for cutting the predesigned areas of the paper substrate is another example of lasers in the fabrication of fluidic devices. In this way, a microfluidic platform was developed using a CO_2 laser and a paper substrate with a hydrophobic surface coating, such as wax paper, palette paper, or parchment paper by Sones and coworkers [32]. In the first step, a silicon-coated surface paper (parchment paper) was spread and positioned on the surface of a laser platform, and then the surface of the paper was patterned by a computer-controlled CO_2 laser cutting and engraving system. After production of the required pattern upon the paper using CorelDraw software, these zones were printed by raster-scanning the laser light over the surface. Finally, to prevent liquid crossing between the channels, silica microparticles were added to patterned regions. In this method, both the speed of scanning and the laser power was accurately controlled to avoid cutting through the parchment paper, instead of the desired surface modification. Although this approach produces platforms with good stability, the instruments used for this procedure are relatively expensive, which limits its application.

11.2.1.6 Ink stamping

This is an easy and convenient procedure, which can be employed without much equipment or training. Due to those features, many investigators have applied this approach with different types of ink and stamps for the fabrication of μPADs.

In this regard, Curto and colleagues reported a simple, one-step and reproducible approach to the construction of μPADs using a PDMS stamp and permanent ink [33]. Briefly, the PDMS stamp, which was treated at 60°C for 8h to control the amount of ink transferred from the PDMS stamp to the paper substrate, was gently applied to the permanent ink-coated stone pad three times. After the inked seal was removed from the indelible ink, it was maintained in the air for 5s to remove any air bubbles formed on top of the PDMS stamp. Lastly, the inked PDMS stamp was placed on the paper substrate and kept there for 3s. Despite its benefits such as low-cost and simplicity, the construction of the PDMS stamp itself may be considered complex.

11.2.1.7 Shaping and cutting of the paper

A paper and nitrocellulose lateral flow fluidic platform was developed using a computer-controlled *x-y* knife tracer, which combined a typical ink pen with a knife plotter, by Fenton and coworkers [34]. Three successive overlapping cuts were used to avoid the ripping of the paper substrate. The advantage was that time for the whole process was only about 60s.

Recently, an easy method with the ability to carry out programmed fluid movement without any active pumping was fabricated using an industrial-cutting device embedded with a knife, and a paper substrate was reported by Giokas and colleagues [35]. For creating the device, the authors carved open channels, which were controlled in terms of length, orientation, and number, onto the paper filter using an industrial-cutting device equipped with a knife. The advantages were multiple repetitions and time-programmable runs.

In another study, a pressure-driven open-channel paper-based microfluidic system was developed by Glavan et al. [36]. In summary, a blueprint pattern was designed onto the surface of omniphobic paper using computer software. The locations of the microchannels were carved using an inexpensive and safe electronic craft cutting/engraving tool, and then the paper substrate was rendered hydrophobic by vapor phase modification with $CF_3(CF_2)_7CH_2CH_2SiCl_3\left(C_{10}{}^F\right)$. After that, a layer of tape with precut holes aligned with the outlets and inlets of the channels was employed to seal the top of the system. Finally, to connect the microchannels to silicone tubing, flangeless ferrules were attached to the system using rings of double-sided adhesive tape. Approximately 10min was required for completing the procedure. Cutting-based techniques are not able to precisely control the size of the channels, without carrying out difficult steps.

11.2.1.8 Lacquer spraying

Nurak and coworkers introduced the use of lacquer for the construction of μPADs [37]. To maintain the paper and iron mask next to each other firmly, a sandwich of the filter paper between a prepatterned iron mask and a magnetic plate was carried out. To create hydrophobic areas upon the surface of the filter paper, the lacquer was sprayed onto the paper, where the hydrophilic areas of paper were protected by the mask. The approach is easy and inexpensive, but there may be some problems with the use of the iron mask.

11.2.1.9 Screen printing

In addition to the physical methods for fabrication of μPADs, screen printing has also attracted some interest. Sameenoi and coworkers constructed simple and low-cost μPADs using the only polystyrene as a hydrophobic material that could be screen printed [16]. In this study, to form three-dimensional hydrophobic boundaries in pre-patterned areas, the polystyrene solution was poured onto the paper using the screen. The added polystyrene solution then penetrated the depth of the paper substrate and formed the desired microchannels. Similarly, Dungchai and colleagues used this procedure for the construction of μPADs in 2011, where a wax solid was used instead of polystyrene and heated to the melting point, and subsequently formed the hydrophobic walls [38]. Screen printing can be utilized for producing small numbers of μPADs since this approach is so common in the printing industry.

11.2.2 Chemical techniques

11.2.2.1 Photolithography

Similar to other mask printing techniques, photolithography patterning also allows the design of patterns onto paper with a hydrophilic zone surrounded by hydrophobic polymeric boundaries. The first μPAD was produced using photolithographic patterning by Whitesides et al. who applied a SU-82010 photoresist to fabricate millimeter-sized channels onto chromatography paper. Briefly, a sheet of chromatography paper was soaked in 2mL of SU-82010 photoresist for 30s and a spinning process was carried out at 2000rpm for 30s. to remove one component of the SU-8 formulation (cyclopentanone). The paper was then heated at 95°C for 5min, and the photoresist and paper substrate were exposed 405nm violet light for 10s through a photomask using a mask aligner. For firm attachment of the photoactivated parts of the resist, the paper was again heated according to the above-described conditions. To remove the unpolymerized photoresist remaining on the paper, the paper was soaked in propylene glycol monomethyl ether acetate solution for about 5min, and then the template was rinsed using propan-2-ol. Lastly, to control the hydrophobicity of the patterned paper, the whole surface was subjected to oxygen plasma for almost 10s. Using this method, a high-resolution microfluidic device was produced, although the complexity of the approach and the high cost of the SU-8 may be limitations.

To overcome these limitations, Whitesides and colleagues utilized an ordinary UV lamp and a hotplate instead of a lithography device for the fast lithographic activation of sheets (FLASH) technique [39]. In the first step, a photoresist was added onto a piece of paper and diffused over the entire surface of the paper using a wooden rolling pin. To evaporate the propylene glycol monomethyl ether acetate in the photoresist formulation, the paper was heated at 130°C for 5–10min using a hotplate. After the temperature of paper reached room temperature, a sticky transparent film and a black paper sheet were applied on both sides of the paper. The functionalized paper was exposed to a 600 W metal halide lamp as a UV light source, and the black and transparent layers were separated from paper and baked on the hotplate at 130°C for 5 min. Finally, the drenching of the paper with acetone for 1 min and washing with acetone and 70% isopropyl alcohol was carried out to remove unpolymerized photoresist as the last steps. This procedure could use sunlight instead of UV light.

In another study, He and coworkers used the combination of hydrophobic silane on paper fibers with intense UV-lithography for the fabrication of μPADs [40]. In this technique, the filter paper was soaked with octadecyltrichlorosilane dissolved in *n*-hexane for 5 min to obtain a hydrophobic filter paper. After that, the filter paper was irradiated with intense UV-light via a template quartz mask. The UV-irradiated zones became hydrophilic and formed hydrophobic barriers, while the covered areas remained extremely hydrophobic.

Because the design of a photomask requires a lot of time and is expensive, some researchers have used an LCD or a digital micromirror to rapidly produce a dynamic photomask. A low-cost and facile approach for the construction of μPADs using dynamic mask photocuring (DMPC) with a stereolithographic three-dimensional printer was reported by He et al. [41]. The whole of the filter paper was soaked in ultraviolet-responsive resin. The functionalized filter paper was then exposed to UV light via a kinetic mask with a simple channel template. After treatment, the UV-exposed areas were converted to hydrophobic walls. In the last step, to remove the paper from the uncured resin, it was rinsed with anhydrous alcohol. The entire time of the procedure was about 2 min.

Songok and coworkers also described a two-step construction process for the design of μPADs employing a UV light and TiO_2 nanoparticles (NPs) [42]. Briefly, they used a rapid, roll-to-roll liquid flame spray method to cover the surface of the filter paper with TiO_2 NPs, creating a hydrophobic surface. Owing to the photocatalytic property of TiO_2, the hydrophilic template was then produced using UV irradiation across a photomask.

Recently, direct laser writing has been developed as an approach that does not require a photomask. Sones and colleagues generated fluidic channels using polymerization of a photopolymer onto the paper via a laser-based direct-writing technique [32]. First, the filter paper was immersed in the light-sensitive polymer dissolved in isopropanol. After the modification, the paper was dried under ambient conditions and then moved beneath the laser spot to form the fluidic channels due to the light-induced photo-polymerization process. The speed of this method may be low because the XY stage requires constant moving in the maskless approach.

11.2.2.2 Plasma treatment

Plasma treatment is used in microfluidic chip bonding. Li and colleagues used a plasma treatment procedure for the construction of μPADs [21]. First, the hydrophobic filter paper was obtained by immersing it in alkyl-ketene-dimer dissolved in *n*-heptane and removed immediately and then placed in the fume hood for evaporation of the heptane. To cure the alkyl-ketene-dimer, the filter paper was heated in an oven at 100°C about 45 min. Next, the hydrophilic pattern was formed by sandwiching highly hydrophobic paper between two metal masks with the desired pattern and then inserted into a vacuum plasma reactor for 15 s. The materials used in this method are cheap and readily available, but the specificity of the metal mask for each pattern may be troublesome and expensive.

More recently, fluorocarbon plasma polymerization has been applied as a one-step rapid method by Kao and coworkers to fabricate μPADs [43]. The filter paper was tightly sandwiched between two metal masks with the required pattern zones, which were fabricated by mechanical cutting of stainless steel sheets, and then the three sandwiched components were placed within a plasma generating system consisting of two powered electrodes. A plasma mixture of an active gas (octafluorocyclobutane) and an inert gas (argon) was then deposited onto the surface of the sandwich under high pressure and formed hydrophobic barriers.

11.2.2.3 Inkjet printing

The integration of paper modification chemistry (sizing) with digital inkjet printing technology, provided a novel construction approach for μPADs, which can be considered as an inkjet printing approach. This method was used by Shen et al. [44]. In their study, the filter paper was printed by a repurposed commercial digital inkjet printer, using alkyl-ketene-dimer (AKD) dissolved in heptane as a hydrophobic ink. To cure the AKD on the cellulose fibers, the treated paper was placed in an oven and heated at 100°C for about 8 min. The μPAD was obtained after the paper was dried under ambient conditions. This method has some advantages, such as being maskless, inexpensive, and simple compared to plasma treatment.

In another study, Maejima and coworkers used an inkjet printing technique for the construction of μPADs [45]. A hydrophobic UV activatable acrylate mixture was coated upon the surface of filter paper, to obtain the desired microfluidic patterns. To form hydrophobic boundaries, the printed paper was irradiated with UV light for about 60 s. Inkjet printing can deposit multiple reagents onto the surface of paper simultaneously, which could be promising for mass fabrication of μPADs.

11.2.2.4 Chemical vapor-phase deposition

Gupta and colleagues designed μPADs using chemical vapor-phase deposition for the first time [46]. A similar procedure was developed for the construction of μPADs applying vapor-phase sedimentation of sheer polymers [47]. In this method, the process began with the sandwiching of the filter paper between a metal mask and a powerful magnet. A discharge sublimation chamber was used to evaporate the monomers and consequently for free radical polymerization using pyrolysis. To form the hydrophobic walls, sedimentation and polymerization of the radical monomers was carried out on the desired area of the paper.

11.2.2.5 Wet etching

A construction technique for μPADs using wet etching of hydrophobic filter paper with a paper-based mask and a patterned template was described by Cai and coworkers [28]. In this technique, by using trimethoxyoctadecylsilane solution as the patterning agent, the naturally hydrophilic filter paper was rendered hydrophobic. After that, a NaOH solution was applied to transfer an aligned paper mask upon the template paper, which permitted etching of the silanized paper by the etching reagent. The zones covered by the mask became hydrophilic, while the uncovered areas remained hydrophobic.

11.2.3 Fabrication techniques for 3D μPADs

Although 2D μPADs have already been developed for healthcare-related diagnostics, environmental monitoring and screening for food safety require low-cost, easy to fabricate, simple, and disposable devices. Some researchers decided to move beyond 2D μPADs, to design 3D μPADs, which could not only perform better than 2D μPADs in terms of speed and efficiency but could also carry out multiplex reactions or multistep preprocessing processes on a single platform. Stacking and origami are two common approaches for 3D μPADs.

11.2.3.1 Stacking technique

Due to the presence of stereoscopic channels within a short Z-dimension inside 3D μPADs, they can carry out tests faster and better compared to 2D μPADs. By combining template layers of paper attached by double-sided sticky tape, Whitesides and coworkers developed a technique for the fabrication of 3D μPADs [48]. The dual-sided sticky tape with pits containing cellulose powder was placed between the patterned filter paper sheets, and not only produced separated channels in the neighboring filter paper sheets but also linked the papers through the holes allowing vertical fluid flow.

Another study, Philips et al. reported the integration of a wax printing procedure with the adhesive spraying technique to design 3D μPADs [49]. Briefly, the filter paper was patterned with hydrophobic barriers using a wax printer according to similar to 2D μPAD fabrication. After spraying an adhesive onto one side of the patterned paper, the second paper substrate was aligned and attached upon the surface of the first patterned paper using a roller. This procedure was repeated to obtain the desired 3D μPADs.

11.2.3.2 Origami

General speaking, the folding of different types of paper to achieve different shapes and structures is called origami. Origami was developed for the fabrication of 3D μPADs by Liu and colleagues in 2011 [50]. First, the required paper layers for the μPADs were patterned and prepared using a photolithography technique on each flat filter paper sheet. Next, the flat patterned filter paper sheets were assembled by a manual folding technique and formed the desired 3D μPADs. Lastly, an aluminum clamp was applied to maintain the folded filter papers in the desired conformation.

11.3 Applications of microfluidic paper-based analytical devices

Both 2D and 3D μPADs have been used for low cost, easy to use, disposable, multi-analyte and semiquantitative assays to diagnose several kinds of diseases. These are especially desirable in developing countries and regions, where technical infrastructure and trained operators are restricted. The reactions include molecular identification, immunological tests, and biochemical assays are all useful in diagnostic studies.

11.3.1 Biochemical detection

Paper-based microfluidic detection has been utilized to assay a wide range of different analytes. Microfluidic paper-based detection systems usually contain two important zones: (1) a sampling zone where the samples enter the system; (2) a detection zone where the reaction between target compounds and immobilized reagents takes place. Different types of chemical reactions, such as enzymatic reactions, precipitation reactions, acid-alkali, and redox reactions can occur within the detection zone and subsequently generate different kinds of signals. For detection of these signals, several techniques have been employed, including chemiluminescence (CL) [51], electrochemiluminescence (ECL) [52], photoelectrochemical (PEC) [53], fluorescent [54], electrochemical [55], or colorimetric [56].

Colorimetric assays are well suited to paper-based platforms and are the most commonly used approach in μPADs because of their features, such as simple operation and a straightforward signal readout. The reaction taking place in the detection zone creates a new color or changes the intensity of the original color, which can be recorded by detector systems, including cameras and scanners, or even with the naked eye. Analyzing the wavelength and intensity of the colors can provide the concentration of the analytes [57]. In this regard, a paper-based colorimetric biosensing microchip was described by Zhou and coworkers to detect both glucose and H_2O_2 in biological samples [58]. First, the filter paper was soaked in 5% cross-linked siloxane 3-aminopropyltriethoxysilane (APTMS) dissolved in ethanol, and a suitable amount of glutaraldehyde (GA) was added to the treated paper to cross-link the APTMS-GA matrix, which appeared with a brick-red color. After this, the prepared filter paper was immersed in different concentration of H_2O_2, and the visual color changed due to the reaction of H_2O_2 with the matrix. A camera was used to record the color change variations of the filter paper and Image J software was used to analyze the photos. For the detection of glucose, the glucose oxidase (GOx) enzyme was added to the paper modified with APTMS-GA complex. After washing and drying of the modified filter paper, a different color change of the paper was generated by the enzymatic reaction between H_2O_2 and glucose (less H_2O_2) and could be measured by comparison with the previous color.

The incorporation of a paper-based colorimetric biosensing platform with a smartphone was reported by Lopez-Ruiz and colleagues to detect pH and the presence of nitrite [59]. A single sampling zone along with seven detection zones with independent channels was patterned onto the surface of filter paper. The Griess reaction was used in the nitrite sensing area and for measurement of pH, phenol red, and chlorophenol red as indicators were embedded in other detection zones. After the solution samples were injected through the inlet of the microfluidic device, they flowed automatically toward the detection areas using capillary force without any extra pumping. The uniform and stable color were detected and recorded by a smartphone when the microfluidic system had dried. This method provided a possibility for simultaneous multianalyte detection using a single platform without any extra processing.

A broad range of NPs possessing higher extinction coefficients compared to typical dyes have been used in paper-based colorimetric analytical systems. The detection of copper Cu^{2+} using μPADs based on the colorimetric sensing of silver NPs (AgNPs) was described by Ratnarathorn et al. [60]. In the first step, UV spectroscopy was utilized for detection of Cu^{2+} based on colorimetric sensing of AgNPs. The surface of the AgNPs was functionalized with -SH groups on homocysteine and dithiothreitol, while the Cu^{2+} ions were selectively absorbed by the $-COOH$ and $-NH_2$ functional groups compared to other ions present in the liquid. Two clear changes occurred in the presence of Cu^{2+}, firstly the plasmon resonance absorption peak at 404 nm was reduced; secondly, a novel red-shifted band at 502 nm emerged. After the addition of Cu^{2+}, the color of the AgNP modified paper changed from yellow to orange and green-brown because of the aggregation of the NPs.

Compared to traditional colorimetric assays and electrochemical methods, paper-based electrochemical microfluidic systems may be better to monitor and scan environments to detect impurities and toxins as well as pathogens due to the need for a low limit of detection [61]. Electrodes were fabricated using a screen printing technique on a microfluidic paper-based platform for detection of bismuth and other heavy metals as described by Tan et al. [62].

Fluorescence measurement is another type of optical method with inherently much higher sensitivity compared to colorimetric approaches. Thom and coworkers developed a paper-based fluorescence microfluidic device for point-of-care diagnosis [63]. In this study, the fluorescence was measured as an output signal and a cell phone with a specific camera was used to image the signal and quantify the assay. After exposure to small-molecule reagents combined with a specific enzyme biomarker, the signal changed from weak fluorescence to strong fluorescence. The digitization of signals obtained from the fluorescence was obtained by imaging the detection zone with a cell phone fitted with a specific camera.

An inexpensive and sensitive biosensor employing the CL technique incorporated into μPADs was reported [64]. Yu and colleagues developed a novel microfluidic paper-based CL analytical system for simultaneous identification and measurement of glucose and uric acid [65]. The liquid samples containing uric acid and glucose traveled different distances within the microfluidic device. By analyzing the distance, the authors demonstrated that uric acid and glucose traveled different distances in the microfluidic platform, allowing them to analyze two samples simultaneously. The patterns on the surface of the paper were designed by a convenient and inexpensive cutting technique. To stabilize the position of the μPADs, a novel device-holder was constructed for the cassette. A black metallic coating containing an injection zone for sample entry blocked the surface of the cassette to prevent the entry of extraneous substances. A holder was utilized to hold the microfluidic platform so that the photomultiplier analyzer and the sampling zone were connected. After the samples were added to the system through the injection sample area, they were transferred toward the CL detection zone by capillary force without any external pressure. To record the CL signals, generated in the sensing areas, a computer was employed.

The benefits of luminescence and electrochemical detection methods include a broad dynamic range of concentrations and high sensitivity. Microfluidic paper-based ECL detection makes these devices attractive with the possibility of spatial and electrical control. A paper-based microfluidic ECL origami-based cell detection device for multiplex cancer cell identification was reported by Wu et al. [52]. In this study, the specific capture of cancer cells was achieved using aptamers that recognized cell surface markers, and it was modified with three-dimensional Au-paper electrodes as an effective signal generation platform. Spongy AuPd alloy nanocomplexes were loaded with concanavalin-A that interacted with mannose residues upon the surface of cancer cells. These catalytic nanolabels reacted with hydrogen peroxide and peroxydisulfate to produce the ECL signal. Four different kinds of cancer cells could be recognized with consistency, accuracy, and reproducibility in optimal conditions. The performance of this system demonstrated simple, efficient, and multiplex detection that may have a role in primary cancer diagnosis and monitoring of clinical treatment.

The use of paper-based ECL microfluidic devices can allow the identification of toxic heavy metals involved in environmental contamination. A 3D microfluidic paper-based analytical system employed ECL nanoprobes for the identification of Pb^{2+} ions and Hg^{2+} ions recognized by oligonucleotides as a rapid, cost-effective, and sensitive technique was reported by Zhang and coworkers [66]. In this method, the desired patterns upon the paper were fabricated using a wax printing process, and the ECL labels used were either carbon nanocrystal-capped silica NPs or $Ru(bpy)_3^{2+}$ – AuNP aggregates. The device detected lead ions and mercury ions based on conformational changes in the DNA strands via the formation of G-quadruplexes or T-Hg-T complexes, respectively.

11.3.2 Immunological detection

Immunoassays can be carried out on paper that has been modified using chemical methods. In these assays, signals are generated when an immunological recognition event takes place and activates a secondary reaction. This method can be applied in clinical assays to identify the presence of humoral antibodies or the presence of antigenic materials, by choosing the appropriate part of the antigen-antibody binding system. These assays can be utilized for determination of *Escherichia coli* O157: H7 [67], goat anti-rabbit IgG [68], red blood cell agglutination [69], rabbit IgG [70], or human chorionic gonadotropin in a commercial pregnancy test strip [71].

In one example, for the identification of IgG antibody anti-hepatitis C virus, a novel multiple immunoassay paper-based microfluidic device was reported by Mu and colleagues [68]. In this study, an industrial punch template served as a cost-effective instrument (approximately $2) to manually design the desired pattern on the surface of the paper at room temperature. The multiple sensing areas were fabricated in a radial shape ("petals") to avoid interference of any contamination by creating air barriers between the detection zones. The solution samples were added to each sensing area directly or before the addition of liquids, and the detection zones were marked with a red dye. Compared with a current ELISA kit, this method has some advantages, such as being cost-effective and needing only low sample consumption.

In another study, acute promyelocytic leukemia cells were detected using an inexpensive electrochemical paper-based cytology system, which was developed by Su et al. [72]. In this method, a three-dimensional Au-coated paper used as a working electrode was functionalized with aptamers to specifically recognize and efficiently capture cancer cells. This system could trap cancer cells with high capacity and good biocompatibility, to maintain the viability of the trapped living cells. This quantitative simple electrochemical detection device had more advantages compared to a colorimetric method since the responses in the latter approach are in the form of "yes" or "no," which are insufficient to diagnose cancer cells accurately.

The inability to store reagents for a long time under refrigeration has been a serious drawback for point of care applications in low resource settings. Since the reproducibility and dependability of a test can be affected by reagent integrity, expensive refrigerators with controlled temperature must be used to store reagents, and preserve their stability. Because the use of paper-based platforms for quantitative assays in POC settings has been growing recently, experiments should be carried out to understand the stability of reagents upon filter paper substrates. In this regard, Wu and coworkers reported an automatic approach to test the long-term activity of reconstituted antibodies, which had been stored upon filter paper, using flow cytometry [73]. The activity of the stored antibodies was measured by evaluating their mean fluorescence intensity to validate this method. The procedure could be used to check the impact of other paper treatment regimes and storage conditions on antibody integrity.

The benefits of optical techniques and EC sensors have been combined in photoelectrochemical (PEC) sensors, which have been widely used for diagnosis in a photovoltaic readout [74]. The fabrication of PEC biosensors, which operate in the visible-light range can not only avoid using UV light but are also able to use sunlight as a low-cost and safe resource.

A sensitive PEC immunoassay sensor containing CdS/TiO_2 hybrid functionalized electrodes in a microfluidic paper-based platform was reported by Wang and colleagues for the detection of carcinoembryonic antigen (a cancer biomarker). This design enhanced the photocurrent by the addition of titanium dioxide (TiO_2) to cadmium sulfide (CdS) quantum dots as a photoelectrochemical biosensor in the visible region [75]. This worked with an efficient overlap of the energy levels between the conduction bands of the CdS and TiO_2. Irradiation caused a rapid electron injection from the excited CdS to TiO_2. This not only prevented the recombination of the electron-hole pairs but also improved the overall efficiency. The sensitivity was substantially increased with the use of glucose oxidase and *N*-(aminobutyl)-*N*-(ethylisoluminol) to modify the AuNPs to magnify the signal.

11.3.3 Molecular detection

Nucleic acid hybridization is the principle underlying many assays and can be carried out on microfluidic paper-based devices. In this regard, Tsai and coworkers developed a microfluidic paper-based colorimetric sensing assay using native 13 nm AuNPs for diagnosis of tuberculosis [76]. In the first step, solid wax was printed onto chromatography paper and heated at 140°C for 2 min using a hot plate to form the hydrophobic walls. Next, oligonucleotide sequences were dissolved in tris-borate buffer at 1.3 nM probe concentration. Then the preprepared standard IS6110 sequence and the unknown human DNA sequences solutions were added to the oligonucleotide probe solutions, and they were denatured at 90°C for 1 min and annealed at ambient temperature for 4 min to complete the hybridization process. A sodium chloride solution and AuNP colloid were then added to the analyte mixture. Lastly, the complex was injected onto the paper with a color standard for image analysis. A smartphone was used to capture and transmit the colorimetric signals. If the target sequences were present in the extracted DNA mixture, hybridization between them and the probes occurred, so there would be fewer ssDNA strands to be taken up by AuNPs, and this would prevent agglomeration occurring when the salt was added. After hybridization, the color of the mixture did not change and remained red, while in the absence of the target sequences, the aggregation of the AuNPs would change to purple color. The aggregation state of AuNPs can be influenced by two important factors: (1) the surface charge of the AuNPs; (2) molecules attached to the surface of the AuNPs. Both of these factors can be tailored by adding the salt solution or linking the biomolecules through electrostatic bonds.

Another platform for molecular diagnostic assays is the use of μPADs fabricated by wax printing to capture and detect DNA hybrids upon the paper. This process can be achieved when carbohydrate-binding modules and ZZ-domains are used to anchor the antibodies onto the surface of the paper. The black lines on the white background serving as hydrophobic walls can be drawn by software and printed using the wax printer. The time for the samples to travel the length of microchannels was 5 min, and after scanning the μPADs, the fluorescence intensity in the detection areas was measured. The limit of detection was equal to or less than 1 pmol in a 15 μL sample volume [77].

In one study, a microfluidic paper electrochemical device was designed for the identification of genotoxic compounds in water, food, or smoke by Mani et al. [78]. In this method, the electrode was fabricated using a screen-printing technique and the desired patterns were printed on the surface of the paper using solid wax and then heated to form hydrophobic barriers. In the presence of DNA, electrochemical oxidation of ruthenium polyvinylpyridine produced the ECL signal. This device could be utilized to detect the existence of genotoxic equivalents in environmental samples.

The analytical endpoint was the identification of DNA damage generated by the agent within the device, utilizing the ECL readout that was evaluated using a camera.

11.3.4 Other detection approaches

Other microfluidic paper-based detection methods have included, spectrophotometric detection of phosphate in a soil solution [79], potentiometric metal ion determination [80], and mass spectroscopy for determination of rhodamine 6G and L-phenylalanine [81]. All the previously mentioned methods can be considered as novel platforms for analysis of substances with implications for the diagnosis of various diseases and environmental contamination.

References

[1] A.W. Martinez, S.T. Phillips, M.J. Butte, G.M. Whitesides, Patterned paper as a platform for inexpensive, low-volume, portable bioassays, Angew Chem Int Ed 46 (8) (2007) 1318–1320.

[2] T. Aid, M. Kaljurand, M. Vaher, Colorimetric determination of total phenolic contents in ionic liquid extracts by paper microzones and digital camera, Anal Methods 7 (7) (2015) 3193–3199.

[3] D.M. Cate, W. Dungchai, J.C. Cunningham, J. Volckens, C.S. Henry, Simple, distance-based measurement for paper analytical devices, Lab Chip 13 (12) (2013) 2397–2404.

[4] A.W. Martinez, S.T. Phillips, G.M. Whitesides, E. Carrilho, Diagnostics for the developing world: microfluidic paper-based analytical devices, ACS Publications, 2009.

[5] D. Yang, J. Ma, Q. Zhang, N. Li, J. Yang, P.A. Raju, et al., Polyelectrolyte-coated gold magnetic nanoparticles for immunoassay development: toward point of care diagnostics for syphilis screening, Anal Chem 85 (14) (2013) 6688–6695.

[6] Y. Gao, A.W. Lam, W.C. Chan, Automating quantum dot barcode assays using microfluidics and magnetism for the development of a point-of-care device, ACS Appl Mater Interfaces 5 (8) (2013) 2853–2860.

[7] X. Mu, X. Xin, C. Fan, X. Li, X. Tian, K.-F. Xu, et al., A paper-based skin patch for the diagnostic screening of cystic fibrosis, Chem Commun 51 (29) (2015) 6365–6368.

[8] W. Zhao, W.-P. Zhang, Z.-L. Zhang, R.-L. He, Y. Lin, M. Xie, et al., Robust and highly sensitive fluorescence approach for point-of-care virus detection based on immunomagnetic separation, Anal Chem 84 (5) (2012) 2358–2365.

[9] Y. Li, X. Yan, X. Feng, J. Wang, W. Du, Y. Wang, et al., Agarose-based microfluidic device for point-of-care concentration and detection of pathogen, Anal Chem 86 (21) (2014) 10653–10659.

[10] F.F. Bier, S. Schumacher, Integration in bioanalysis: technologies for point-of-care testing, in: Molecular diagnostics, Springer, 2013, pp. 1–14.

[11] J. Sun, Y. Xianyu, X. Jiang, Point-of-care biochemical assays using gold nanoparticle-implemented microfluidics, Chem Soc Rev 43 (17) (2014) 6239–6253.

[12] E. Carrilho, A.W. Martinez, G.M. Whitesides, Understanding wax printing: a simple micropatterning process for paper-based microfluidics, Anal Chem 81 (16) (2009) 7091–7095.

[13] C. Renault, J. Koehne, A.J. Ricco, R.M. Crooks, Three-dimensional wax patterning of paper fluidic devices, Langmuir 30 (23) (2014) 7030–7036.

[14] S.A. Klasner, A.K. Price, K.W. Hoeman, R.S. Wilson, K.J. Bell, C.T. Culbertson, Paper-based microfluidic devices for analysis of clinically relevant analytes present in urine and saliva, Anal Bioanal Chem 397 (5) (2010) 1821–1829.
[15] L. Yu, Z.Z. Shi, Microfluidic paper-based analytical devices fabricated by low-cost photolithography and embossing of Parafilm®, Lab Chip 15 (7) (2015) 1642–1645.
[16] Y. Sameenoi, P.N. Nongkai, S. Nouanthavong, C.S. Henry, D. Nacapricha, One-step polymer screen-printing for microfluidic paper-based analytical device (μPAD) fabrication, Analyst 139 (24) (2014) 6580–6588.
[17] J. Olkkonen, K. Lehtinen, T. Erho, Flexographically printed fluidic structures in paper, Anal Chem 82 (24) (2010) 10246–10250.
[18] P. Spicar-Mihalic, B. Toley, J. Houghtaling, T. Liang, P. Yager, E. Fu, CO_2 laser cutting and ablative etching for the fabrication of paper-based devices, J Micromech Microeng 23 (6) (2013), 067003.
[19] J. Nie, Y. Liang, Y. Zhang, S. Le, D. Li, S. Zhang, One-step patterning of hollow microstructures in paper by laser cutting to create microfluidic analytical devices, Analyst 138 (2) (2013) 671–676.
[20] Z. Nie, C.A. Nijhuis, J. Gong, X. Chen, A. Kumachev, A.W. Martinez, et al., Electrochemical sensing in paper-based microfluidic devices, Lab Chip 10 (4) (2010) 477–483.
[21] X. Li, J. Tian, T. Nguyen, W. Shen, Paper-based microfluidic devices by plasma treatment, Anal Chem 80 (23) (2008) 9131–9134.
[22] D.A. Bruzewicz, M. Reches, G.M. Whitesides, Low-cost printing of poly (dimethylsiloxane) barriers to define microchannels in paper, Anal Chem 80 (9) (2008) 3387–3392.
[23] Y. He, Y. Wu, X. Xiao, J. Fu, G. Xue, A low-cost and rapid microfluidic paper-based analytical device fabrication method: flash foam stamp lithography, RSC Adv 4 (109) (2014) 63860–63865.
[24] K. Abe, K. Suzuki, D. Citterio, Inkjet-printed microfluidic multianalyte chemical sensing paper, Anal Chem 80 (18) (2008) 6928–6934.
[25] C. Renault, X. Li, S.E. Fosdick, R.M. Crooks, Hollow-channel paper analytical devices, Anal Chem 85 (16) (2013) 7976–7979.
[26] P.D. Haller, C.A. Flowers, M. Gupta, Three-dimensional patterning of porous materials using vapor phase polymerization, Soft Matter 7 (6) (2011) 2428–2432.
[27] Y. Jiang, Study on fabrication of microfluidic paper-based analytical devices and manipulation of microfluidic flow in paper-based channels using a hand-held corona treater (Master thesis), ZheJiang University, HangZhou, China, 2014.
[28] L. Cai, C. Xu, S. Lin, J. Luo, M. Wu, F. Yang, A simple paper-based sensor fabricated by selective wet etching of silanized filter paper using a paper mask, Biomicrofluidics 8 (5) (2014), 056504.
[29] Y. Lu, W. Shi, L. Jiang, J. Qin, B. Lin, Rapid prototyping of paper-based microfluidics with wax for low-cost, portable bioassay, Electrophoresis 30 (9) (2009) 1497–1500.
[30] T. Songjaroen, W. Dungchai, O. Chailapakul, W. Laiwattanapaisal, Novel, simple and low-cost alternative method for fabrication of paper-based microfluidics by wax dipping, Talanta 85 (5) (2011) 2587–2593.
[31] T. Kawase, H. Sirringhaus, R.H. Friend, T. Shimoda, Inkjet printed via-hole interconnections and resistors for all-polymer transistor circuits, Adv Mater 13 (21) (2001) 1601–1605.
[32] C. Sones, I. Katis, P. He, B. Mills, M. Namiq, P. Shardlow, et al., Laser-induced photopolymerisation for creation of paper-based fluidic devices, Lab Chip 14 (23) (2014) 4567–4574.

[33] V.F. Curto, N. Lopez-Ruiz, L.F. Capitan-Vallvey, A.J. Palma, F. Benito-Lopez, D. Diamond, Fast prototyping of paper-based microfluidic devices by contact stamping using indelible ink, RSC Adv 3 (41) (2013) 18811–18816.

[34] E.M. Fenton, M.R. Mascarenas, G.P. López, S.S. Sibbett, Multiplex lateral-flow test strips fabricated by two-dimensional shaping, ACS Appl Mater Interfaces 1 (1) (2008) 124–129.

[35] D.L. Giokas, G.Z. Tsogas, A.G. Vlessidis, Programming fluid transport in paper-based microfluidic devices using razor-crafted open channels, Anal Chem 86 (13) (2014) 6202–6207.

[36] A.C. Glavan, R.V. Martinez, E.J. Maxwell, A.B. Subramaniam, R.M. Nunes, S. Soh, et al., Rapid fabrication of pressure-driven open-channel microfluidic devices in omniphobic RF paper, Lab Chip 13 (15) (2013) 2922–2930.

[37] T. Nurak, N. Praphairaksit, O. Chailapakul, Fabrication of paper-based devices by lacquer spraying method for the determination of nickel(II) ion in waste water, Talanta 114 (2013) 291–296.

[38] W. Dungchai, O. Chailapakul, C.S. Henry, A low-cost, simple, and rapid fabrication method for paper-based microfluidics using wax screen-printing, Analyst 136 (1) (2011) 77–82.

[39] A.W. Martinez, S.T. Phillips, B.J. Wiley, M. Gupta, G.M. Whitesides, FLASH: a rapid method for prototyping paper-based microfluidic devices, Lab Chip 8 (12) (2008) 2146–2150.

[40] Q. He, C. Ma, X. Hu, H. Chen, Method for fabrication of paper-based microfluidic devices by alkylsilane self-assembling and UV/O_3-patterning, Anal Chem 85 (3) (2013) 1327–1331.

[41] Y. He, W.-B. Wu, J.-Z. Fu, Rapid fabrication of paper-based microfluidic analytical devices with desktop stereolithography 3D printer, RSC Adv 5 (4) (2015) 2694–2701.

[42] J. Songok, M. Tuominen, H. Teisala, J. Haapanen, J. Makela, J. Kuusipalo, et al., Paper-based microfluidics: fabrication technique and dynamics of capillary-driven surface flow, ACS Appl Mater Interfaces 6 (22) (2014) 20060–20066.

[43] P.-K. Kao, C.-C. Hsu, One-step rapid fabrication of paper-based microfluidic devices using fluorocarbon plasma polymerization, Microfluid Nanofluid 16 (5) (2014) 811–818.

[44] X. Li, J. Tian, G. Garnier, W. Shen, Fabrication of paper-based microfluidic sensors by printing, Colloids Surf B: Biointerfaces 76 (2) (2010) 564–570.

[45] K. Maejima, S. Tomikawa, K. Suzuki, D. Citterio, Inkjet printing: an integrated and green chemical approach to microfluidic paper-based analytical devices, RSC Adv 3 (24) (2013) 9258–9263.

[46] P. Kwong, M. Gupta, Vapor phase deposition of functional polymers onto paper-based microfluidic devices for advanced unit operations, Anal Chem 84 (22) (2012) 10129–10135.

[47] G. Demirel, E. Babur, Vapor-phase deposition of polymers as a simple and versatile technique to generate paper-based microfluidic platforms for bioassay applications, Analyst 139 (10) (2014) 2326–2331.

[48] A.W. Martinez, S.T. Phillips, G.M. Whitesides, Three-dimensional microfluidic devices fabricated in layered paper and tape, Proc Natl Acad Sci U S A 105 (50) (2008) 19606–19611.

[49] G.G. Lewis, M.J. DiTucci, M.S. Baker, S.T. Phillips, High throughput method for prototyping three-dimensional, paper-based microfluidic devices, Lab Chip 12 (15) (2012) 2630–2633.

[50] H. Liu, R.M. Crooks, Three-dimensional paper microfluidic devices assembled using the principles of origami, J Am Chem Soc 133 (44) (2011) 17564–17566.
[51] L. Ge, S. Wang, S. Ge, J. Yu, M. Yan, N. Li, et al., Electrophoretic separation in a microfluidic paper-based analytical device with an on-column wireless electrogenerated chemiluminescence detector, Chem Commun 50 (43) (2014) 5699–5702.
[52] L. Wu, C. Ma, L. Ge, Q. Kong, M. Yan, S. Ge, et al., Paper-based electrochemiluminescence origami cyto-device for multiple cancer cells detection using porous AuPd alloy as catalytically promoted nanolabels, Biosens Bioelectron 63 (2015) 450–457.
[53] L. Ge, P. Wang, S. Ge, N. Li, J. Yu, M. Yan, et al., Photoelectrochemical lab-on-paper device based on an integrated paper supercapacitor and internal light source, Anal Chem 85 (8) (2013) 3961–3970.
[54] M.M. Gong, P. Zhang, B.D. MacDonald, D. Sinton, Nanoporous membranes enable concentration and transport in fully wet paper-based assays, Anal Chem 86 (16) (2014) 8090–8097.
[55] W. Dungchai, O. Chailapakul, C.S. Henry, Electrochemical detection for paper-based microfluidics, Anal Chem 81 (14) (2009) 5821–5826.
[56] H. Li, D. Han, G. Pauletti, A. Steckl, Blood coagulation screening using a paper-based microfluidic lateral flow device, Lab Chip 14 (20) (2014) 4035–4041.
[57] M.S. Khan, X. Li, W. Shen, G. Garnier, Thermal stability of bioactive enzymatic papers, Colloids Surf B: Biointerfaces 75 (1) (2010) 239–246.
[58] M. Zhou, M. Yang, F. Zhou, Paper based colorimetric biosensing platform utilizing cross-linked siloxane as probe, Biosens Bioelectron 55 (2014) 39–43.
[59] N. Lopez-Ruiz, V.F. Curto, M.M. Erenas, F. Benito-Lopez, D. Diamond, A.J. Palma, et al., Smartphone-based simultaneous pH and nitrite colorimetric determination for paper microfluidic devices, Anal Chem 86 (19) (2014) 9554–9562.
[60] N. Ratnarathorn, O. Chailapakul, C.S. Henry, W. Dungchai, Simple silver nanoparticle colorimetric sensing for copper by paper-based devices, Talanta 99 (2012) 552–557.
[61] E.J. Maxwell, A.D. Mazzeo, G.M. Whitesides, Paper-based electroanalytical devices for accessible diagnostic testing, MRS Bull 38 (4) (2013) 309–314.
[62] S.N. Tan, L. Ge, W. Wang, Paper disk on screen printed electrode for one-step sensing with an internal standard, Anal Chem 82 (21) (2010) 8844–8847.
[63] N.K. Thom, G.G. Lewis, K. Yeung, S.T. Phillips, Quantitative fluorescence assays using a self-powered paper-based microfluidic device and a camera-equipped cellular phone, RSC Adv 4 (3) (2014) 1334–1340.
[64] J. Yu, S. Wang, L. Ge, S. Ge, A novel chemiluminescence paper microfluidic biosensor based on enzymatic reaction for uric acid determination, Biosens Bioelectron 26 (7) (2011) 3284–3289.
[65] J. Yu, L. Ge, J. Huang, S. Wang, S. Ge, Microfluidic paper-based chemiluminescence biosensor for simultaneous determination of glucose and uric acid, Lab Chip 11 (7) (2011) 1286–1291.
[66] M. Zhang, L. Ge, S. Ge, M. Yan, J. Yu, J. Huang, et al., Three-dimensional paper-based electrochemiluminescence device for simultaneous detection of Pb^{2+} and Hg^{2+} based on potential-control technique, Biosens Bioelectron 41 (2013) 544–550.
[67] S. Reinholt, A. Sonnenfeldt, A. Naik, M. Frey, A. Baeumner, Developing new materials for paper-based diagnostics using electrospun nanofibers, Anal Bioanal Chem 406 (14) (2014) 3297–3304.
[68] X. Mu, L. Zhang, S. Chang, W. Cui, Z. Zheng, Multiplex microfluidic paper-based immunoassay for the diagnosis of hepatitis C virus infection, Anal Chem 86 (11) (2014) 5338–5344.

[69] X. Yang, O. Forouzan, T.P. Brown, S.S. Shevkoplyas, Integrated separation of blood plasma from whole blood for microfluidic paper-based analytical devices, Lab Chip 12 (2) (2012) 274–280.

[70] R. Gerbers, W. Foellscher, H. Chen, C. Anagnostopoulos, M. Faghri, A new paper-based platform technology for point-of-care diagnostics, Lab Chip 14 (20) (2014) 4042–4049.

[71] A. Apilux, Y. Ukita, M. Chikae, O. Chailapakul, Y. Takamura, Development of automated paper-based devices for sequential multistep sandwich enzyme-linked immunosorbent assays using inkjet printing, Lab Chip 13 (1) (2013) 126–135.

[72] M. Su, L. Ge, S. Ge, N. Li, J. Yu, M. Yan, et al., Paper-based electrochemical cyto-device for sensitive detection of cancer cells and in situ anticancer drug screening, Anal Chim Acta 847 (2014) 1–9.

[73] G. Wu, J. Srivastava, M.H. Zaman, Stability measurements of antibodies stored on paper, Anal Biochem 449 (2014) 147–154.

[74] P. Wang, L. Ge, S. Ge, J. Yu, M. Yan, J. Huang, A paper-based photoelectrochemical immunoassay for low-cost and multiplexed point-of-care testing, Chem Commun 49 (32) (2013) 3294–3296.

[75] Y. Wang, H. Liu, P. Wang, J. Yu, S. Ge, M. Yan, Chemiluminescence excited photoelectrochemical competitive immunosensing lab-on-paper device using an integrated paper supercapacitor for signal amplication, Sens Actuators B: Chem 208 (2015) 546–553.

[76] T.-T. Tsai, S.-W. Shen, C.-M. Cheng, C.-F. Chen, Paper-based tuberculosis diagnostic devices with colorimetric gold nanoparticles, Sci Technol Adv Mater 14 (4) (2013) 044404.

[77] A.M. Rosa, A.F. Louro, S.A. Martins, J. Inácio, A.M. Azevedo, P. DMF, Capture and detection of DNA hybrids on paper via the anchoring of antibodies with fusions of carbohydrate binding modules and ZZ-domains, Anal Chem 86 (9) (2014) 4340–4347.

[78] V. Mani, K. Kadimisetty, S. Malla, A.A. Joshi, J.F. Rusling, Paper-based electrochemiluminescent screening for genotoxic activity in the environment, Environ Sci Technol 47 (4) (2013) 1937–1944.

[79] B.M. Jayawardane, W. Wongwilai, K. Grudpan, S. Kolev, M. Heaven, D. Nash, et al., Evaluation and application of a paper-based device for the determination of reactive phosphate in soil solution, J Environ Qual 43 (3) (2014) 1081–1085.

[80] G. Lisak, J. Cui, J. Bobacka, Paper-based microfluidic sampling for potentiometric determination of ions, Sens Actuators B: Chem 207 (2015) 933–939.

[81] W. Liu, S. Mao, J. Wu, J.-M. Lin, Development and applications of paper-based electrospray ionization-mass spectrometry for monitoring of sequentially generated droplets, Analyst 138 (7) (2013) 2163–2170.

CHAPTER

Smartphone-based microfluidic devices

12

Akbar Hasanzadeh[a,b,*]

[a]*Department of Medical Nanotechnology, Faculty of Advanced Technologies in Medicine, Iran University of Medical Sciences, Tehran, Iran*

[b]*Advances Nanobiotechnology and Nanomedicine Research Group (ANNRG), Iran University of Medical Sciences, Tehran, Iran*

[*]*Corresponding author. E-mail: akbarhasanzadeh16@gmail.com*

12.1 Introduction

Software and hardware development have led to the advancement of smartphone technology which has affected every inhabitant of the world [1, 2]. In the late 1990s, with the entry of smartphones into the wide consumer market, commercial smartphones have been transformed into hand-held computers. Smartphones were rapidly adopted all over the world when people started to use Apple iPhone products in 2007. Based on statistics, it is anticipated that the number of smartphone users will increase from 2.5 billion in 2016 to 3.8 billion in 2021 [3]. Nowadays, smartphones can play the role of computers with the advantages of being easy-to-use, large memory, sufficient battery, audio and USB ports, touch screens, cheap, portable, multifunctional (taking photos, playing songs, and finding directions). Recently, smartphones have been combined with microfluidic devices, so-called MS^2, and can act as mobile diagnostic tools, which can analyze primary information rapidly and on-site [4, 5]. Microfluidic systems with reaction chambers and channels in the length scale of micrometers can manipulate fluidic samples with volumes of microliters [6]. Due to the advantages of microfluidic devices, consisting of batch processing, well-controlled microenvironment, high-throughput testing, reduced sample consumption, these systems have attracted much interest for diagnostic applications. Besides the aforementioned merits of MS^2, they still have some drawbacks, such as being expensive, relatively bulky, and not easy to handle, compared to traditional diagnostic systems. Both industry and scientific communities have continued to study the combination of microfluidic devices and smartphones, in the fields of environmental and food safety monitoring, disease diagnosis, and routine health tests [7, 8].

Biomedical Applications of Microfluidic Devices. https://doi.org/10.1016/B978-0-12-818791-3.00014-0

12.2 Utilization of MS^2 for biomedical diagnosis

The detection of blood-borne pathogens (e.g., malaria) using microscopy-based diagnostic methods is challenging in some developing regions and low resource settings. Moreover, polymerase chain reaction (PCR) or enzyme-linked immunosorbent assay (ELISA), which are the traditional approaches for detecting protein or nucleic acid biomarkers, suffer from some restrictions such as the need for specialized and expensive equipment and are time-consuming and laborious processes. To this end, MS^2 can provide a route to create novel and easier techniques for biomedical diagnostics [9].

12.3 Detection of pathogens using MS^2

One of the most common approaches in medical diagnosis and health checking is the detection and counting of human cells or pathogen cells. A broad range of infectious diseases and cancers can be diagnosed if the presence of pathogens or abnormal cells is observed using a microscope as the gold standard test. For the direct detection of bloodborne pathogens, using a smartphone-based microscope could be a low cost, portable approach, which could not only perform as well as the current microscopic system but could also improve pathogen identification, especially in resource-limited countries [10]. An innovative smartphone-based microscope was integrated with thin glass capillaries, which could detect the presence of *Loa loa* microfilariae (mf) in blood by measuring the motion of mf instead of morphology or molecular biomarkers. This device was fabricated by D'Ambrosio and his coworkers [11]. To measure the number of moving mf within 2.59 μL of blood, they used a single field-of-view (FOV). Additional FOVs could be observed over the length of the thin glass capillary through moving the capillary using a servo-motor. The quantification of this approach allowed five FOVs to be analyzed in less than 2 min, and the specificity and sensitivity of this method were found to be 94% and 100%, respectively

The combination of a paper-based microfluidic dot-ELISA system and a smartphone as a point-of-care (POC) diagnostic device to identify influenza A (Flu A) virus in the blood, was developed as a self-operating, portable, and low-cost system by Wu and colleagues. The reaction module and the reagent storage reservoir were embedded in a low-cost paper-based microfluidic chip. The integration of an absorbent pad and nitrocellulose (NC) membrane formed the reaction module, which was equipped with a specific monoclonal antibody for each experiment used for immunoassay-based identification. For storage and release of the reagents, the storage module consisted of two reagent chambers with distribution channels. The distributed reagents moved through the NC membrane at a controllable speed towards the absorbent pad under the effects of gravity and capillary force without any external pressure. After images of the NC membrane were captured using a smartphone camera, they were processed by a smart algorithm of a custom software application, which was designed using Java to run on smartphones. They showed that a low-cost, easy-to-handle, transportable, and sensitive paper-based microfluidic system could be constructed with the aid of a smartphone to detect Flu A as opposed to more traditional methods. Due to the ability of the smartphone to capture and analyze images using custom application software, providing data display and transmission, in combination with a paper-based microfluidic diagnostic system, this approach could be easily adapted to detect other pathogens [12].

Amplification of nucleic acids provides a highly specific, sensitive, and rapid assay method which can be applied to identify a broad spectrum of pathogens related to infectious diseases [13]. In this regard, Qiu et al. integrated a smartphone with a microfluidic-based convection PCR in a POC setting to detect influenza A (H1N1) virus. Briefly, the rapid amplification of the nucleic acids was carried out by using convection PCR in a capillary tube with an ordinary heating block. To create a constant temperature gradient all over the capillary tube, the bottom of the tube was heated using a resistive heater, which was used a 5V power supply, whereas the terminal end of the tube was held at a constant temperature. The existence of the stable temperature gradient across the capillary tube produced a continuous circulatory stream, which caused transport of the reagents through the tube containing areas at different temperatures by the PCR stages, denaturing, annealing, and extension. Taqman probes tagged with FAM dye (carboxyfluorescein) were used for real-time identification. To illuminate the reagent for fluorescence excitation, a light-emitting diode was placed at the bottom of the capillary tube. A smartphone was used to capture the fluorescence images with its camera for real-time fluorescence identification and was also used to process the images and interpret the data by an intelligent custom algorithm running on the smartphone with Java. As a result, they demonstrated that compared to traditional PCR and real-time methods, the microfluidic convection real-time PCR equipped with a smartphone was a portable, simple and easy-to-use device that could successfully identify Influenza A (H1N1) virus with a concentration of 1.0 TCID 50/mL with lower costs and shorter time (less than 30 min) [14].

The integration of Mie scattering into microfabricated optical waveguides or "optofluidic channels" could produce a microbead immunoagglutination assay in a lab-on-a-chip format in which appended target antigens bound with antibody-conjugated microbeads as a state-of-the-art sensitive detection system [15]. Stemple and his coworkers fabricated a new smartphone-based optofluidic lab-on-a-chip to detect histidine-rich protein 2 (HRP-2), a *Plasmodium falciparum* (malaria) specific antigen, as a model pathogen in human whole blood, which was diluted to 10%. HRP-2 and antibody-conjugated microbeads reacted together within the PDMS-based lab-on-a-chip. A smartphone with a white LED flash and a camera acted as the only light source and detector in this assay. A series of lenses and mirrors were used in this assay to deliver LED light to the optofluidic channels within the microchip. To measure Mie scattering from the sample, the reaction channel was positioned at a 45-degree angle. A smartphone camera as the detector received the scattered light intensity, caused by the immunoagglutination between HRP-2 and the antibody-conjugated microbeads. The whole assay time and the limit of detection (LOD) were nearly 10 min and 1 pg/mL in 10% whole human blood, respectively. This portable and easy-to-use system not only could detect HRP-2 successfully with high sensitivity, but was also able to be used for identification of several pathogens in blood with good sensitivity [16].

One of the most significant ways to manage the health risk of sexually transmitted diseases (STDs), which are often transferred by sexual intercourse (but not exclusively) such as HIV and syphilis. Early diagnosis is important for both mothers and pregnant women where it can affect the children [17]. For simultaneous identification of HIV, syphilis and control samples, Laksanasopin and coworkers designed a novel handheld ELISA system, which consisted of a smartphone and a disposable microfluidic cassette with several detection regions. In this assay, two types of metal nanoparticles, gold and silver, were utilized as the signal amplification elements. Specific antibodies were located within multiple detection zones of the microfluidic cassette to capture the target antigens. Targeted antigens were detected in blood samples by creating a manual negative pressure in the microfluidic cassette to move the reagents for the ELISA assay. Photodetectors and LEDs were attached to a microcontroller to measure the optical density absorbance (read-out test). The optical density results were analyzed by a smartphone, which was connected to the microcontroller and powered by the audio jack interface. To carry out the assay, about 2 μL blood was obtained from the samples, and the results of this assay were obtained within 15 min. The results of this triple analysis, the sensitivity of 92%–100% and specificity of 79%–100%, were comparable with the gold standard laboratory-based HIV ELISA tests [18].

12.4 Analysis of genes

Molecular diagnostic often involves nucleic acid amplification. Recently, microfluidic devices have been used as a point of care and home genetic diagnosis platforms [19, 20]. Due to the advantages of PCR nucleic acid-based diagnostics, including quantification ability, high sensitivity and specificity, many researchers have started to developed microfluidic chips for PCR [21–23]. Despite the abovementioned advantages of PCR, the high electricity consumption for thermal cycling restricts its use in many areas of the world [24]. To address this problem, a solar-powered quantitative PCR system, consisting of a solar cell and a microfluidic device, was developed by Jiang et al. [25]. In this system, the solar cell allowed the required thermal cycling by obtaining energy from natural sources. Three ring-shaped temperature regions were embedded within the device to cycle the experimental sample. To measure and display the temperature of the zones, a smartphone was connected to a microcontroller, which helped to control the on-chip thermocouples. This system not only demonstrated major advantages, such as high throughput, high reaction speeds and low cross-contamination, compared to the standard PCR method but also decreased the power consumption to nearly 80 mW. Besides, only about 30 min was needed for this system to identify nucleic acid sequences in human skin biopsies.

Although the use of solar-power based PCR devices is promising for nucleic acid diagnosis, some obstacles remain including the complexity of the system and the accuracy of thermal cycling. To overcome these limitations, a loop-mediated isothermal amplification (LAMP) approach that acted as a handheld nucleic acid testing platform was introduced by Liu and coworkers [26]. This system, the so-called Gene-Z system, did not need to use any thermal cycling for nucleic acid amplification. The polymer microfluidic chip contained an array of reaction wells, which were designed along with the appropriate PCR reagents for detection of bacteria, in the Gene-Z system. In this system, an aluminum heater was used to heat the microfluidic chip to the desired temperatures. To prevent the cross-over of optical signals between the wells, embedded shell-structured reaction wells were employed. For gathering the fluorescence signals, 64 polymeric optical fibers and an equal number of green LEDs were positioned on top of the aluminum heater. After converting the fluorescence signals to an electrical voltage, this voltage was measured by a photodiode attached to the microcontroller. Both the heater and the LEDs were monitored by a smartphone. An IPod Touch in addition to the mentioned tasks, gathered and processed the information from the microcontroller and reported the data via Wi-Fi. This inexpensive rapid PCR device with low consumption of reagents could identify two different nucleic acid sequences from two different pathogens within 8 min.

In another study, a paper microfluidic chip was combined with a smartphone to identify the nucleic acids of *Salmonella typhimurium* by Fronczek et al. [27] in a rapid, user-friendly, compact, one-step detection device without the need for amplification. *S. typhimurium* cells in water were transferred to 10% poultry packaging liquid, and the samples were loaded onto the paper chips. These were for incubated for 3 min for cell lysis, and the paper chips were eluted by addition of buffer. In the last step, the specified zones within the paper channels were filled with 3 μL of Qubit fluorescent intercalating dye. To measure the fluorescence emitted from the paper chip, a smartphone was modified with a fluorescence microscope, which consisted of a dichroic mirror, a blue LED, 2 bandpass filters and two 10× objective lenses. A rapid assay was possible (only 5 min) using this user-friendly device. Different values of LOD were obtained when different kinds of paper were used; nitrocellulose paper and cellulose paper showed 10^4 and 10^3 CFU/mL LOD, respectively.

12.5 Analysis of food safety and environmental contamination using MS^2

12.5.1 Identification of heavy metal pollution

Rain and running water are the two most common sources of pollution, in particular, heavy metals such as cobalt, copper, cadmium, mercury, vanadium, chromium, manganese, zinc, nickel, lead, molybdenum, iron, selenium, and arsenic. These elements may be leached out of natural geological formations or else can be industrial waste products, and can eventually enter into water designed for human consumption. Accumulation of heavy metals at high concentrations can cause a range of health problems such as cancer. Identification of pollution associated with heavy metals is as critical as the detection of other pathogenic agents to reduce health risks to the wider population. Hence, portable and inexpensive methods with a good ability to detect toxic concentrations of heavy metals are required. Although atomic absorption spectroscopy (heavy metal quantitative measurement) and "Heavy Metal Water Test Kit" (heavy metal qualitative analysis) are employed for this purpose, the former suffers from complexity and is time-consuming, while the latter is not able to precisely quantify heavy metals [8, 28]. Recently, a novel class of heavy metal detection devices, MS^2, could be a portable, easy-to-use method for rapid and quantitative identification of heavy metals.

Three dimensional (3D) paper-based microfluidic systems have been investigated for heavy metal detection with advantages, such as low-cost and structural simplicity. The MS^2 system 3D paper-based microfluidic device coupled with a smartphone is not only able to decrease the time and costs but can also exactly quantify the heavy metals [29]. Wang and coworkers could identify four different heavy metals (Cu, Ni, Cd, and Cr) using an integrated 3D multilayer paper-based microfluidic chip equipped with a smartphone for colorimetric sensing. To fabricate the 3D paper-based microfluidic chip with multiple detection zones, they joined together four patterned paper strips including hydrophilic and hydrophobic channels, with three double-sided adhesive tapes between the sheets. In the next step, four different water samples were injected into the microfluidic device through each inlet, and then the liquid samples were allowed to diffuse into the microfluidic chip by capillary force without external pumping. After the samples arrived at the preplaced metal-selective chromogenic reagents, they reacted together and created the desired changes in colors. To detect and process the concentration of heavy metals, colorimetric images were captured and analyzed by the smartphone. The detections limits were 0.29, 0.33, 0.35, and 0.19 ppm for Cu, Ni, Cd, and Cr, respectively. Although the LODs in this method were similar to those from commercial atomic absorption spectroscopy, the smart-phone based method had benefits, such as low-cost, rapid detection and being user-friendly [30].

In another study, Li and colleagues developed the 3D paper-based microfluidic chip to detect six different metal ions (Fe, Ni, Cr, Cu, Al, and Zn) simultaneously with help of a smartphone. Briefly, the 3D paper-based microfluidic chip consisted of a patterned paper layer with different detection zones. Liquid samples were introduced into the microfluidic chip and were distributed to the channels by capillary force without pumping. The samples were pretreated by crossing the pretreatment zones before they reached the detection zones and underwent the chromogenic reactions. They showed that by designing a circuitous flow route with an L-shaped structure, not only was the accuracy of delivery of the chromogenic reagents ensured but also color uniformity and reproducibility was improved. They used a LED lamp and a smartphone to capture the images. The LODs of Fe, Ni, Cu, Zn, Cr, and Al were 0.2, 0.3, 0.03, 0.04, 0.1, and 0.08 ppm, respectively.

Electrochemical (EC) detection has high stability, good quantification without any sensitivity to ambient light, making it suitable for microfluidic chips, compared to optical-based detection The MS^2 system typically uses a camera to take images or capture fluorescence signals. Recently, some researchers have used a USB instead of a camera to capture the information from MS^2s. An EC sensor contained within the microfluidic chip, with an EC signal processor and a smartphone, was designed by Unyoung and coworkers to identify arsenic. Samples of contaminated water were added into the plastic-based microfluidic system, which was fabricated with an ink-based three-electrode platform. To measure the arsenic concentration, a voltammetry experiment was run using the EC processer. The smartphone as detector and processor was attached to the EC analyzer using a USB cable. Approximately 1 ppb of arsenic was the LOD (an important groundwater contaminant). Due to the advantages of EC-based MS^2 technology, including the ability to be incorporated with electronics, low-cost and portability, they are promising to be used in deprived regions, especially undeveloped countries [31].

12.5.2 Identification of bacterial contaminants

Concerns related to the quality and safety of water and food have increased in both well-developed and developing societies [32]. Polluted water and food sources contaminated with some types of bacteria and inorganic agents can threaten human life. Thus, developing systems, which can detect contaminants in food and water with high precision and rapidity, is important in today's world. Although some typical traditional approaches can detect pathogens in food and water, such as microscope-based systems, nitrite assays, and rapid diagnostic test strip (RDTs) are available, they are often large and expensive which prevents their widespread use. The optical features of smartphones, which can help to design accurate and inexpensive microscopic assays, have been employed to overcome the limitations of traditional microscopy-based methods. One of the first advances in this field was provided when a miniature microscope, which was able to capture images in both fluorescence and bright-field modes was developed for connecting to a smartphone by Breslauer and coworkers [33]. The miniaturization of optical microscopy has provided some innovative approaches to create portable systems for the detection of water and food contaminants. *Escherichia coli* (*E. coli*) can contaminate food and drinking water causing disease and damaging public health, so a portable smart phone based *E. coli* identification and screening device were developed by Zhu and coworkers [34]. In summary, liquid samples containing *E. coli* were added into glass capillaries, which were premodified with antibodies against *E. coli* and acted as microfluidic channels in a smartphone-based fluorescence imaging system. The second group of antibodies was conjugated to quantum dots (inorganic nanocrystals with unique optical and chemical features), which were dispersed into the capillaries to produce the fluorescence signals. In this study, ultraviolet light-emitting diodes (UV-LEDs) were used to excite the fluorescently conjugated antibodies attached to *E. coli*. The smartphone camera located at the bottom of the glass capillary tubes captured the emission from the quantum dots through an additional lens. The concentration of *E. coli* was measured in the samples by analyzing the fluorescent emissions from the capillaries. This test could be carried out in 2h. The LOD was almost 5–10CFU/mL in buffer solution, and a comparable LOD was found in fat-free milk as a complex liquid sample containing proteins and other potentially interfering substances. The specificity of this system also was assessed for different bacterial species (e.g., *Salmonella*), where they observed similar performance. Comparing with standard methods, such as PCR, mass spectroscopy, flow cytometry or ELISA assays, this lightweight, portable, the cost-effective, and the efficient platform has several advantages.

Park and coworkers introduced a portable, handheld and easy-to-use optical diagnostic device (integrating a paper-based microfluidic platform with a smartphone) to reduce the costs of typical optical-based microfluidic devices. They used this system for the detection of *S. typhimurium* in water by Mie scattering. Microbeads conjugated with anti-*S. typhimurium* and anti-*E. coli* antibodies were preloaded into the channels of the microfluidic device. The targeted pathogens were recognized when the paper-based microfluidic chip was dipped into the bacterial solutions and immunoagglutination was triggered. By locating a smartphone at an optimized angle and a suitable distance from the paper device, the intensity of light scattering caused by immunoagglutination could be correlated with the target pathogen concentration. The smartphone used ambient light to capture the images and analyzed them with a simple image-processing algorithm. The analysis time for this system was less than 90s and the detection limit was at the single-cell-level. Paper-based microfluidics using cellulose fibers are a cost-effective and easy-to-use way to prevent the interference of external contaminating particles such as dust within the system [35].

In addition to the previously mentioned methods for detection of pathogens in food and water, colorimetric assays are also used this field. The reaction products from the chromogenic reagents absorb light at a characteristic wavelength which is quantified to provide the concentration of targeted pathogens.

A smartphone-based multilayered microfluidic colorimetric assay was developed by Chen and coworkers to detect 2,2,4,4-tetrabromodiphenyl ether (BDE-47), a common environmental contaminant in foodstuffs. The microfluidic platform consisted of three layers. The first was a layer with chambers in which the sample was loaded, the second layer was equipped with channels, and the third layer was composed of PDMS and black carbon and acted as an electrode. Through a USB cable, the smartphone-powered an Arduino controller, which controlled the electrodes. These electrodes carried out an electrolytic reaction to produce gaseous bubbles with a volume change to drive the liquid flow so that no pumps were required. The colorimetric signal was the quantitative readout generated by the detection zones and captured using the smartphone and transferred to a computer server for postanalysis. The authors reported that this colorimetric-based microfluidic assay was not only faster (about 15min) than the conventional ELISA kits (at least 2h), but also needed a lower amount of sample [36].

12.5.3 Tests for pH, nitrate and nitrite

The pH of water is a simple indicator of palatability and safety for drinking, swimming, and other activities. For drinking water, the pH should be between 6.5 and

9.5 pH. For instance, one of the common ways to identify the presence of bacteria in the water is the evaluation of pH, because the acidic condition often occurs when water is contaminated with bacteria [37, 38]. Furthermore, nitrate and nitrite (a reduction product of nitrate) should be measured in food and water, because both ions are associated with agricultural processes and septic waste, and therefore, can be considered as indicators of contamination. Nitrate comes from fertilizer used in the countryside and the suburbs where it can contaminate groundwater, while although nitrite is a common food preservative it can also be seen as a contaminant [39].

A cost-effective paper-based microfluidic platform was integrated with a smartphone by Lopez-Ruiz and coworkers for the simultaneous detection of nitrite and measurement of pH in liquid samples [38]. Seven detection zones were embedded in a microfluidic chip. Three detection zones determined the pH value, three zones were designed to detect the concentration of nitrite, and one zone acted as a blank area. The Griess reagent was preloaded in three nitrite detection areas, and also phenol red and chlorophenol red were preloaded as chromogenic reagents into the pH detection zones. A smartphone with an Android application was utilized to capture and analysis the images. The efficiency and reproducibility of the system were checked by using two different cell phones, which showed similar results. Nine samples with different concentrations of nitrite and pH values were tested to evaluate the performance of the system. A resolution of 0.51% at 4.0 mg/L and a LOD of 52 mg/L were obtained for nitrite test. For the pH test, the resolution gained was 0.04 pH units, an accuracy of 0.09 pH units and a mean squared error of 0.167. Both the nitrite and pH results were better than the results of commercial pH and nitrite measurement methods.

Although a USB cable can act as a connector between an Android smartphone and a microfluidic chip for rapid EC detection, the use of iOS (Apple iPhone) instead of an Android cell phone prevents the use of a micro-USB interface because there is no place on an iPhone to connect a USB cable. To overcome this obstacle, audio jacks have been developed to connect a microfluidic-device to an iPhone for an EC assay. To determine the concentration of nitrate in solution samples, an EC sensing paper-based microfluidic system connected a smartphone was introduced by Wang et al. Briefly, this device consisted of a smartphone connected to the microfluidic chip by an audio jack connector, which conveyed signals between the circuit in the channels and the cell phone. The EC detector was a paper-based microfluidic platform with a circuit board for monitoring the EC reaction. The total time of the assay was about 1 min with 0.2 ppm limit of detection [40].

12.6 Applications of MS^2 for routine clinical testing

Many diseases are diagnosed too late due to the lack of rapid easily-performed diagnostic assays. Not only could these devices identify primary symptoms rapidly, but they also do not require expensive and complex equipment. For example, assessing routine health tests can lead to better and earlier diagnosis of some diseases. For instance, serum cholesterol measurement can provide early diagnosis of heart disease, pH monitoring in saliva can prevent enamel decalcification, monitoring of sweat can reduce the risk of dehydration, urine analysis can detect diabetes, and serum vitamin D is involved with several diseases [41–44]. More traditional clinical laboratory assays could be replaced by MS^2s as cost-effective, handheld and easy-to-use alternatives.

A paper-based microfluidic platform combined with a smartphone was described by Chun and coworkers for glucose detection in blood samples [45]. The paper-based device was fabricated using two paper layers connected by double-sided adhesive tape. Firstly, a sample loading zone and a detection area containing glucose oxidase (GOx), horseradish peroxidase (HRP) and chromogenic reagents, were embedded in the upper layer. The bottom paper layer containing the microfluidic channels was then attached to the upper layer by double-sided adhesive tape. After injection of the glucose solution samples into the loading zone, they traveled through the microfluidic channels towards the detection zone by capillary force without external pressure. In the presence of H_2O_2 produced by the GOx enzyme acting on glucose, the second HRP enzyme converted the chromogenic reagent to a blue color as the signal readout. The color change was recorded and processed by the smartphone. The device was placed in a box to reduce signal interference from environmental light. To evaluate the performance of the system, different concentrations of glucose in water (0–20 mM) and human serum (5–17 mM) were tested. The detection limit was almost 0.3 mM, which was less than the cutoff concentration of glucose in serum (~7 mM) needed for evaluation of diabetes. This system could be effective for glucose measurement in blood.

The detection of cholesterol in blood or plasma (e.g., using test strips) has drawbacks, being relatively expensive and unable to analyze and store data easily. The common test strip devices, such as the pregnancy test strip, include dry reagents providing identification of target agents by creating color changes or forming lines. Another limitation is that the result is observed with the naked eye, which introduces errors and reduces the accuracy of the results. The use of a smartphone combined with test strips dramatically decreases the risk of mistakes. A cell phone accessory and software application using a portable test strip was developed by Oncescu et al. to determine cholesterol levels in whole blood based on colorimetric sensing [46]. In this study, a series of filter papers were implanted into the test strip to isolate plasma from whole blood. After that, the isolated plasma was driven to the reaction pad. The smartphone not only was used as a light source but was also used to capture and process the images. The authors showed that the accuracy for cholesterol levels was within 1.8% between 140 and 400 mg/dL and the total time of the assay was about 60 s. The maximum difference between the test results from this novel device and the CardioChek PA system was less than 5.5%. The vitamin D levels and pH values in sweat and saliva were measured by the same research group. They used colorimetric signal identification and a disposable test strip with a smartphone as a unified MS^2 system for detection of these indicators. The accuracy was obtained within 0.2 pH units for pH measurement in saliva and sweat. The vitamin D test results were comparable to those from conventional ELISA kits, and the system was able to measure the physiological levels of vitamin D. MS^2 systems can act as a noninvasive real-time assay for detection of vitamin D levels and pH values in saliva and sweat [47, 48].

Bioluminescence and chemiluminescence signal readouts have higher sensitivity, rapidity, and efficiency compared to commercial colorimetric approaches [49]. The combination of a 3D printed microfluidic platform with a smartphone was used together with bioluminescence and chemiluminescence detection for the measurement of cholesterol and bile acids in biological fluids by Roda et al. [50]. Two different analyses were used in this study as a proof-of-principle: chemiluminescence analysis was used to detect cholesterol levels and a bioluminescence assay for the detection of total bile acids. In this report, the sample cartridge consisted of a blood-filtering pad, which was inserted in the device and attached to a reaction zone via a microfluidic channel. Another microfluidic channel was used to connect a separate 15 μL storage chamber containing the BL-CL reagents to the reaction zone. The 3α-hydroxyl steroid dehydrogenase enzyme was coupled to cholesterol esterase/cholesterol oxidase enzymes along with H_2O_2-horseradish peroxidase within a nitrocellulose disk, which was located in the reaction chamber. During the test, after injection of 15 μL of the sample from the inlet into the cartridge, the solution was automatically driven toward the reaction chamber. The cartridge was placed into an adaptor joined to the smartphone. To record the luminescence signals, the smartphone camera was employed. The total bile acids and total cholesterol had limits of detection about 0.5 μmol/L and 20 mg/dL, respectively. The total time of the assay was about 3 min.

Notwithstanding the high sensitivity of chemiluminescence assays, there are still difficulties with the control of the reaction time and the signal levels that prevent their wide application [51]. To address these limitations, electrochemiluminescence methods can generate an electrical potential which may be more reliable compared to chemiluminescence readouts [52]. An electrochemiluminescence sensing device including a smartphone and a paper-based microfluidic chip was introduced by Delaney and coworkers [53, 54]. By using a smartphone, this platform was able to control both the photonic detection and the EC excitation.

In conclusion, MS^2s using different sensing methods can create an easy-to-use and disposable device for routine clinical tests, although additional developments are necessary for improved control of the reaction sensitivity, reliability, reproducibility, and stability.

References

[1] X. Meng, H. Huang, K. Yan, X. Tian, W. Yu, H. Cui, et al., Smartphone based hand-held quantitative phase microscope using the transport of intensity equation method, Lab Chip 17 (1) (2017) 104–109.

[2] D. Calabria, C. Caliceti, M. Zangheri, M. Mirasoli, P. Simoni, A. Roda, Smartphone-based enzymatic biosensor for oral fluid L-lactate detection in one minute using confined multilayer paper reflectometry, Biosens Bioelectron 94 (2017) 124–130.

[3] A. Holst, Number of smartphone users worldwide from 2016 to 2021, 2019, Available from: https://www.statista.com/statistics/330695/number-of-smartphone-users-worldwide/.

[4] A. Solanas, C. Patsakis, M. Conti, I.S. Vlachos, V. Ramos, F. Falcone, et al., Smart health: a context-aware health paradigm within smart cities, IEEE Commun Mag 52 (8) (2014) 74–81.
[5] D. Erickson, D. O'Dell, L. Jiang, V. Oncescu, A. Gumus, S. Lee, et al., Smartphone technology can be transformative to the deployment of lab-on-chip diagnostics, Lab Chip 14 (17) (2014) 3159–3164.
[6] D.R. Reyes, D. Iossifidis, P.-A. Auroux, A. Manz, Micro total analysis systems. 1. Introduction, theory, and technology, Anal Chem 74 (12) (2002) 2623–2636.
[7] X. Mao, T.J. Huang, Microfluidic diagnostics for the developing world, Lab Chip 12 (8) (2012) 1412–1416.
[8] K. Yang, H. Peretz-Soroka, Y. Liu, F. Lin, Novel developments in mobile sensing based on the integration of microfluidic devices and smartphones, Lab Chip 16 (6) (2016) 943–958.
[9] A. Moody, P. Chiodini, Methods for the detection of blood parasites, Clin Lab Haematol 22 (4) (2000) 189–201.
[10] X. Liu, T.-Y. Lin, P.B. Lillehoj, Smartphones for cell and biomolecular detection, Ann Biomed Eng 42 (11) (2014) 2205–2217.
[11] M. D'Ambrosio, M. Bakalar, S. Bennuru, C. Reber, A. Skandarajah, L. Nilsson, et al., Point-of-care quantification of blood-borne filarial parasites with a mobile phone microscope, Sci Transl Med 7 (2015) 286re4.
[12] D. Wu, J. Zhang, F. Xu, X. Wen, P. Li, X. Zhang, et al., A paper-based microfluidic Dot-ELISA system with smartphone for the detection of influenza A, Microfluid Nanofluid 21 (3) (2017) 43.
[13] Y.M. Park, Y.D. Han, K.R. Kim, C. Zhang, H.C. Yoon, An immunoblot-based optical biosensor for screening of osteoarthritis using a smartphone-embedded illuminometer, Anal Methods 7 (15) (2015) 6437–6442.
[14] 12. X. Qiu, S. Ge, P. Gao, K. Li, S. Yang, S. Zhang, et al., A smartphone-based point-of-care diagnosis of H1N1 with microfluidic convection PCR, Microsyst Technol 23 (7) (2017) 2951–2956.
[15] B.C. Heinze, J.R. Gamboa, K. Kim, J.-Y. Song, J.-Y. Yoon, Microfluidic immunosensor with integrated liquid core waveguides for sensitive Mie scattering detection of avian influenza antigens in a real biological matrix, Anal Bioanal Chem 398 (6) (2010) 2693–2700.
[16] C.C. Stemple, S.V. Angus, T.S. Park, J.-Y. Yoon, Smartphone-based optofluidic lab-on-a-chip for detecting pathogens from blood, J Lab Autom 19 (1) (2014) 35–41.
[17] M. Genç, W.J. Ledger, Syphilis in pregnancy, Sex Transm Infect 76 (2) (2000) 73–79.
[18] T. Laksanasopin, T.W. Guo, S. Nayak, A.A. Sridhara, S. Xie, O.O. Olowookere, et al., A smartphone dongle for diagnosis of infectious diseases at the point of care, Sci Transl Med 7 (273) (2015). 273re1–re1.
[19] P. Yager, T. Edwards, E. Fu, K. Helton, K. Nelson, M.R. Tam, et al., Microfluidic diagnostic technologies for global public health, Nature 442 (7101) (2006) 412.
[20] Z. Chen, M.G. Mauk, J. Wang, W.R. Abrams, P.L. Corstjens, R.S. Niedbala, et al., A microfluidic system for saliva-based detection of infectious diseases, Ann N Y Acad Sci 1098 (1) (2007) 429–436.
[21] C.D. Chin, V. Linder, S.K. Sia, Commercialization of microfluidic point-of-care diagnostic devices, Lab Chip 12 (12) (2012) 2118–2134.
[22] P. Yager, G.J. Domingo, J. Gerdes, Point-of-care diagnostics for global health, Annu Rev Biomed Eng 10 (2008).

[23] Z. Chen, S. Qian, W.R. Abrams, D. Malamud, H.H. Bau, Thermosiphon-based PCR reactor: experiment and modeling, Anal Chem 76 (13) (2004) 3707–3715.

[24] F. Ahmad, S.A. Hashsham, Miniaturized nucleic acid amplification systems for rapid and point-of-care diagnostics: a review, Anal Chim Acta 733 (2012) 1–15.

[25] L. Jiang, M. Mancuso, Z. Lu, G. Akar, E. Cesarman, D. Erickson, Solar thermal polymerase chain reaction for smartphone-assisted molecular diagnostics, Sci Rep 4 (2014) 4137.

[26] C. Liu, M.G. Mauk, H.H. Bau, A disposable, integrated loop-mediated isothermal amplification cassette with thermally actuated valves, Microfluid Nanofluid 11 (2) (2011) 209–220.

[27] C.F. Fronczek, T. San Park, D.K. Harshman, A.M. Nicolini, J.-Y. Yoon, Paper microfluidic extraction and direct smartphone-based identification of pathogenic nucleic acids from field and clinical samples, RSC Adv 4 (22) (2014) 11103–11110.

[28] J.M. Matés, J.A. Segura, F.J. Alonso, J. Márquez, Roles of dioxins and heavy metals in cancer and neurological diseases using ROS-mediated mechanisms, Free Radic Biol Med 49 (9) (2010) 1328–1341.

[29] A.W. Martinez, S.T. Phillips, G.M. Whitesides, Three-dimensional microfluidic devices fabricated in layered paper and tape, Proc Natl Acad Sci U S A 105 (50) (2008) 19606–19611.

[30] H. Wang, Y.-J. Li, J.-F. Wei, J.-R. Xu, Y.-H. Wang, G.-X. Zheng, Paper-based three-dimensional microfluidic device for monitoring of heavy metals with a camera cell phone, Anal Bioanal Chem 406 (12) (2014) 2799–2807.

[31] U. Kim, B. Demaree, J. VanderGiessen, M. Reynolds, K. Perricone, J. Seubert, et al. (Eds.), Electrochemical detection of arsenic via a microfluidic sensor and mobile interface towards affordable, rapid, and point-of-use water monitoring, 2013 IEEE 15th international conference on e-health networking, applications and services (Healthcom 2013), IEEE, 2013.

[32] V. Murray, G. Lau, Drinking water safety: guidance to health and water professionals and other health protection issues on water safety, 2011.

[33] D.N. Breslauer, R.N. Maamari, N.A. Switz, W.A. Lam, D.A. Fletcher, Mobile phone based clinical microscopy for global health applications, PLoS One 4 (7) (2009), e6320.

[34] H. Zhu, U. Sikora, A. Ozcan, Quantum dot enabled detection of *Escherichia coli* using a cell-phone, Analyst 137 (11) (2012) 2541–2544.

[35] T. San Park, W. Li, K.E. McCracken, J.-Y. Yoon, Smartphone quantifies Salmonella from paper microfluidics, Lab Chip 13 (24) (2013) 4832–4840.

[36] A. Chen, R. Wang, C.R. Bever, S. Xing, B.D. Hammock, T. Pan, Smartphone-interfaced lab-on-a-chip devices for field-deployable enzyme-linked immunosorbent assay, Biomicrofluidics 8 (6) (2014), 064101.

[37] C. Shadbolt, T. Ross, T. McMeekin, Differentiation of the effects of lethal pH and water activity: food safety implications, Lett Appl Microbiol 32 (2) (2001) 99–102.

[38] N. Lopez-Ruiz, V.F. Curto, M.M. Erenas, F. Benito-Lopez, D. Diamond, A.J. Palma, et al., Smartphone-based simultaneous pH and nitrite colorimetric determination for paper microfluidic devices, Anal Chem 86 (19) (2014) 9554–9562.

[39] Z. Usydus, J. Szlinder-Richert, L. Polak-Juszczak, K. Komar, M. Adamczyk, M. Malesa-Ciecwierz, et al., Fish products available in Polish market—assessment of the nutritive value and human exposure to dioxins and other contaminants, Chemosphere 74 (11) (2009) 1420–1428.

[40] X. Wang, M.R. Gartia, J. Jiang, T.-W. Chang, J. Qian, Y. Liu, et al., Audio jack based miniaturized mobile phone electrochemical sensing platform, Sens Actuators B 209 (2015) 677–685.

[41] N. West, J. Hughes, M. Addy, The effect of pH on the erosion of dentine and enamel by dietary acids in vitro, J Oral Rehabil 28 (9) (2001) 860–864.

[42] R. Morgan, M. Patterson, M. Nimmo, Acute effects of dehydration on sweat composition in men during prolonged exercise in the heat, Acta Physiol Scand 182 (1) (2004) 37–43.

[43] B.D. Malhotra, A. Chaubey, Biosensors for clinical diagnostics industry, Sens Actuators B 91 (1-3) (2003) 117–127.

[44] M.F. Holick, Sunlight and vitamin D for bone health and prevention of autoimmune diseases, cancers, and cardiovascular disease, Am J Clin Nutr 80 (6) (2004) 1678S–1688S.

[45] H.J. Chun, Y.M. Park, Y.D. Han, Y.H. Jang, H.C. Yoon, Paper-based glucose biosensing system utilizing a smartphone as a signal reader, Biochip J 8 (3) (2014) 218–226.

[46] V. Oncescu, M. Mancuso, D. Erickson, Cholesterol testing on a smartphone, Lab Chip 14 (4) (2014) 759–763.

[47] S. Lee, V. Oncescu, M. Mancuso, S. Mehta, D. Erickson, A smartphone platform for the quantification of vitamin D levels, Lab Chip 14 (8) (2014) 1437–1442.

[48] V. Oncescu, D. O'Dell, D. Erickson, Smartphone based health accessory for colorimetric detection of biomarkers in sweat and saliva, Lab Chip 13 (16) (2013) 3232–3238.

[49] A. Roda, P. Pasini, M. Mirasoli, E. Michelini, M. Guardigli, Biotechnological applications of bioluminescence and chemiluminescence, Trends Biotechnol 22 (6) (2004) 295–303.

[50] A. Roda, E. Michelini, L. Cevenini, D. Calabria, M.M. Calabretta, P. Simoni, Integrating biochemiluminescence detection on smartphones: mobile chemistry platform for point-of-need analysis, Anal Chem 86 (15) (2014) 7299–7304.

[51] S. Wang, L. Ge, X. Song, J. Yu, S. Ge, J. Huang, et al., Paper-based chemiluminescence ELISA: lab-on-paper based on chitosan modified paper device and wax-screen-printing, Biosens Bioelectron 31 (1) (2012) 212–218.

[52] Y. Xu, Z. Lv, Y. Xia, Y. Han, B. Lou, E. Wang, Highly porous magnetite/graphene nanocomposites for a solid-state electrochemiluminescence sensor on paper-based chips, Anal Bioanal Chem 405 (11) (2013) 3549–3558.

[53] J.L. Delaney, E.H. Doeven, A.J. Harsant, C.F. Hogan, Reprint of: use of a mobile phone for potentiostatic control with low cost paper-based microfluidic sensors, Anal Chim Acta 803 (2013) 123–127.

[54] J.L. Delaney, C.F. Hogan, J. Tian, W. Shen, Electrogenerated chemiluminescence detection in paper-based microfluidic sensors, Anal Chem 83 (4) (2011) 1300–1306.

CHAPTER

Targeted delivery of nucleic acids using microfluidic systems 13

Masoumehossadat Hosseini[a,b,*], Navid Rabiee[c], and Mojtaba Bagherzadeh[c]

[a]*Faculty of Chemistry and Petroleum Sciences, Department of Chemistry, Shahid Beheshti University, Tehran, Iran*

[b]*Soroush Mana Pharmed, Golrang Pharmaceutical Investment Co (GPI), Golrang Industrial Group (GIG), Tehran, Iran*

[c]*Department of Chemistry, Sharif University of Technology, Tehran, Iran*

**Corresponding author. E-mail: Hosseini7@ymail.com*

13.1 Introduction

Since the discovery of DNA, the delivery of nucleic acids into cells and tissues has become a possible therapeutic option, particularly for emerging diseases. Since nucleic acid-based drugs are highly sensitive to external conditions and their overall stability is low, one of the most important factors contributing to the efficacy and effectiveness of these drugs is the question of their effective transfer into the targeted cells and tissue. There have been several studies recently aimed at the targeted delivery of nucleic acids to cells and tissues carried out by many researchers around the world. One approach for the delivery of nucleic acids to target cells is the use of microfluidic devices, which may pave the way for targeted gene therapy. First, we explore nucleic acid structures in this chapter of the book, and then, with the knowledge of their chemical structure, we introduce an efficient tool known as microfluidic systems. In fact, these systems are now a mature technology that can overcome many of the barriers and limitations in nucleic acid transport. In this chapter of the book, we cover how nucleic acids can be combined with microfluidics for effective transfer into biological organisms. In addition, many other fluidic systems such as microfluidic, nanofluidic, and optofluidic devices have been employed to manipulate and disassemble biomedical components in biological sample complexes [1].

Since nucleic acids are equally important but are less stable than other biochemical or chemical drugs, the search for a reliable pathway for their efficient transfer into target cells is an important task. Microfluidic devices and fluidic systems are powerful techniques for this purpose. In fact, microfluidic systems can act as a miniaturized laboratory on a chip.

Biomedical Applications of Microfluidic Devices. https://doi.org/10.1016/B978-0-12-818791-3.00009-7

13.2 Structure of nucleic acids

Nucleic acids are chemical organic compounds taking the form of biopolymers. They are ubiquitous in living cells, in particular deoxyribonucleic acid (DNA) [2, 3] and ribonucleic acid (RNA). Nucleic acids including DNA and RNA are essential to all life forms. They consist of many nucleotide monomers linked together in a long chain. The nucleotides contain three components: a phosphate group, a sugar with five carbons, and a nitrogen-containing heterocyclic base. The sugar can be in two forms depending on the type of nucleic acid: the sugar in DNA structure is derived from deoxyribose, while in RNA it is derived from ribose [4, 5]. All the nitrogen bases are similar for both DNA and RNA structures, except that thymine, is used in DNA, while uracil is used in RNA. Two complementary nucleic acid strands are present in DNA that intertwine with each other to form the double helix. RNA structures generally have only a single-stranded chain. Nucleic acid molecules are usually without branches, and can be either linear or circular when the ends are joined together. Some examples of circular double-stranded DNA are bacterial chromosomes, plasmids, mitochondrial DNA, and chloroplast DNA. On the other hand, the chromosomes in the eukaryotic nucleus usually contain DNA in the linear form. We can categorize the molecules of life (DNA and RNA) in terms of a rising series of chemical structures: primary structure, secondary structure, tertiary structure, and quaternary structure.

13.2.1 Primary structure

The simplest, most elementary and basic nucleic acid structure is a completely linear polymer with bases linked by phosphodiester internucleotide bonds. In this structure, the phosphate is connected to the carbohydrate group in the 5′ position with the phosphate of the next nucleotide attached to the 3′ carbon atom. In DNA the four nitrogen bases are Adenine (A), Guanine (G), Cytosine (C), and Thymine (T). In RNA the bases are Adenine (A), Guanine (G), Cytosine (C), and Uracil (U) [6].

13.2.2 Secondary structure

In this class of structure it is necessary to distinguish between DNA and RNA molecules in order to make the concept of secondary structure understandable. In the case of DNA the secondary structure is formed from complementary binding of one strand to the other by hydrogen bonds formed between two matching nitrogen bases. Because of the special structure of these bases, purines (A, G) form hydrogen bonds with pyrimidines (C, T, or U). The secondary structure of DNA molecule arises by the wrapping of two complementary strands of polynucleotides around each other to form a double helix. This helix structure is the secondary structure of DNA. In addition to hydrogen bonds formed between the matching nitrogen bases, other factors involved in the secondary structure of DNA, which tend to stabilize the structure are stacking interactions using Van der Waals forces and hydrophobic interactions between the aligned strands. Most data about double-stranded nucleic acids have been obtained from x-ray diffraction studies. According to the Watson and Crick model, there can be other spatial conformations. Some types of molecular structures are known as A-DNA, B-DNA, and Z-DNA.

All of these structures have common characteristics. They all spiral in a right-handed or clockwise direction, and have the same axis. If there is a mismatch between pairs of nucleotide bases it affects the structure of the phosphate ester framework, and the central axis becomes deformed. The two ends of the spiral are chemically and structurally similar. Nonparallel bidirectional structures are important for single-stranded nucleic acids, such as t-RNA.

A small number of polynucleotides have been observed where double helices or multiple helices possess aligned strands. These structures do not follow the Watson and Crick base-pairing rules [7, 8].

13.2.3 The tertiary structure of nucleic acids

The tertiary structure in tRNA is formed by interactions with hydrogen bonds. This class of nucleic acid has the position of each atom in three-dimensional space defined by molecular interactions. As mentioned before, three kinds of DNA exist named A-DNA, B-DNA, and Z-DNA [9]. According to the type of orientation and interaction in space, these structures can be formed. The factors that govern the tertiary structure are: helix length, number of bases in each strand, difference in size [10].

The tertiary structure is different between RNA and DNA because of the presence of different bases. In RNA, t-RNA an example of the tertiary structure of nucleic acids because it can take up particular conformations like the cloverleaf structure [11].

In DNA it is more difficult to understand the tertiary structure but it is important to understand DNA folding within the double helix.

13.2.4 The quaternary structure of nucleic acids

Some nucleic acids have complex quaternary structures. These can take three forms: spherical, circular, or linear, and can form three-dimensional, two-dimensional, or one-dimensional frameworks. The three-dimensional framework is the newest type of nucleic acid spatial structure which was first described in 1996 by the Mirkin group at Northwestern University. Actually spherical nucleic acids (SNAs) can be thought of as a class of nanoparticles, which have a dense spherical framework composed of DNA or RNA. Since the RNA and DNA have similar structures they can provide SNAs with special physical and chemical properties. Because of the exclusively three-dimensional structure of SNAs, they are fundamentally different from the linear nucleic acids found in nature.

SNAs can enter human cells and tissues with relative ease; this is different from normal RNA and DNA molecules that do not have this ability. Therefore, SNAs can be used to design drugs to treat various diseases such as diabetes mellitus. The choice of SNAs as a vehicle can allow conjugation and connection with various chemical compounds. This conjugation can alter the chemical and physical properties in order to affect the orientation and rotation of DNA and RNA molecules, as well as oligonucleotides, which can help to increase the flexibility of SNAs.

RNA can also form complex 3D structures. RNA structures are also caused by Watson-Crick pairing between complementary bases. One 3D structure of RNA produces so-called aptamers that are able to specifically identify and bind to proteins, other nucleic acids, or even small-molecule ligands.

The simplest structure for nucleic acids is the linear form, which consists of nucleotide strands without any warping. It is important to know the structural form of nucleic acids in order to use them in treatment. The spatial structure for nucleic acids can determine their function even as much as their sequence.

13.3 Structures of natural and artificial nucleic acids

The following section discusses the structures and backbone of nucleic acids. We classified nucleic acids into four categories in order to distinguish them chemically.

13.3.1 DNA chemical structure

The first genetic molecule to be discovered was DNA that was discovered to carry the hereditary information encoded in the chromosomes. By determining the DNA chemical structure and base sequence, the genetic properties, and heritable storage of this biomolecule could be understood. Since the 1940s, research into DNA structure has been carried out on a massive scale. In terms of chemical structure, as already mentioned, the structural units of DNA are nucleotides, which contain phosphate groups, deoxyribose sugars and the most important nitrogenous bases (C, A, G, T), which are heterocyclic organic compounds [12].

The fundamental principle of DNA structure is based on the polynucleotide helical double-stranded chain [2].

For the first time ever in 2018, Zeraati et al. discovered a new form of DNA that had been present in our body cells without anyone noticing. This research team from the Kinghorn Centre for Clinical Trials at the Garvan Institute of Medical Research in Sydney described a new type of DNA structure, which was distinct from the ordinary common double-stranded structure. This structure was called an intercalated motif (i-motif) with a four-stranded knot-like structure and was found to be present in human cells. Details of this research were published June 2018 in Nature Chemistry [13] with the discovery of this new form of DNA i-motif, the previous results of some laboratory studies (in silico and in vitro) were confirmed. This discovery had a strong effect on investigations into the artificial and laboratory structures of DNA. In fact, for many years, scientists had been working on various possible forms of DNA molecules, such as triple helices or cruciform structures, with some interesting laboratory results. Examples of these DNA structures include the discovery of G-Quadruplex DNA in 2013 [14]. The i-motif structure had first been observed about two decades ago in artificial laboratory conditions [15], but it was widely believed that it would probably never be found in nature.

One of the most important factors in gene regulation is to control the level of DNA methylation, and this idea has become known as epigenetics. The discovery of factors that govern the methylation or hypomethylation of the CpG islands (CGI) is crucial in helping to address this issue. Therefore, knowing the exact structure of DNA and the factors that influence its structural changes can be helpful in this direction. In 2018, a research team provided evidence for the genomic effects of secondary G-quadruplex (G4) DNA structures, and their effects on the methylation of CGI [16]. This team demonstrated that the presence of the G4 structure is strongly associated with CGI hypomethylation within the human genome. They showed that these G4 sites were occupied by DNA methyltransferase 1 (DNMT1), based on biophysical observations, and also that DNMT1 had a higher binding affinity for G4s than duplex structures, hemimethylated or single-stranded DNA. However, biochemical assays also showed that the G4 structure inhibited DNMT1 enzymatic activity rather than the DNA base sequence. Based on these data, it was shown that G4 DNMT1 formation protected specific CGIs from methylation and inhibited local methylation.

Therefore, knowing the exact structure and mechanism of nucleic acids is crucial to devise treatments for some genetic diseases caused by defective gene expression, and sometimes even for the prevention of these diseases.

According to these and other studies, there may be various types of weird shapes that serve some unknown biological function, and in the future it may be proven that there are more complex and interesting structures of inherited DNA molecules, and therefore applications in the field of medical treatment may emerge [17, 18].

13.3.2 RNA chemical structure

RNA is one of the most basic biochemical molecules, and differs from DNA by employing uracil as a base instead of thymine. These molecules play an important and vital role in regulating, preserving and retaining the genomes of all living organisms [19–21].

There is only one strand in the RNA polymeric molecule. The variety of RNA molecules can be classified into mRNA (messenger), tRNA (transfer), and rRNA (ribosomal). This makes RNA interesting because these molecules may be used in nucleic acid therapy. On the one hand, for the proper selection of RNA molecules for the targeted treatment of many diseases, and on the other hand, finding suitable strategies for the targeted delivery of these molecules to the desired tissues.

13.3.3 Aptamer chemical structures

Aptamers are synthetic single-stranded sequences of RNA or DNA that are folded into secondary and tertiary structures with extraordinary specificity for recognizing and binding to other molecules. Actually aptamers are small sequences of RNA or DNA molecules about 25–80 nucleotides in length. The first aptamers were described in 1990. Compared to antibodies their unique characteristics could make them more effective than antibodies. Aptamers are generally screened and selected through the systematic evolution of ligands by exponential enrichment (SELEX) laboratory procedure. Using this process, aptamers can be designed to bind to almost any target moiety (from small inorganic minerals to proteins and complete cells).

After aptamers have been selected, they can be multiplied using the polymerase chain reaction (PCR) to produce large amounts of sequences with high purity. The simple chemical structure of aptamers makes them useful to bind to various targets. Eventually, because of the stability of aptamers compared to antibodies they can be used under harsher conditions (such as high temperature). Many studies and discoveries on the use of aptamers are ongoing, like medical diagnosis and treatment. Owing to their simple and synthetic structure, in addition to their wide variety of applications aptamers have been widely studied by researchers. Here we discuss some applications of aptamers, which show their advantages:

(1) Aptamers are produced in vitro by a synthetic chemical process.
(2) Aptamers can identify a wide range of target molecules such as: proteins, peptides, amino acids, drugs, metal ions, or even whole cells.
(3) Chemical modification of aptamers is relatively easy.

The use of aptamers as diagnostic tools, therapeutics, bio-imaging agents, and drug delivery vehicles has been reported.

13.3.4 Peptide nucleic acids

Peptide nucleic acids (PNAs) is a completely synthetic class of nucleic acids which is different from DNA, RNA or aptamers, which all have sugar and phosphate in their backbone. PNAs have a peptide backbone, which connects the nucleotide bases within their structure.

The amide bond in the PNA structure is neutral in charge, which is different from RNA and DNA which both have negative charges due to the phosphate group in their structure. Neutrally charged biomolecules can interact with cells much easier than those with negative charges. Peptide nucleic acids were first introduced by Nielsen et al., in 1991 [22].

Recently, artificial nucleic acids such as peptide nucleic acids have become of interest in medical treatment. Owing to the favorable physicochemical characteristics of peptide nucleic acids, several researchers have used this backbone in modified antisense oligonucleotides [23, 24].

A study by a research team led by Dorota Gryko and Joanna Trylska reported the biological and therapeutic effects of peptide nucleic acids. They showed that the conjugation of peptide nucleic acids to vitamin B_{12} could inhibit the growth of *Escherichia coli* bacteria [25]. For this purpose they conjugated a peptide nucleic acid to vitamin B_{12} with a suitable linker. This team showed that vitamin B_{12} could selectively deliver PNA to Gram-negative bacteria, because vitamin B_{12} is an essential coenzyme in *E. coli*. Application of vitamin B_{12} as a carrier could be expanded to cover other antisense oligonucleotides like 2′OMe RNA and locked nucleic acids which are modified forms of RNA, that could be delivered to *E. coli* and *Salmonella typhimurium* cells [26].

One of the most important advantages of PNA technology is their capacity for targeted delivery to the desired tissue [27]. For instance, this has been accomplished using cell-penetrating peptides (CPPs) which are able to cross the cell membrane [28–35]. .Because of the easier cellular uptake of PNAs [36–40], in the last few years, researchers have looked for other pathways for the targeted delivery of PNAs [41].

13.3.5 Locked nucleic acids (LNA)

The term locked nucleic acid (LNA) refers to a type of nucleic acid with properties that make them useful as complementary RNA or DNA oligonucleotides [42, 43].

The named locked nucleic acid comes from the special structure of this type of nucleic acid wherein the conformation of the nucleic acids according to the Watson-Crick principle, the ribose rings are locked. There is an additional bridge using a methylene group that connects the 2′ oxygen and the 4′ carbon of the ribose ring.

LNA oligonucleotides have been employed in nucleic acid-based therapies both in vivo and in vitro, because of their unprecedented thermal stability and remarkable features. LNAs have been used as oligonucleotides for siRNA in preclinical studies [44]. LNAs have also been used as LNA aptamers [45, 46], and LNA oligonucleotides [47].

13.4 Therapeutic potential of nucleic acids

There are now many different types of RNA molecules including messenger RNA (mRNA), transfer RNA (tRNA), ribosomal RNA (rRNA), antisense RNA (asRNA), double-stranded RNA (dsRNA), guide RNA (gRNA), microRNA (miRNA), noncoding RNA (ncRNA), precursor miRNA (pre-miRNA), primary miRNA (pri-miRNA), short-hairpin RNA (shRNA), small interfering RNA (siRNA), small RNA (sRNA), and long noncoding RNA (lncRNA). Many of these nucleic acids play an important role in the pathogenesis and treatment of several diseases, such as neurodegenerative disease, cardiovascular disease, cancer, and autoimmune diseases, proper delivery techniques could be effective in devising new treatments. Nucleic acids can be used as vaccines, drugs, or imaging agents, and suitable tools for their transfer into target tissues or cells have attracted the attention of many researchers.

In the following section, a new technique called microfluidics for nucleic acid transfer is discussed. Studies in recent years have shown that nucleic acids can be a powerful tool for the treatment of certain diseases. Infact some of these nucleic acid-based drugs can act by binding to an active site of a protein, an enzyme or a receptor (druggable targets) in order to activate, or inhibit their function [48, 49]. The use of nucleic acids in gene therapy is based on inhibiting the translation of RNA and reducing the expression of some target protein that has been associated with an illness [50]. Bioengineered RNAs (BERAs) including different kinds of nucleic acid scaffolds and their analogs have been tested in animal models of some diseases. In one study in rates, it was demonstrated that a bioengineered miR-34a prodrug could suppress subcutaneous xenograft tumor growth (human NSCLC A549 lung cancer cells) in a dose-dependent manner. Furthermore, the BERAs did not demonstrate any toxicity.

In the following section, we will divide therapeutic nucleic acids into two categories: DNA-based approaches and RNA-based approaches [51].

13.4.1 DNA-based approaches

After much effort in recent years, a new generation of nucleic acid-based drugs has been commercialized by the pharmaceutical industry and finally entered into clinical treatment. DNA drugs can be used as vaccines or as drugs for some recalcitrant or newly emerging diseases such as influenza, cancer and HIV. In the meantime, there are also drugs that can affect the progress of diseases by affecting DNA molecules. The first drug to treat a rare form of genetic blindness (Leber's congenital amaurosis) operates via altering DNA, and was approved by the FDA in December under the name of Luxturna (Voretigene neparvovec) [52–54]. Luxturna provides a working copy of the RPE65 gene into retinal cells to replace lost gene function [55].

13.4.1.1 Plasmid DNA

A plasmid is a double-stranded circular small DNA molecule inside a cell, and is physically separate from the chromosomal DNA molecules and can function independently. Basically, plasmids are relatively common in gene therapy, due to their low immunogenicity and the low risk of developing heritable mutations.

For years, after it was discovered that disease called AIDS was caused by the HIV virus, it was thought to be a death sentence. Although HIV is one of deadliest types of viruses in the world, effective treatments have now been found, and vaccines are continuously being investigated. Gene therapy and DNA vaccination belong to a new group of molecular therapies that use nucleic acids as therapeutic and preventive agents. A DNA vaccine can be constructed from plasmids, which carry a gene for one of the five proteins of the HIV virus [56, 57]. Many years ago it was shown that an immune response could be generated by injection of DNA into mice [58–61]. A review on DNA vaccines about 8 years ago emphasized that plasmids can induce immunity against a dreaded pathogen [62–64]. Experiments were carried out on animals and humans showing promising results in special situations. Preclinical trials on animals achieved good results, and clinical trials on humans are in progress. Plasmid-based vaccines and therapies are under study in humans for a wide range of diseases, and some have already been approved for animals.

In addition to studies on HIV, other clinical trials have also been initiated for the treatment of some cancers, and after many years of effort and study some interesting results have been obtained [65, 66]. Actually DNA vaccines are able to activate the immune system against cancer [67]. To date, the latest DNA vaccine has been tested as a personalized medicine in which DNA from the patient's own tumor is sequenced, and then inserted into a plasmid for immunization [65]. .It should be noted that in the case of other DNA vaccines, preclinical studies and phase I and II clinical trials are underway. Advances in nucleic acid transfer technology have allowed the delivery of DNA vaccines using physical methods like sonoporation, DNA tattooing, electropermeabilization, or gene gun propelled particles. These techniques are required due to the lack of DNA transport to the nucleus after simple injection [68–74]. Moreover the spatial structure of DNA with its double-stranded structure stimulates the innate immune response [75, 76]. Another characteristic of DNA vaccines is that they can produce immunological memory, which is not possible for antibodies or small molecules drugs [77, 78].

In recent years many innovative approaches to DNA vaccines have been reported. These include: (1) Chimeric DNA vaccines [79]; (2) Neoantigen DNA vaccines [80]; and (3) Polyepitope DNA vaccines [81]. More effective tumor treatment could be obtained by the combination of DNA vaccines with other therapies, because the effectiveness of DNA vaccine against some tumors is not sufficient when used alone [82].

13.4.1.2 Oligonucleotides and antisense oligonucleotides

Oligonucleotides are chains consisting of a small number (around 20) of nucleotide bases. The mechanism of action of synthetic oligonucleotides is that they prevent the transcription of genes involved in disease processes. One mechanism uses oligonucleotides to target a gene by disruption of the transcription process of the faulty gene. Among 22 new drugs that were approved by the FDA in 2016, three of them were oligodeoxynucleotide (ODN)-based therapeutics. DEFITELIO is a drug for patients who are at risk of developing liver vein occlusion and thus requiring a bone marrow transplant. EXONDYS 51 is a medication for Duchenne's muscular dystrophy. SPINRAZA is a medicine for the treatment of patients with spinal muscular atrophy. The currently ODN approvals show that the potential of DNA drugs has been well demonstrated by researchers over the last few years. Over 100 companies have introduced hundreds of ODN programs in recent years. In 2017 FDA published an article about the approved oligonucleotides with therapeutic applications [83]. A potential new approach to HIV therapy was provided by the use of FANA antisense oligonucleotides as an anti-HIV-1 therapeutic agent with dual mechanisms and a self-delivery function [84]. The researchers designed and demonstrated 2′-deoxy-2′-fluoroarabinonucleotide (FANA) antisense oligonucleotides (ASOs) targeting highly conserved regions in the HIV-1genome. Carrier-free cellular internalization of these modified ASOs occurred within 3h with and potent suppression of HIV-1 replication. In vitro mechanistic studies showed that the inhibitory effect of FANA ASOs was due to the activation of RNase H1. These promising results have encouraged researchers to further investigate oligonucleotides as therapeutic agents [85].

13.4.2 RNA-based approaches

Until several decades ago, the market for drugs used to treat various diseases was limited to pharmaceuticals, peptides, monoclonal antibodies, and recombinant proteins. With the approval of the first nucleotide drug by the FDA, this new generation of drugs has attracted the attention of researchers and pharmacists. RNA-based drugs are faced with some difficulties such as intrinsic immunogenicity, unstable structure, and the need for a vehicle for drug delivery to the cells. Researchers were able to overcome these problems by applying chemical modifications to their structure and using different carriers. Various categories of RNA-based drugs are currently undergoing clinical trials, including interfering RNA, antisense oligonucleotides, and aptamers. Recent studies have shown that a large proportion of DNA is not used for encoding proteins, but rather is transcribed into noncoding RNAs (ncRNAs). Both coding and noncoding RNAs can have therapeutic potential. Prior to the 1980s, RNA was only viewed as a medium for transferring genetic information from DNA to proteins. But with the discovery of RNA enzymes in the early 1980s, and RNA interference in the late 1990s, this attitude has changed. [86–88]. RNAs have now been proposed to be used as drugs in the treatment of diseases such as genetic abnormalities, viral infections, and various types of cancer [89]. RNA therapies also include a wide spectrum of applications that do not fall within the scope of gene therapy. In fact in the last few years some RNA-based drugs have provided impressive therapeutic results [90]. Researchers are investigating RNA as new drugs in conjunction with newly discovered RNA biology. RNA drugs needs to overcome two major barriers: weak pharmacological properties because of its low stability in the presence of RNase enzymes, and a lack of suitable strategies for delivery of RNA. Some RNA drugs have been approved by the FDA for neurodegenerative diseases, such as nusinersen (Spinraza) and eteplirsen (Exondys 51) [91]. Interestingly, recent reports have suggested that RNA-based drugs have a higher therapeutic potential compared to DNA-based drugs. RNA-based drugs could also be used for the treatment of cardiovascular disease [92].

13.4.2.1 Small interfering RNAs

One class of double-stranded RNA is small interfering RNAs (siRNA), also known as short interfering RNAs and silencing RNA. They consist of 20–25 base pairs and in similar manner to miRNA they act through RNA interference (RNAi). The siRNAs were first discovered in 1998 and due to their therapeutic potential, the discovery was awarded the Nobel Prize in physiology or medicine in 2006 [93]. Gene silencing involves the interaction of a siRNA with the cognate genomic DNA sequence, which neutralizes the expression of the targeted mRNA molecules by RNA interference (RNAi) [94]. The discovery of microRNAs and RNA interference (RNAi) has trigged a new look at RNAs for treatment of diseases [95]. .The first small interfering RNA-based drug approved by FDA was called patisiran, used to treat polyneuropathy in patients with hereditary transthyretin-mediated amyloidosis. Patisiran is the newest and latest siRNA drug approved by the FDA in August 2018 after 20 years of efforts by researchers and its market value is now between $345,000 and $450,000 a year [96–98]. One of therapeutic application of RNA is also RNA vaccines which have been tested in vivo [99–101]. In addition, there other disease such as various cancers, eye, and heart diseases which are being tested in clinical trials using RNA-based drugs.

In recent years, there has been rapid progress in RNAi-based therapy by optimization of the chemical structure of the siRNAs. In one recent study, a Canadian research group synthesized a particular type of novel siRNA that was modified at the 2′ and 4′ and as well as 3′ position by attaching OMe and F groups onto the ribose ring. They found that the effect of 4′-OMe or 4′-F substitution on the sugar to produce a chemically modified siRNA could be effective at gene silencing, especially when also modified at the 3′-position [104]. In fact, this group expanded the chemical modification toolkit for gene silencing and paved the way for further investigations toward other gene targets. Because of the impressive results obtained from 2′,4′-modified oligonucleotides in recent years; many investigators have paid more attention to this point. Another example of this is the 2′ modification of ribose by OMe substitution, which can provide nuclease resistance, and improve the thermal stability and RNAi activity [105]. New FDA-approved therapeutic agents have been produced by chemical modification of the structure of siRNA. Macugen (Pegaptanib) is an antiangiogenic drug against neovascular age-related macular degeneration. This was a 2-F/OMe-modified 28-mer antiVEGF RNA aptamer [106, 107]. Mipomersen (Kynamro) and Nusinersen (Spinraza) are types of 2-*O*-(2-methoxyethyl)-(2-MOE) modified antisense oligonucleotides which are used as drugs for familial hypercholesterolemia, and spinal muscular atrophy, respectively [108]. A GalNAc-siRNA conjugate is able to specifically target liver cells that express the asialoglycoprotein receptor [109–112]. High-throughput screening and drug discovery efforts for RNAi-drugs and siRNA can be facilitated by re-engineering RNA molecules in order to discover new therapeutic agents [113]

13.4.2.2 Short hairpin RNAs (shRNA)

Another kind of RNA interference which is applied for posttranscriptional gene silencing is the short hairpin (shRNA) [114, 115]. As its name implies the shape of this molecule is similar to a hairpin and this structure facilitates the function of this molecule. In contrast to other RNA types shRNA is produced in the nucleus of the cell. In recent years some shRNAs have been studied for their therapeutic potential in clinical trial phases. Some therapeutic applications of shRNAs have been proposed for prostate cancer, melanoma, and neurodegenerative disorders. Until now, few therapeutic uses of shRNA have been reported, and are limited to pre-clinical animal studies, largely because appropriate tools for its targeted delivery to the desired tissue do not exist.

13.4.2.3 microRNAs (miRNAs)

MicroRNAs (miRNA) have a short chain length of 19–23 nucleotides and act to control gene expression by inhibiting mRNA translation and destroying the mRNAs. The miRNAs bind to the complementary ends of mRNAs (3′-*UTR*, 3′-untranslated region). The biogenesis of microRNAs involves two stages, a primary miRNA is first cleaved to a precursor miRNA, which is then cleaved to the mature miRNA, which is finally incorporated into the RISC complex [116–120]. Studies on miRNAs began in 1993, and while only 5 papers were published in 2001, by 2008, this number had reached 3500 articles in the PubMed database [121–124]. In 2018 Chinese researchers investigated a miRNA called miR495, which interacts with the UBE2C-ABCG2/ERCC1 axis which is involved in nonsmall cell lung cancer (NSCLC). Their findings showed that miR-495 interacts with its substrate UBE2C by binding to the 3′-UTR, and UBE2C binds to the promoters of ABCG2 and ERCC1 to modulate their transcriptional activity. The miR495-UBE2CABCG2/ERCC1 axis could reverse cisplatin resistance by regulating the drug resistance genes ABCG2 and ERCC1 in NSCLC cells [125]. Another research team worked on miR-502-3p and found its expression could be induced by niacin thus changing the sensitivity of human adipocytes [126].. Another research team in China found that microRNA-298 could reverse multidrug resistance to antiepileptic drugs in vitro through suppressing MDR1/P-gp gene expression [127]. In recent years, miRNAs that are able to alter the expression of the relevant protein by regulating the expression of genes at the posttranscriptional level have received much more attention from researchers. A study from several research teams in Germany in 2019 estimated the total number of active human miRNAs in nucleic acids research [128]. MicroRNAs can act either as an anticancer agent or as a tumor suppressor agent depending on the function of their targeted genes [129]. Researchers found in a recent study using pigs that microRNAs could play a therapeutic role in cardiac repair after myocardial infarction [130].

13.4.2.4 Antisense oligonucleotides (ASOs)

One strategy for treatment of genetic disorders is antisense therapy. Genetic disorders result in multiple diseases caused by a variation in the genetic sequences due to different reasons including mutations. Antisense molecules are nucleic acids that specifically bind to complementary nucleic acid sequences via Watson-Crick pairing. Antisense oligonucleotides (ASOs) have become well-known therapeutic agents, and are now important in medicinal chemistry and molecular biology. Unlike chemical drugs that target proteins themselves, the target molecule of antisense RNA drugs is the mRNA sequence that comes from the gene associated with the disease. Many diseases, such as cancer, inflammatory, infectious diseases, and genetic defects, can be treated by antisense drugs, which prevent the translation of mRNA to its protein. In fact, by preventing the formation of the defective protein, ASOs can be very effective with few side effects. These drugs, by their specificity for a specific sequence of the desired mRNA, prevent its translation to the protein. Given the fact that the nature of the binding of RNA to its target is clear, the design of antisense oligonucleotides more straightforward [131]. The first drug in this class was VITRAVENE (fomivirsen, Ionis Pharmaceuticals—formerly Isis) which was approved in 1998 for treatment of a kind of eye infection called CMV, in patients infected by the HIV virus [132].

Approximately 15 years after the discovery of the first drug, a second ASO drug called KYNAMRO (mipomersen, Ionis Pharmaceuticals) was approved by the FDA in 2013 for the treatment of a disease called familial hypercholesterolemia [133]. Furthermore, alicaforsen was developed by Atlantic Pharmaceuticals, which is an

ASO targeting ICAM-1 in order to treat pouchitis in patients with inflammatory bowel disease, and received FDA approval in January 2017 [134]. ASO drugs have been tested for the reversal of protein mutation in Huntington's disease patients. The most commonly used antisense oligonucleutide agents have been for the treatment of neurological disorders [135]. Tables 13.1 and 13.2 summarize the production of ASO drugs. *MOE*, antisense oligonucleotide methoxy ethyl [136–138].

Since the some of these nucleic acids (DNA and RNA) are naturally present in the human body, artificially modified forms such as PNA and LNA are biologically similar and may have fewer side effects. DNA and RNA are biocompatible and biodegradable because of their biological properties. However DNA and RNA have unstable structures and their half-life is short. Nucleic acid analogs such as PNA and LNA have a longer half-life compared to DNA and RNA. Nucleic acids and their analogs have been used to treat bone diseases, and for bone regeneration. Previously scientists and doctors used simple biological materials as a scaffold for repairing damaged tissues. However, most biomaterials have some limitations and disadvantages for use in bone tissue engineering. Some of these limitations are, low precision, high molecular weight, and complicated structures. Nucleic acids and nucleic acid analogs likely do not suffer from these limitations. Given the fact that biological scaffolds are not mechanically strong or sufficiently long-lasting, pure nanocarriers have been designed to deliver functional nucleic acid sequences which could be useful for the repair and regeneration of bone tissue. As biomaterials and other bone repair methods using seeded cells have some limitations such as the low cell survival rate and uncertain safety, functional nucleic acids have attracted some attention. For example, in the repair of bone tissues, the use of growth factors such as insulin-like growth factor, vascular endothelial growth factor or platelet-derived growth factor has some problems. These include the fact that they cannot easily be attached to biomaterial scaffolds, and on the other hand their transport to the damaged area at a high enough concentration for a long time is difficult. A better choice may to use gene therapy to trigger the expression of growth factors at the desired location within the damaged bone.

There are various mechanisms for the delivery of different nucleic acid molecules, which may experience different fates when they encounter cells. Some nucleic acids such as plasmid DNA can easily be taken up by cells, and its mechanism is automatic. The mechanism of small interfering RNAs and micro RNAs is by binding to the corresponding gene sequence when they enter into the cells. Gene therapy is a toolkit of therapeutic approaches that can treat diseases by repairing and eliminating genetic defects. In the past, gene therapy was reliant on a vector to transfer the nucleic acid agent into the cell, but now there are other approaches. The first clinical trial of gene therapy was undertaken by the National Institutes of Health of the United States in 1990. The genes on the chromosomes are the physical and functional units that control the working of the body. They are specific sequences of bases that encode the amino acids that make up the actual proteins. Although genes are important, the proteins perform the vital functions and make up the majority of cellular structures. Genetic diseases occur when genes are altered in such a way that

Table 13.1 Some examples of RNA drugs which are approved or in phase III trials [102, 103].

Drug	Developer	Target	Indication	Status
Patisiran	Alnylam	TTR	Hereditary ATTR amyloidosis	Approved
QPI-1002	Quark	p53	Delayed graft function	Phase III
QPI-1007	Quark	Caspase 2	Nonarteritic anterior ischemic optic neuropathy	Phase III
Tivanisiran	Sylentis/PharmaMar	TRPV1	Moderate to severe dry eye	Phase III
Fitusiran	Sanofi/Alnylam	Antithrombin	Hemophilia A and hemophilia B	Phase III
Givosiran	Alnylam	ALAS1	Acute hepatic porphyrias	Phase III
Inclisiran	The Medicines Company/Alnylam	PCSK9	Hypercholesterolemia	Phase III

Table 13.2 Examples of ASO drugs.

ASO drug	Chemistry structure	Disease	Situation
Eteplirsen	Morpholino	Duchenne muscular dystrophy	FDA approved
Inotersen	ASO MOE gapmer	familial amyloid polyneuropathy	FDA approved
Nusinersen	ASO, full 2′-MOE	spinal muscular atrophy	FDA approved
RG6042	ASO MOE gapmer	Huntington disease	Phase 3 clinical trial
WVE-210201	Stereopure ASO	Duchenne muscular dystrophy	Phase 1 clinical trial
WVE-120102	Stereopure ASO	Huntington disease	Phase 1/2 clinical trial
WVE-120101	Stereopure ASO	Huntington disease	Phase 1/2 clinical trial
IONIS MAPTRx	ASO MOE gapmer	Alzheimer's disease	Phase 1/2 clinical trial
IONIS-SOD1Rx	ASO MOE gapmer	amyotrophic lateral sclerosis	Phase 1 clinical trial
BIIB078	ASO MOE	amyotrophic lateral sclerosis	Phase 1 clinical trial
ATXN3 ASO	ASO MOE gapmer	spinocerebellar ataxia	Preclinical development
ATXN2 ASO	ASO MOE gapmer	spinocerebellar ataxia	Preclinical development

encoded proteins cannot perform their natural function. Gene therapy is a technique for correcting the defective genes that are responsible for a disease.

13.4.2.5 An overview of fluidic and microfluidic systems

Because of the wide variety of pharmaceuticals and drugs, many methods have been used to deliver them to the damaged or target tissues to treat diseases. One of these classes of pharmaceuticals is nucleic acids. Nowadays effective nucleic acid delivery is a challenging topic in pharmacology and medical treatment. Some common methods of transporting chemicals and drugs have drawbacks, including the need for high concentrations of chemicals or expensive drugs to achieve a therapeutic effect. Nucleic acids are classified as expensive drugs, but they are also among the most effective types of drugs for the treatment of many diseases. Therefore, the need for new nucleic acid delivery techniques is increasing.

One of the novel strategies for the efficient and targeted delivery of nucleic acids is the application of fluidic systems, such as microfluidic and nanofluidic devices. Microfluidics is the design and science of a device that manipulates very small amounts of fluid, with a volume much smaller than one drop. We will provide brief overview of the use of fluidic systems. In 1957, for the first time, fluidic systems were studied by Billy M. Horton of the Harry Diamond Laboratories [139]. This researcher found that the direction of flue gas could be guided by a tool with high power similar to a pair of bellows. This simulation led him to present a theory of flow interactions, which stated that by separating one liquid flow within different fluid flows, it could be amplified. After the study of fluidic systems began in the early years, a variety of new high-technology uses have emerged. Among the applications of fluidic systems, they can be used in computer systems, mechanics, medical fields, and so forth. Following much research using fluidic systems, researchers have come up with fluidic systems at smaller scales, including microfluidics and even nanofluidics.

The main components of microfluidic technology include a device with one or more channels (less than 1 mm in diameter) and a pump like a syringe or a peristaltic pump, in order to conduct fluid flow [140].

Microfluidic systems have recently attracted much attention because they have many advantages due to their miniature structure and the fact that the surface-to-volume ratio in microfluidic systems is increased. The following are the advantages of this method: (1) Less need to use high quantities of reagents; (2) Heat transfer and high mass transfer; (3) Increased accuracy and processing efficiency due to predictable liquid flow at a small scale [141].

Some nano-complexes (NC) that can carry nucleic acids can be produced and transferred using microfluidic systems via an electrostatic coupling mechanism [142].

Microfluidic devices include microchannels that are less than a millimeter in diameter, on the micron scale. For comparison, a human hair is about 100 μm thick.

Microfluidic systems consisting of microfibers can be used as tools for controlled drug/gene delivery [143, 144]. Microfluidics have demonstrated outstanding performance for the fabrication or formulation of various pharmaceutical substances and therapeutics, particularly for gene and cell therapy, and can address current and future biological production challenges.

13.5 Mechanisms in microfluidic systems

We need to first understand the mechanism of operation of microfluidic systems. There are two general mechanisms for microfluidic systems: (1) pressure-driven flow, and (2) electrokinetically driven flow.

The mechanism of action in many microfluidics is that, when injecting a particulate suspension into a microfluidic channel, several forces are applied to the suspended particles which determine the movement of the particles along the mainstream and lateral directions. In the mainstream, the force created by the velocity difference between the particles and the liquid, is called the viscous tensile force, and causes the particles to accelerate to near the velocity of the surrounding fluid. In fact, the wall of the channel slows down the movement of adjacent particles, thereby causing the fluid flow to decrease. The fluid phases are first moved by various driving forces to enter the microfluidic channels. The most common driving force used for fluid movement is the pressure resulting from the difference in relative pressure between the inlet and outlet of the flow channel. The required pressure can also be provided by the use of air pressure [145]. Static air pressure is an external mechanical force with a special capability that can be controlled by a pressure regulator. One reason why microfluidic systems have become a useful tool, is that the liquids can be driven by their own internal capillary forces, and this has the advantage of eliminating the need for any external mechanical forces [146].

13.6 Applications of microfluidic systems to nucleic acid transfection

One of application for microfluidic system is called DNA chips. In general, there are two main kinds of fluid control. One is continuous-flow microfluidics and the other is digital (or droplet-based) microfluidics, which have been discussed in the literature [147] and previously in this book.

In this section, the targeted delivery of nucleic acids by fluidic systems is discussed. Since the process of production of nanocarriers (NC) is difficult, it has resulted in a new approach to improving the quality of the NC, by using emulsions and hydrodynamic flow concentration in microfluidics devices [148–150].

The advantages of using microfluidic systems include: (1) The obtained NCs are smaller and more uniform; (2) They have better stability than with bulk mixing; (3) Higher transfer efficiency is achieved than with bulk mixing; and (4) By using microfluidic systems, the cytotoxicity of the NCs is lower than those from bulk mixing [151].

As discussed above, the unique properties of these systems can prevent the undesired mixing of liquids under multilayer flow. In 2016 one research group compared the highly effective and positive effects of pDNA/cationic liposome (CL) lipoplexes with enhanced transfection efficiency in the presence and absence of microfluidic systems [152]. In this experiment, the electrostatic assembly of plasmid DNA and cationic liposomes was investigated in two forms: (1) bulk-mixing (BM) and (2) microfluidic devices with $R \pm 1.5$. The use of microfluidics resulted in the production of smaller lipoplexes with less resistance and stacking of the multiple layers, and performed better than standard BM assembled polyplexes, with increased transfection efficiency. What makes nucleic acids more efficient in microfluidic systems is that by using quantum dot-Forster resonance energy transfer, they can release their cargo more slowly inside the cells, which may increase the number of nucleic acid molecules in the cell [153]. Under the hydrodynamic flow concentration, nucleic acids are concentrated by the cationic polymer and the lipid, and flow together into a narrow stream where rapid mixing is achieved by diffusion at the interface within microseconds [153]. Using microfluidic techniques to prepare the smaller NCs, they could transfect the cells in a more reproducible manner compared to their bulk mixed counterparts without causing any toxicity. A technique called microfluidic drifting devices have been developed to achieve three-dimensional hydrodynamic focusing in a single-layer microdynamic hydrodynamic device [150].

Overall, there are three general steps for the effective delivery of nucleic acids into cells: (1) formation of a nucleic acid complex with specific reagents which is called the packaging step; (2) the nucleic acid complex adheres to the cell surface and then undergoes endocytosis into endosomes; (3) the nucleic acids inside the lysosomes are released into the cells. Each of these steps is time consuming and the number of transfer steps is high. As a result, finding a suitable method for targeted delivery of nucleic acids is an important issue that has become a major goal for researchers. Electrostatic forces are responsible for forming a complex between negatively charged nucleic acids and positively charged polyamine polymers and these polyplexes were reported in 2017 [154]. There are many advantages for the use of cell surface engineering for bio-orthogonal mediated nucleic acid delivery. One example is the preparation of complexes using microfluidic technology and siRNAs, where the time required can be decreased to less than 1 min using a bio-orthogonal transfection strategy in a microfluidic device with a flow rate of 0.8 μL/min. The increased efficiency and reliability gained with microfluidic technology is promising [154]

Researchers have recently devised a new technique known as optofluidics, involving the integration of microfluidics with optics as tools. The technique has not only merged the two technologies to create greater efficacy in the delivery of nucleic acids, but has also successfully combined this approach with nanopores on optofluidic chips to simultaneously provide the sensitivity of nanoelectronics and optical nanoparticles [155]. In one research paper, it was shown that nanopore-optofluidic devices could function as an effective tool for single-chip manipulation of nucleic acids. The researchers used this technique to gain precise control over the delivery of particles into the microfluidic channels [156]. This platform was designed so that it could be used to control a number of specific particle parameters for further measurement, either for sorting the downstream fluid, or for purifying different molecules after their identification. In addition, the system allows the user to perform a reset according to the need of the program. The channels of the microfluidic system were constructed with T-shaped connections. In this device, the T-junctions with a focusing current were used to generate a nucleic acid delivery vector using a microfluidic drop generator.

In one study, it was demonstrated that the nanocarriers formed using a microfluidic device were taken up by cells in about 5 h with 90% cell viability and an overall 60% transfection efficiency. However, when the bulk particle method was compared there was 75% cell viability and only 40% transfection efficiency [157, 158].

The electroporation method has been widely studied for targeted and effective nucleic acid delivery into cells and tissues. The integration of electroporation methodology and microfluidic technology has been called microfluidic electroporation and has been investigated for cellular analysis and delivery as reported by Tao Geng and Chang Lu. Several methods have recently been developed to efficiently deliver nucleic acids into cells via passage through the cell membrane barrier. One method that is very effective is electroporation or electropermeabilization. Molecules and ions are able to penetrate and pass through the cell membrane by passing through temporary pores created by a small electric current. It has been shown that this method is more efficient compared to other methods of nucleic acid delivery, and has good reproducibility [159, 160]. The integration of electroporation techniques and microfluidic systems has overcome overcame many of the barriers preventing nucleic acid transfer [161–163].

Providing a precise and reliable mechanism for the electroporation transfer method of nucleic acids is difficult. However, there are two hypotheses: a pore hypothesis and an electromechanical instability hypothesis [164–168]. Electroporation-based microfluidics has been explored for delivering small interfering RNAs (siRNA), small molecule chemical drugs, and large biomolecules such as DNA and proteins into cells [169, 170].

Nonviral vectors are one of the most common methods for gene transfer and nucleic acid delivery. A research team focused on a novel method of gene transfer using nonviral vectors in the form of a small microfluidic chip. In this study researchers used a microfluidic platform for transfection, and eventually obtained a microfluidic platform for the high throughput screening of nonviral gene delivery vectors [171]. In fact, these researchers created a small lab on a chip using microfluidic systems for nucleic acid transfer as a reliable tool. The researchers investigated the trapping of cells in the microfluidic device, and by using a spatiotemporally tunable microenvironment they could optimize the transfection protocols. This enabled the researchers to compare the results of transfection using two commercially available lipid vectors with different concentrations of lipid/DNA complexes in real-time. In this study, the use of microfluidic systems was a powerful tool for the simultaneous evaluation of five different transfection conditions, not only saving sample consumption but also enabling more precise control of the cell behavior. The results proved that it could be used as a reliable and useful tool for high-throughput cell analysis on a small scale, enabling gene delivery vectors to be screened and optimized between different doses and combinations of lipid-DNA species.

One of the barriers to drug delivery is the vascular endothelium, which acts as an obstacle to drug delivery by strictly governing the transport of small molecules and solutes. Therefore, advances in techniques for drug transport across the endothelial barrier are required to improve many systemic therapies. In one study, it was shown that the permeability of the vascular endothelium to magnetic particles was increased if an external magnetic field was employed. In this study, iron oxide nanoparticles were observed to bind to the endothelial cells, and were then able to activate the intracellular transport pathway to pass into the tissue. Given the limitations of drug delivery, especially nucleic acids, the need for targeted and effective delivery of drugs to target cells is acute. One of the most promising drug delivery techniques is employing magnetic nanoparticles [172–174]. Magnetic nanoparticles were used to investigate the structural and functional changes of vascular endothelial cells under laboratory conditions using endothelialized microfluidic channels [175]. In this study, the enhancement of vascular permeability was investigated by placing the external magnets in order to target the magnetic nanoparticles to the vascular endothelium.

Microfluidic systems were also used for the transfer of siRNAs by encapsulation into nonionic surfactant vesicles (NISV) for delivery of these RNAs into cancer cells [176]. siRNAs are often used for gene silencing, but an efficient pathway for their transfer into the target cells and tissue is still required [177]. Various types of NISV formulations were synthesized via microfluidic mixing, and the potential of NISV for the delivery of siRNAs targeting green fluorescent protein (GFP) into A549 cells was evaluated. The different formulations of NISV were monodisperse and small (< 60 nm) that is desirable for delivery to tumors site by increased permeability [178]. The stability of these cationic NISV prepared with different surfactants via the microfluidics method were investigated [179] and their ability for siRNA delivery was assessed. The cationic charge on the most effective NISV was provided by the cationic lipid called didodecyldimethylammonium bromide (DDAB). This formulation had some advantages because it created a bilayer structure in the NISV with a positive charge in order to bind siRNA drugs by electrostatic interactions. To prove the efficacy of these surfactants, they were compared with commercial cationic lipids. It was necessary to dissolve the required lipid components in the desired ratios with a maximum lipid concentration of 10 mg/mL in ethanol. The lipid phase was injected into one inlet channel of the microfluidic device using a disposable syringe, and the other inlet was aqueous buffer (sterile RNase-free water). The CNs were formulated at a 3:1 volume flow ratio between the aqueous and lipid phases, and an overall flow rate of 12 mL/min at 50°C. The obtained CN were collected from the outlet stream of the microfluidic channel and were directly diluted with sterile RNase-free water to decrease the final ethanol content in the preparation to 6.25% (v/v) solution. For the first time these researchers could develop CNs prepared by microfluidics for siRNA transfection [176].

13.7 Future prospects for microfluidic systems related to nucleic acids

In the field of nucleic acids, microfluidic systems, can not only play an important role in the transport of nucleic acids, but also in their preparation and purification. As such, microfluidics has attracted the attention of many researchers in recent years. For instance, a study by a Korean research team can be cited. They employed a novel technique by integrating finger-actuated microfluidic pumps and valves in order to purify nucleic acids [180]. In this experiment the use of valves and pumps first defined the flow paths, and the distributed the liquid into these channels. Furthermore it produced constant and stable flow in the microfluidic device. As a proof of concept, their results showed some advantages for the use of microfluidic systems for nucleic acid purification, as demonstrated by the purification of synthetic DNA from hepatitis B virus (HBV).

13.8 Conclusions

As nucleic acids are particularly unstable, the development of effective nucleic acid delivery systems for clinical applications and especially for gene therapy, is important. However, the advent of new microfluidic systems for nucleic acid transfer has improved the effectiveness of the transfer process. There are limitations to this approach, as with other modes of gene delivery, and the main barrier is the scaling up of these devices to operate at high transmission rates. Despite these limitations, new microfluidic systems, sometimes integrated with a variety of different techniques, have opened a new avenue for nucleic acid transfer, purification, and amplification. This encourages researchers to use this approach on a wider scale in the future.

References

[1] L.A. Fraser, Y.W. Cheung, A.B. Kinghorn, W. Guo, S.C.C. Shiu, C. Jinata, et al., Microfluidic technology for nucleic acid aptamer evolution and application, Adv Biosyst 3 (5) (2019) 1900012.

[2] C.A. Kaiser, M. Krieger, H. Lodish, A. Berk, Molecular cell biology, WH Freeman, 2007.

[3] J.D. Watson, A. Berry, DNA: the secret of life, Knopf, 2009.

[4] L.A. Moran, R.A. Horton, K.G. Scrimgeour, M.D. Perry, Principles of biochemistry, Academic Press, USA, 2014.

[5] W. Saenger, Principles of nucleic acid structure, Springer Science & Business Media, 2013.

[6] B.G. Barrell, B.F.C. Clark, Handbook of nucleic acid sequences, Academic Press, USA, 1974.

[7] W.A. Baase, W.C. Johnson Jr., Secondary structure of nucleic acids in the folded chromosome from *E. coli*, Nucleic Acids Res 3 (11) (1976) 3123–3132.

[8] A. Sedova, N.K. Banavali, Geometric patterns for neighboring bases near the stacked state in nucleic acid strands, Biochemistry 56 (10) (2017) 1426–1443.
[9] R.E. Dickerson, H.R. Drew, B.N. Conner, R.M. Wing, A.V. Fratini, M.L. Kopka, The anatomy of a-, b-, and z-DNA, Science 216 (4545) (1982) 475–485.
[10] T. McKee, J.R. McKee, Biochemistry: an introduction, WCB/McGraw-Hill, 1999.
[11] Y. Itoh, S.-I. Sekine, S. Suetsugu, S. Yokoyama, Tertiary structure of bacterial selenocysteine tRNA, Nucleic Acids Res 41 (13) (2013) 6729–6738.
[12] A. Ghosh, M. Bansal, A glossary of DNA structures from A to Z, Acta Crystallogr D: Biol Crystallogr 59 (4) (2003) 620–626.
[13] M. Zeraati, D.B. Langley, P. Schofield, A.L. Moye, R. Rouet, W.E. Hughes, et al., I-motif DNA structures are formed in the nuclei of human cells, Nat Chem 10 (6) (2018) 631.
[14] G. Biffi, D. Tannahill, J. McCafferty, S. Balasubramanian, Quantitative visualization of DNA G-quadruplex structures in human cells, Nat Chem 5 (3) (2013) 182.
[15] A.T. Phan, M. Guéron, J.-L. Leroy, The solution structure and internal motions of a fragment of the cytidine-rich strand of the human telomere, J Mol Biol 299 (1) (2000) 123–144.
[16] S.-Q. Mao, A.T. Ghanbarian, J. Spiegel, S.M. Cuesta, D. Beraldi, M. Di Antonio, et al., DNA G-quadruplex structures mold the DNA methylome, Nat Struct Mol Biol 25 (10) (2018) 951.
[17] R.D. Wells, Non-B DNA conformations, mutagenesis and disease, Trends Biochem Sci 32 (6) (2007) 271–278.
[18] M. Zeraati, A.L. Moye, J.W. Wong, D. Perera, M.J. Cowley, D.U. Christ, et al., Cancer-associated noncoding mutations affect RNA G-quadruplex-mediated regulation of gene expression, Sci Rep 7 (1) (2017) 708.
[19] T.R. Cech, J.A. Steitz, The noncoding RNA revolution—trashing old rules to forge new ones, Cell 157 (1) (2014) 77–94.
[20] G.F. Joyce, RNA evolution and the origins of life, Nature 338 (6212) (1989) 217.
[21] P.A. Sharp, The centrality of RNA, Cell 136 (4) (2009) 577–580.
[22] P.E. Nielsen, M. Egholm, R.H. Berg, O. Buchardt, Sequence-selective recognition of DNA by strand displacement with a thymine-substituted polyamide, Science 254 (5037) (1991) 1497–1500.
[23] A. Ghosal, P.E. Nielsen, Potent antibacterial antisense peptide–peptide nucleic acid conjugates against *Pseudomonas aeruginosa*, Nucleic Acid Ther 22 (5) (2012) 323–334.
[24] P.E. Nielsen, Antisense peptide nucleic acids, Curr Opin Mol Ther 2 (3) (2000) 282–287.
[25] M. Róownicki, Z. Dąbrowska, M. Wojciechowska, A.J. Wierzba, K. Maximova, D. Gryko, et al., Inhibition of *Escherichia coli* growth by vitamin B12–peptide nucleic acid conjugates, ACS Omega 4 (1) (2019) 819–824.
[26] M. Giedyk, A. Jackowska, M. Równicki, M. Kolanowska, J. Trylska, D. Gryko, Vitamin B 12 transports modified RNA into *E. coli* and *S. typhimurium* cells, Chem Commun 55 (6) (2019) 763–766.
[27] C. Avitabile, A. Accardo, P. Ringhieri, G. Morelli, M. Saviano, G. Montagner, et al., Incorporation of naked peptide nucleic acids into liposomes leads to fast and efficient delivery, Bioconjug Chem 26 (8) (2015) 1533–1541.
[28] E. Brognara, E. Fabbri, G. Montagner, J. Gasparello, A. Manicardi, R. Corradini, et al., High levels of apoptosis are induced in human glioma cell lines by co-administration of peptide nucleic acids targeting miR-221 and miR-222, Int J Oncol 48 (3) (2016) 1029–1038.

[29] E. Fabbri, A. Manicardi, T. Tedeschi, S. Sforza, N. Bianchi, E. Brognara, et al., Modulation of the biological activity of microRNA-210 with peptide nucleic acids (PNAs), ChemMedChem 6 (12) (2011) 2192–2202.
[30] D. Hnedzko, D.W. McGee, Y.A. Karamitas, E. Rozners, Sequence-selective recognition of double-stranded RNA and enhanced cellular uptake of cationic nucleobase and backbone-modified peptide nucleic acids, RNA 23 (1) (2017) 58–69.
[31] J. Hu, D.R. Corey, Inhibiting gene expression with peptide nucleic acid (PNA)–peptide conjugates that target chromosomal DNA, Biochemistry 46 (25) (2007) 7581–7589.
[32] A. Manicardi, E. Fabbri, T. Tedeschi, S. Sforza, N. Bianchi, E. Brognara, et al., Cellular uptakes, biostabilities and anti-miR-210 activities of chiral arginine-PNAs in leukaemic K562 cells, Chembiochem 13 (9) (2012) 1327–1337.
[33] M. Mondhe, A. Chessher, S. Goh, L. Good, J.E. Stach, Species-selective killing of bacteria by antimicrobial peptide-PNAs, PLoS One 9 (2) (2014), e89082.
[34] A.F. Saleh, A. Arzumanov, R. Abes, D. Owen, B. Lebleu, M.J. Gait, Synthesis and splice-redirecting activity of branched, arginine-rich peptide dendrimer conjugates of peptide nucleic acid oligonucleotides, Bioconjug Chem 21 (10) (2010) 1902–1911.
[35] Y. Turner, G. Wallukat, P. Säälik, B. Wiesner, S. Pritz, J. Oehlke, Cellular uptake and biological activity of peptide nucleic acids conjugated with peptides with and without cell-penetrating ability, J Peptide Sci 16 (1) (2010) 71–80.
[36] A. Baek, Y.M. Baek, H.-M. Kim, B.-H. Jun, D.-E. Kim, Polyethylene glycol-engrafted graphene oxide as biocompatible materials for peptide nucleic acid delivery into cells, Bioconjug Chem 29 (2) (2018) 528–537.
[37] K.R. Beavers, T.A. Werfel, T. Shen, T.E. Kavanaugh, K.V. Kilchrist, J.W. Mares, et al., Porous silicon and polymer nanocomposites for delivery of peptide nucleic acids as anti-microRNA therapies, Adv Mater 28 (36) (2016) 7984–7992.
[38] A. Bertucci, H. Lülf, D. Septiadi, A. Manicardi, R. Corradini, L. De Cola, Intracellular delivery of peptide nucleic acid and organic molecules using zeolite-L nanocrystals, Adv Healthcare Mater 3 (11) (2014) 1812–1817.
[39] A. Bertucci, E.A. Prasetyanto, D. Septiadi, A. Manicardi, E. Brognara, R. Gambari, et al., Combined delivery of temozolomide and anti-miR221 PNA using mesoporous silica nanoparticles induces apoptosis in resistant glioma cells, Small 11 (42) (2015) 5687–5695.
[40] H. Pansuwan, B. Ditmangklo, C. Vilaivan, B. Jiangchareon, P. Pan-In, S. Wanichwecharungruang, et al., Hydrophilic and cell-penetrable pyrrolidinyl peptide nucleic acid via post-synthetic modification with hydrophilic side chains, Bioconjug Chem 28 (9) (2017) 2284–2292.
[41] J. Gasparello, A. Manicardi, A. Casnati, R. Corradini, R. Gambari, A. Finotti, et al., Efficient cell penetration and delivery of peptide nucleic acids by an argininocalix [4] arene, Sci Rep 9 (1) (2019) 3036.
[42] R.N. Veedu, J. Wengel, Locked nucleic acid as a novel class of therapeutic agents, RNA Biol 6 (3) (2009) 321–323.
[43] R.N. Veedu, J. Wengel, Locked nucleic acids: promising nucleic acid analogs for therapeutic applications, Chem Biodivers 7 (3) (2010) 536–542.
[44] M.B. Thayer, J.M. Lade, D. Doherty, F. Xie, B. Basiri, O.S. Barnaby, et al., Application of locked nucleic acid oligonucleotides for siRNA preclinical bioanalytics, Sci Rep 9 (1) (2019) 3566.
[45] M.R. Jakobsen, J. Haasnoot, J. Wengel, B. Berkhout, J. Kjems, Efficient inhibition of HIV-1 expression by LNA modified antisense oligonucleotides and DNAzymes targeted to functionally selected binding sites, Retrovirology 4 (1) (2007) 29.

[46] I. Lebars, T. Richard, C. Di Primo, J.-J. Toulmé, LNA derivatives of a kissing aptamer targeted to the trans-activating responsive RNA element of HIV-1, Blood Cell Mol Dis 38 (3) (2007) 204–209.
[47] J.S. Jepsen, M.D. Sørensen, J. Wengel, Locked nucleic acid: a potent nucleic acid analog in therapeutics and biotechnology, Oligonucleotides 14 (2) (2004) 130–146.
[48] S.J. Dixon, B.R. Stockwell, Identifying druggable disease-modifying gene products, Curr Opin Chem Biol 13 (5–6) (2009) 549–555.
[49] E.B. Fauman, B.K. Rai, E.S. Huang, Structure-based druggability assessment—identifying suitable targets for small molecule therapeutics, Curr Opin Chem Biol 15 (4) (2011) 463–468.
[50] K. Sridharan, N.J. Gogtay, Therapeutic nucleic acids: current clinical status, Br J Clin Pharmacol 82 (3) (2016) 659–672.
[51] S.A. Gorski, J. Vogel, J.A. Doudna, RNA-based recognition and targeting: sowing the seeds of specificity, Nat Rev Mol Cell Biol 18 (4) (2017) 215.
[52] H. Ledford, FDA advisers back gene therapy for rare form of blindness, Nat News 550 (7676) (2017) 314.
[53] J.M. Wilson, Interview with Jean Bennett, MD, PhD, Hum Gene Ther Clin Dev 29 (1) (2018) 7–9.
[54] H. Ameri, Prospect of retinal gene therapy following commercialization of voretigene neparvovec-rzyl for retinal dystrophy mediated by RPE65 mutation, J Curr Ophthalmol 30 (1) (2018) 1.
[55] S. Russell, J. Bennett, A.M. Maguire, K.A. High, Voretigene neparvovec-rzyl for the treatment of biallelic RPE65 mutation-associated retinal dystrophy, Expert Opin Orphan Drugs 6 (8) (2018) 457–464.
[56] B. Ferraro, M.P. Morrow, N.A. Hutnick, T.H. Shin, C.E. Lucke, D.B. Weiner, Clinical applications of DNA vaccines: current progress, Clin Infect Dis 53 (3) (2011) 296–302.
[57] K.H. Khan, DNA vaccines: roles against diseases, Germs 3 (1) (2013) 26.
[58] E.F. Fynan, R.G. Webster, D.H. Fuller, J.R. Haynes, J.C. Santoro, H.L. Robinson, DNA vaccines: protective immunizations by parenteral, mucosal, and gene-gun inoculations, Proc Natl Acad Sci U S A 90 (24) (1993) 11478–11482.
[59] D.-C. Tang, M. DeVit, S.A. Johnston, Genetic immunization is a simple method for eliciting an immune response, Nature 356 (6365) (1992) 152.
[60] J.B. Ulmer, J.J. Donnelly, S.E. Parker, G.H. Rhodes, P.L. Felgner, V. Dwarki, et al., Heterologous protection against influenza by injection of DNA encoding a viral protein, Science 259 (5102) (1993) 1745–1749.
[61] B. Wang, M.G. Agadjanyan, V. Srikantan, K.E. Ugen, W. Hall, M.H. Kaplan, et al., Molecular cloning, expression, and biological characterization of an HTLV-II envelope glycoprotein: HIV-1 expression is permissive for HTLV-II-induced cell fusion, AIDS Res Hum Retrovir 9 (9) (1993) 849–860.
[62] D.A. Hokey, D.B. Weiner (Eds.), DNA vaccines for HIV: challenges and opportunities, Springer seminars in immunopathology, Springer, 2006.
[63] J. Rice, C.H. Ottensmeier, F.K. Stevenson, DNA vaccines: precision tools for activating effective immunity against cancer, Nat Rev Cancer 8 (2) (2008) 108.
[64] D.J. Laddy, J. Yan, A.S. Khan, H. Andersen, A. Cohn, J. Greenhouse, et al., Electroporation of synthetic DNA antigens offers protection in nonhuman primates challenged with highly pathogenic avian influenza virus, J Virol 83 (9) (2009) 4624–4630.
[65] M.E. Gatti-Mays, J.M. Redman, J.M. Collins, M. Bilusic, Cancer vaccines: enhanced immunogenic modulation through therapeutic combinations, Hum Vaccines Immunother 13 (11) (2017) 2561–2574.

[66] J. Martin-Liberal, M.O. de Olza, C. Hierro, A. Gros, J. Rodon, J. Tabernero, The expanding role of immunotherapy, Cancer Treat Rev 54 (2017) 74–86.
[67] S. Amara, V. Tiriveedhi, The five immune forces impacting DNA-based cancer immunotherapeutic strategy, Int J Mol Sci 18 (3) (2017) 650.
[68] J.J. Suschak, J.A. Williams, C.S. Schmaljohn, Advancements in DNA vaccine vectors, non-mechanical delivery methods, and molecular adjuvants to increase immunogenicity, Hum Vaccines Immunother 13 (12) (2017) 2837–2848.
[69] L. Lambricht, A. Lopes, S. Kos, G. Sersa, V. Préat, G. Vandermeulen, Clinical potential of electroporation for gene therapy and DNA vaccine delivery, Expert Opin Drug Deliv 13 (2) (2016) 295–310.
[70] S. Jorritsma, E. Gowans, B. Grubor-Bauk, D. Wijesundara, Delivery methods to increase cellular uptake and immunogenicity of DNA vaccines, Vaccine 34 (46) (2016) 5488–5494.
[71] Y. Liu, J. Yan, P.J. Santangelo, M.R. Prausnitz, DNA uptake, intracellular trafficking and gene transfection after ultrasound exposure, J Control Release 234 (2016) 1–9.
[72] J.H. van den Berg, K. Oosterhuis, T.N. Schumacher, J.B. Haanen, A.D. Bins, Intradermal vaccination by DNA tattooing, in: DNA vaccines, Springer, 2014, pp. 131–140.
[73] D.L. Doolan, Malaria methods and protocols, Springer Science & Business Media, 2002.
[74] D.L. Miller, S.V. Pislaru, J.F. Greenleaf, Sonoporation: mechanical DNA delivery by ultrasonic cavitation, Somat Cell Mol Genet 27 (1–6) (2002) 115–134.
[75] D. Ori, M. Murase, T. Kawai, Cytosolic nucleic acid sensors and innate immune regulation, Int Rev Immunol 36 (2) (2017) 74–88.
[76] C.-K. Tang, G.A. Pietersz, Intracellular detection and immune signaling pathways of DNA vaccines, Expert Rev Vaccines 8 (9) (2009) 1161–1170.
[77] A. Lopes, K. Vanvarenberg, V. Préat, G. Vandermeulen, Codon-optimized P1A-encoding DNA vaccine: toward a therapeutic vaccination against P815 Mastocytoma, Mol Ther Nucleic Acids 8 (2017) 404–415.
[78] S. Denies, L. Cicchelero, I. Polis, N.N. Sanders, Immunogenicity and safety of xenogeneic vascular endothelial growth factor receptor-2 DNA vaccination in mice and dogs, Oncotarget 7 (10) (2016) 10905.
[79] F. Riccardo, E. Bolli, M. Macagno, M. Arigoni, F. Cavallo, E. Quaglino, Chimeric DNA vaccines: an effective way to overcome immune tolerance, in: Cancer vaccines, Springer, 2014, pp. 99–122.
[80] C.A. Brennick, M.M. George, W.L. Corwin, P.K. Srivastava, H. Ebrahimi-Nik, Neoepitopes as cancer immunotherapy targets: key challenges and opportunities, Immunotherapy 9 (4) (2017) 361–371.
[81] J. Bae, R. Prabhala, A. Voskertchian, A. Brown, C. Maguire, P. Richardson, et al., A multiepitope of XBP1, CD138 and CS1 peptides induces myeloma-specific cytotoxic T lymphocytes in T cells of smoldering myeloma patients, Leukemia 29 (1) (2015) 218.
[82] I. Melero, D.M. Berman, M.A. Aznar, A.J. Korman, J.L.P. Gracia, J. Haanen, Evolving synergistic combinations of targeted immunotherapies to combat cancer, Nat Rev Cancer 15 (8) (2015) 457.
[83] C.A. Stein, D. Castanotto, FDA-approved oligonucleotide therapies in 2017, Mol Ther 25 (5) (2017) 1069–1075.
[84] M. Takahashi, H. Li, J. Zhou, P. Chomchan, V. Aishwarya, M.J. Damha, et al., Dual mechanisms of action of self-delivering, anti-HIV-1 FANA oligonucleotides as a potential new approach to HIV therapy, Mol Ther Nucleic Acids 17 (2019) 615–625.

[85] C.C. Muth, ASO therapy: hope for genetic neurological diseases, JAMA 319 (7) (2018) 644–646.
[86] A. Fire, S. Xu, M.K. Montgomery, S.A. Kostas, S.E. Driver, C.C. Mello, Potent and specific genetic interference by double-stranded RNA in *Caenorhabditis elegans*, Nature 391 (6669) (1998) 806.
[87] C. Guerrier-Takada, K. Gardiner, T. Marsh, N. Pace, S. Altman, The RNA moiety of ribonuclease P is the catalytic subunit of the enzyme, Cell 35 (3) (1983) 849–857.
[88] K. Kruger, P.J. Grabowski, A.J. Zaug, J. Sands, D.E. Gottschling, T.R. Cech, Self-splicing RNA: autoexcision and autocyclization of the ribosomal RNA intervening sequence of Tetrahymena, Cell 31 (1) (1982) 147–157.
[89] I. Melnikova, RNA-based therapies, Nature Publishing Group, 2007.
[90] J. Chen, J. Xie, Progress on RNAi-based molecular medicines, Int J Nanomedicine 7 (2012) 3971.
[91] R.S. Finkel, E. Mercuri, B.T. Darras, A.M. Connolly, N.L. Kuntz, J. Kirschner, et al., Nusinersen versus sham control in infantile-onset spinal muscular atrophy, N Engl J Med 377 (18) (2017) 1723–1732.
[92] D. Lu, T. Thum, RNA-based diagnostic and therapeutic strategies for cardiovascular disease, Nat Rev Cardiol 1 (2019).
[93] Bernards R. The nobel prize in physiology or medicine for 2006 for the discovery of RNA interference. 2006.
[94] S. Saurabh, A.S. Vidyarthi, D. Prasad, RNA interference: concept to reality in crop improvement, Planta 239 (3) (2014) 543–564.
[95] A. Wittrup, J. Lieberman, Knocking down disease: a progress report on siRNA therapeutics, Nat Rev Genet 16 (9) (2015) 543.
[96] D. Al Shaer, O. Al Musaimi, F. Albericio, B.G. de la Torre, 2018 FDA Tides Harvest, Pharmaceuticals 12 (2) (2019) 52.
[97] C. Morrison, Alnylam prepares to land first RNAi drug approval, Nature Publishing Group, 2018.
[98] U.S. Food & Drug Administration, FDA approves first-of-its kind targeted RNA-based therapy to treat a rare disease, 2018.
[99] W.S. Park, N. Miyano-Kurosaki, M. Hayafune, E. Nakajima, T. Matsuzaki, F. Shimada, et al., Prevention of HIV-1 infection in human peripheral blood mononuclear cells by specific RNA interference, Nucleic Acids Res 30 (22) (2002) 4830–4835.
[100] M.A. McNamara, S.K. Nair, E.K. Holl, RNA-based vaccines in cancer immunotherapy, J Immunol Res 2015 (2015).
[101] M.A. Martínez, A. Gutiérrez, M. Armand-Ugón, J. Blanco, M. Parera, J. Gómez, et al., Suppression of chemokine receptor expression by RNA interference allows for inhibition of HIV-1 replication, AIDS 16 (18) (2002) 2385–2390.
[102] A. Mullard, 2017 FDA drug approvals, Nature Publishing Group, 2018.
[103] A. Mullard, FDA approves landmark RNAi drug, Nature Publishing Group, 2018.
[104] E. Malek-Adamian, J. Fakhoury, A.E. Arnold, S. Martínez-Montero, M.S. Shoichet, M.J. Damha, Effect of sugar 2′,4′-modifications on gene silencing activity of small interfering RNA duplexes, Nucleic Acid Ther 29 (4) (2019) 187–194.
[105] J.M. Harp, D.C. Guenther, A. Bisbe, L. Perkins, S. Matsuda, G.R. Bommineni, et al., Structural basis for the synergy of 4′-and 2′-modifications on siRNA nuclease resistance, thermal stability and RNAi activity, Nucleic Acids Res 46 (16) (2018) 8090–8104.
[106] X. Shen, D.R. Corey, Chemistry, mechanism and clinical status of antisense oligonucleotides and duplex RNAs, Nucleic Acids Res 46 (4) (2017) 1584–1600.

[107] F. Guo, Q. Li, C. Zhou, Synthesis and biological applications of fluoro-modified nucleic acids, Org Biomol Chem 15 (45) (2017) 9552–9565.
[108] K. El Harchaoui, F. Akdim, E.S. Stroes, M.D. Trip, J.J. Kastelein, Current and future pharmacologic options for the management of patients unable to achieve low-density lipoprotein-cholesterol goals with statins, Am J Cardiovasc Drugs 8 (4) (2008) 233–242.
[109] D.J. Foster, C.R. Brown, S. Shaikh, C. Trapp, M.K. Schlegel, K. Qian, et al., Advanced siRNA designs further improve in vivo performance of GalNAc-siRNA conjugates, Mol Ther 26 (3) (2018) 708–717.
[110] J.L. Willoughby, A. Chan, A. Sehgal, J.S. Butler, J.K. Nair, T. Racie, et al., Evaluation of GalNAc-siRNA conjugate activity in pre-clinical animal models with reduced asialoglycoprotein receptor expression, Mol Ther 26 (1) (2018) 105–114.
[111] J.K. Nair, H. Attarwala, A. Sehgal, Q. Wang, K. Aluri, X. Zhang, et al., Impact of enhanced metabolic stability on pharmacokinetics and pharmacodynamics of GalNAc–siRNA conjugates, Nucleic Acids Res 45 (19) (2017) 10969–10977.
[112] M.M. Janas, M.K. Schlegel, C.E. Harbison, V.O. Yilmaz, Y. Jiang, R. Parmar, et al., Selection of GalNAc-conjugated siRNAs with limited off-target-driven rat hepatotoxicity, Nat Commun 9 (1) (2018) 723.
[113] M. Egli, M. Manoharan, Re-engineering RNA molecules into therapeutic agents, Acc Chem Res 52 (4) (2019) 1036–1047.
[114] P.J. Paddison, A.A. Caudy, E. Bernstein, G.J. Hannon, D.S. Conklin, Short hairpin RNAs (shRNAs) induce sequence-specific silencing in mammalian cells, Genes Dev 16 (8) (2002) 948–958.
[115] T.R. Brummelkamp, R. Bernards, R. Agami, A system for stable expression of short interfering RNAs in mammalian cells, Science 296 (5567) (2002) 550–553.
[116] M. Li, J. Li, X. Ding, M. He, S.-Y. Cheng, microRNA and cancer, AAPS J 12 (3) (2010) 309–317.
[117] M. Kim, A.L. Kasinski, F.J. Slack, MicroRNA therapeutics in preclinical cancer models, Lancet Oncol 12 (4) (2011) 319–321.
[118] M. Negrini, M.S. Nicoloso, G.A. Calin, MicroRNAs and cancer—new paradigms in molecular oncology, Curr Opin Cell Biol 21 (3) (2009) 470–479.
[119] T. Tran, M. Montano, MicroRNAs: mirrors of health and disease, in: Translating microRNAs to the clinic, Elsevier, 2017, pp. 1–15.
[120] C. Kanellopoulou, S. Monticelli (Eds.), A role for microRNAs in the development of the immune system and in the pathogenesis of cancer, in: Seminars in cancer biology, Elsevier, 2008.
[121] I. Büssing, F.J. Slack, H. Großhans, Let-7 microRNAs in development, stem cells and cancer, Trends Mol Med 14 (9) (2008) 400–409.
[122] W.C. Cho, MicroRNAs in cancer—from research to therapy, Biochim Biophys Acta Rev Cancer 1805 (2) (2010) 209–217.
[123] W.C. Cho, MicroRNAs: potential biomarkers for cancer diagnosis, prognosis and targets for therapy, Int J Biochem Cell Biol 42 (8) (2010) 1273–1281.
[124] E. Giovannetti, A. Erozenci, J. Smit, R. Danesi, G.J. Peters, Molecular mechanisms underlying the role of microRNAs (miRNAs) in anticancer drug resistance and implications for clinical practice, Crit Rev Oncol Hematol 81 (2) (2012) 103–122.
[125] J. Guo, D. Jin, Y. Wu, L. Yang, J. Du, K. Gong, et al., The miR 495-UBE2C-ABCG2/ERCC1 axis reverses cisplatin resistance by downregulating drug resistance genes in cisplatin-resistant non-small cell lung cancer cells, EBioMedicine 35 (2018) 204–221.

[126] E. Montastier, D. Beuzelin, F. Martins, L. Mir, M.-A. Marqués, C. Thalamas, et al., Niacin induces miR-502-3p expression which impairs insulin sensitivity in human adipocytes, Int J Obes 1 (2018).
[127] Y. Xie, Y. Shao, X. Deng, M. Wang, C. Yinghui, MicroRNA-298 reverses multidrug resistance to antiepileptic drugs by suppressing MDR1/P-gp expression in vitro, Front Neurosci 12 (2018) 602.
[128] J. Alles, T. Fehlmann, U. Fischer, C. Backes, V. Galata, M. Minet, et al., An estimate of the total number of true human miRNAs, Nucleic Acids Res 47 (7) (2019) 3353–3364.
[129] M.D. Wouters, D.C. van Gent, J.H. Hoeijmakers, J. Pothof, MicroRNAs, the DNA damage response and cancer, Mutat Res Fundam Mol Mech Mutagen 717 (1–2) (2011) 54–66.
[130] K. Gabisonia, G. Prosdocimo, G.D. Aquaro, L. Carlucci, L. Zentilin, I. Secco, et al., MicroRNA therapy stimulates uncontrolled cardiac repair after myocardial infarction in pigs, Nature 569 (7756) (2019) 418.
[131] C.F. Bennett, E.E. Swayze, RNA targeting therapeutics: molecular mechanisms of antisense oligonucleotides as a therapeutic platform, Annu Rev Pharmacol Toxicol 50 (2010) 259–293.
[132] B.G. Katzung, Basic and clinical pharmacology, McGraw-Hill Education, 2017.
[133] E. Wong, G.T. Mipomersen, A novel antisense oligonucleotide inhibitor for the management of homozygous familial hypercholesterolemia, Pharm Ther 39 (2014) 119–122.
[134] V. Jairath, R. Khanna, B.G. Feagan, Alicaforsen for the treatment of inflammatory bowel disease, Expert Opin Investig Drugs 26 (8) (2017) 991–997.
[135] C.D. Wurster, A.C. Ludolph, Antisense oligonucleotides in neurological disorders, Ther Adv Neurol Disord 11 (2018). 1756286418776932.
[136] D.R. Scoles, P. Meera, M.D. Schneider, S. Paul, W. Dansithong, K.P. Figueroa, et al., Antisense oligonucleotide therapy for spinocerebellar ataxia type 2, Nature 544 (7650) (2017) 362.
[137] D.R. Scoles, E.V. Minikel, S.M. Pulst, Antisense oligonucleotides. A primer, Neural Genet 5 (2) (2019), e323.
[138] L.R. Moore, G. Rajpal, I.T. Dillingham, M. Qutob, K.G. Blumenstein, D. Gattis, et al., Evaluation of antisense oligonucleotides targeting ATXN3 in SCA3 mouse models, Mol Ther Nucleic Acids 7 (2017) 200–210.
[139] J.J. McKetta Jr., Encyclopedia of chemical processing and design: volume 27—hydrogen cyanide to ketones dimethyl (acetone), CRC Press, 1987.
[140] G.M. Whitesides, The origins and the future of microfluidics, Nature 442 (7101) (2006) 368–373.
[141] J.M. Ottino, S. Wiggins, Introduction: mixing in microfluidics, The Royal Society, 2004.
[142] P.M. Valencia, O.C. Farokhzad, R. Karnik, R. Langer, Microfluidic technologies for accelerating the clinical translation of nanoparticles, Nat Nanotechnol 7 (10) (2012) 623.
[143] Y. Jun, E. Kang, S. Chae, S.-H. Lee, Microfluidic spinning of micro-and nano-scale fibers for tissue engineering, Lab Chip 14 (13) (2014) 2145–2160.
[144] S.Y. Chew, J. Wen, E.K. Yim, K.W. Leong, Sustained release of proteins from electrospun biodegradable fibers, Biomacromolecules 6 (4) (2005) 2017–2024.
[145] K.W. Bong, S.C. Chapin, D.C. Pregibon, D. Baah, T.M. Floyd-Smith, P.S. Doyle, Compressed-air flow control system, Lab Chip 11 (4) (2011) 743–747.
[146] H. Gu, F. Rong, B. Tang, Y. Zhao, D. Fu, Z. Gu, Photonic crystal beads from gravity-driven microfluidics, Langmuir 29 (25) (2013) 7576–7582.

[147] H.E. Keith, A. Rasooly, Lab on a chip technology, in: Fabrication and microfluidics, Caister Academic Press, 2009.

[148] C.L. Grigsby, Y.-P. Ho, C. Lin, J.F. Engbersen, K.W. Leong, Microfluidic preparation of polymer-nucleic acid nanocomplexes improves nonviral gene transfer, Sci Rep 3 (2013) 3155.

[149] A.T.-H. Hsieh, N. Hori, R. Massoudi, P.J.-H. Pan, H. Sasaki, Y.A. Lin, et al., Nonviral gene vector formation in monodispersed picolitre incubator for consistent gene delivery, Lab Chip 9 (18) (2009) 2638–2643.

[150] M. Lu, Y.-P. Ho, C.L. Grigsby, A.A. Nawaz, K.W. Leong, T.J. Huang, Three-dimensional hydrodynamic focusing method for polyplex synthesis, ACS Nano 8 (1) (2014) 332–339.

[151] Y.-P. Ho, C.L. Grigsby, F. Zhao, K.W. Leong, Tuning physical properties of nanocomplexes through microfluidics-assisted confinement, Nano Lett 11 (5) (2011) 2178–2182.

[152] T.A. Balbino, J.M. Serafin, A.A. Malfatti-Gasperini, C.L. de Oliveira, L.P. Cavalcanti, M.B. de Jesus, et al., Microfluidic assembly of pDNA/cationic liposome lipoplexes with high pDNA loading for gene delivery, Langmuir 32 (7) (2016) 1799–1807.

[153] M.L. Schipper, G. Iyer, A.L. Koh, Z. Cheng, Y. Ebenstein, A. Aharoni, et al., Particle size, surface coating, and PEGylation influence the biodistribution of quantum dots in living mice, Small 5 (1) (2009) 126–134.

[154] P.J. O'Brien, S. Elahipanah, D. Rogozhnikov, M.N. Yousaf, Bio-orthogonal mediated nucleic acid transfection of cells via cell surface engineering, ACS Central Sci 3 (5) (2017) 489–500.

[155] S. Liu, Y. Zhao, J.W. Parks, D.W. Deamer, A.R. Hawkins, H. Schmidt, Correlated electrical and optical analysis of single nanoparticles and biomolecules on a nanopore-gated optofluidic chip, Nano Lett 14 (8) (2014) 4816–4820.

[156] M. Rahman, M. Stott, M. Harrington, Y. Li, M. Sampad, L. Lancaster, et al., On demand delivery and analysis of single molecules on a programmable nanopore-optofluidic device, Nat Commun 10 (1) (2019) 1–7.

[157] S. Damiati, U.B. Kompella, S.A. Damiati, R. Kodzius, Microfluidic devices for drug delivery systems and drug screening, Genes 9 (2) (2018) 103.

[158] J.H. Tsui, W. Lee, S.H. Pun, J. Kim, D.-H. Kim, Microfluidics-assisted in vitro drug screening and carrier production, Adv Drug Deliv Rev 65 (11 – 12) (2013) 1575–1588.

[159] C.A. Jordan, E. Neumann, A.E. Sowers, Electroporation and electrofusion in cell biology, Springer Science & Business Media, 2013.

[160] D. Chang, Guide to electroporation and electrofusion, Academic Press, 1991.

[161] M. Fox, D. Esveld, A. Valero, R. Luttge, H. Mastwijk, P. Bartels, et al., Electroporation of cells in microfluidic devices: a review, Anal Bioanal Chem 385 (3) (2006) 474.

[162] S. Movahed, D. Li, Microfluidics cell electroporation, Microfluid Nanofluid 10 (4) (2011) 703–734.

[163] W.G. Lee, U. Demirci, A. Khademhosseini, Microscale electroporation: challenges and perspectives for clinical applications, Integr Biol 1 (3) (2009) 242–251.

[164] S. Ho, G.S. Mittal, Electroporation of cell membranes: a review, Crit Rev Biotechnol 16 (4) (1996) 349–362.

[165] J. Teissie, M. Golzio, M. Rols, Mechanisms of cell membrane electropermeabilization: a minireview of our present (lack of?) knowledge, Biochim Biophys Acta Gen Subj 1724 (3) (2005) 270–280.

[166] C. Chen, S. Smye, M. Robinson, J. Evans, Membrane electroporation theories: a review, Med Biol Eng Comput 44 (1–2) (2006) 5–14.

[167] J.C. Weaver, Y.A. Chizmadzhev, Theory of electroporation: a review, Bioelectrochem Bioenerg 41 (2) (1996) 135–160.

[168] J.-M. Escoffre, T. Portet, L. Wasungu, J. Teissié, D. Dean, M.-P. Rols, What is (still not) known of the mechanism by which electroporation mediates gene transfer and expression in cells and tissues, Mol Biotechnol 41 (3) (2009) 286–295.

[169] S. le Gac, I. Van Uitert, Electroporation in microfluidic devices, in: Handbook of electroporation, Springer, 2018.

[170] C. Sun, Z. Cao, M. Wu, C. Lu, Intracellular tracking of single native molecules with electroporation-delivered quantum dots, Anal Chem 86 (22) (2014) 11403–11409.

[171] E. Giupponi, R. Visone, P. Occhetta, F. Colombo, M. Rasponi, G. Candiani, Development of a microfluidic platform for high-throughput screening of non-viral gene delivery vectors, Biotechnol Bioeng 115 (3) (2018) 775–784.

[172] A.J. El Haj, J.R. Glossop, H.S. Sura, M.R. Lees, B. Hu, S. Wolbank, et al., An in vitro model of mesenchymal stem cell targeting using magnetic particle labelling, J Tissue Eng Regen Med 9 (6) (2015) 724–733.

[173] G. Bao, S. Mitragotri, S. Tong, Multifunctional nanoparticles for drug delivery and molecular imaging, Annu Rev Biomed Eng 15 (2013) 253–282.

[174] Y. Namiki, T. Namiki, H. Yoshida, Y. Ishii, A. Tsubota, S. Koido, et al., A novel magnetic crystal–lipid nanostructure for magnetically guided in vivo gene delivery, Nat Nanotechnol 4 (9) (2009) 598.

[175] Y. Qiu, S. Tong, L. Zhang, Y. Sakurai, D.R. Myers, L. Hong, et al., Magnetic forces enable controlled drug delivery by disrupting endothelial cell-cell junctions, Nat Commun 8 (1) (2017) 1–10.

[176] M.A. Obeid, A. Elburi, L.C. Young, A.B. Mullen, R.J. Tate, V.A. Ferro, Formulation of nonionic surfactant vesicles (NISV) prepared by microfluidics for therapeutic delivery of siRNA into cancer cells, Mol Pharm 14 (7) (2017) 2450–2458.

[177] C. Zhou, Y. Mao, Y. Sugimoto, Y. Zhang, N. Kanthamneni, B. Yu, et al., SPANosomes as delivery vehicles for small interfering RNA (siRNA), Mol Pharm 9 (2) (2012) 201–210.

[178] P. Yingchoncharoen, D.S. Kalinowski, D.R. Richardson, Lipid-based drug delivery systems in cancer therapy: what is available and what is yet to come, Pharmacol Rev 68 (3) (2016) 701–787.

[179] M.A. Obeid, I. Khadra, A.B. Mullen, R.J. Tate, V.A. Ferro, The effects of hydration media on the characteristics of non-ionic surfactant vesicles (NISV) prepared by microfluidics, Int J Pharm 516 (1–2) (2017) 52–60.

[180] J. Park, J.-K. Park, Integrated microfluidic pumps and valves operated by finger actuation, Lab Chip 19 (18) (2019) 2973–2977.

CHAPTER

Microfluidics: Future perspectives

14

Arefeh Ebadati[a,b,*]

[a]*Department of Medical Nanotechnology, Faculty of Advanced Technologies in Medicine, Iran University of Medical Sciences, Tehran, Iran*

[b]*Oncopathology Research Center, Iran University of Medical Sciences, Tehran, Iran*

**Corresponding author. E-mail: arefeh.e@gmail.com*

14.1 Introduction

The use of microfluidics has rapidly expanded within many scientific disciplines today, and in future is expected to continue to bolster progress in many sciences. Given the number of lucrative commercialized microfluidic devices and reputable scientific articles discussing microfluidics, the importance of this field can be further appreciated.

Infact, the art of miniaturizing new devices, assays, and technologies, due to their ease of use, improved rapidity, and more accurate results, is crucial to the future of clinical science, engineering, and chemistry. The results of this breakthrough have provided some new and exciting ideas for advancing a number of scientific endeavors [1, 2].

For this reason, in this chapter, we intend to survey the future prospects and offer suggestions for improvement and resolution of problems in this field.

14.2 Future prospective in biology and health

As the discovery of microelectromechanical systems (MEMS) and microfluidic systems, these technologies have been widely used in a variety of topics including healthcare.

The use of biosensor-based diagnostic kits, which are capable of detecting targeted biomarkers requiring only 10 μL of sample volume, is one of the major achievements of MEMS in the health care field. However, there are some limitations in the industrial manufacture of BioMEMS due to the need for building clean rooms containing high-end equipment, as well as well-trained operators for their implementation. It is expected that these problems will be largely overcome in the future by increased funding from government agencies, affiliated laboratories, universities, and industrial companies. However, the production of more efficient and

Biomedical Applications of Microfluidic Devices. https://doi.org/10.1016/B978-0-12-818791-3.00004-8

cost-effective microfluidic devices also depends on the comprehensive collaboration between scientists to form and sustain knowledge-based bodies of expertise [2, 3].

Other diagnostic microfluidic applications, such as circulating tumor cell (CTC) detection, also have limitations which are expected to overcome in the future.

For example, the development and improvement of the ability to handle an increased number of clinical specimens, as well as the ability to segregate cells such as CTC-coated platelets or CTC-neutrophils, are important areas for better understanding of cancer progression. In addition, increasing the ability of these systems to detect cancer in its early stages by the introduction of new compounds for CTC detection with higher biocompatibility is a goal for future studies. It is anticipated that by overcoming problems in this area, microfluidic systems could play a growing role in the early detection of cancer in the near future [4, 5].

The discovery of innovative materials for the fabrication of microfluidic systems is an essential need in the field that has yet to be achieved on a large scale.

One new avenue for microfluidics technology is the development of sperm inspection systems. In order to determine sperm quality, microfluidic systems are only able to evaluate limited parameters at present. Comprehensive research to provide definitive evidence of the status of male fertility by analyzing sperm motility and functionality is another prospective application in this area. Microfluidic technology could have a significant on the lives of ordinary by providing sperm analysis systems equipped with smartphones that can be used at home for analysis of sperm quality thereby improving the chances of parenthood [6].

The future of microfluidic systems in the field of health care is not limited to diagnosis. Providing guidance for drug discovery efforts and monitoring the progress of drug treatment in individual patients is also important.

An extensive collaboration between physicians and biologists with nanotechnologists and microfluidic engineers will allow the design of more specific drug carriers, which can be combined with peptides, antibodies, or nucleic acids to improve the specific delivery of drugs to the target tissues. It is also to be expected that with ongoing research and by solving the challenges lying ahead, the mass production of these devices by industrial companies will transform them from sophisticated laboratory constructions into everyday consumer products [7]. This will dramatically increase the public perception of high technology in the same way as has happened with silicon-microprocessor based electronic devices.

In addition to the use of microfluidic systems in the diagnosis of diseases, there is a clear need for their use in the field of tissue engineering. Despite recent advances in tissue engineering in the reconstruction of skin and other tissues, there are still many problems due to the fundamental difference in the complexity and function of the laboratory models compared to living human skin and organs. Research in 2017 showed that the combination of induced pluripotent stem cell (IPSC) and microfluidic systems could be a solution to the future of tissue engineering. In this study, a skin-on-a-chip technology was used to solve some problems due to increased physiological interaction with a controlled environment, increased barrier function, and immune cell involvement [8].

14.3 Future prospectives in chemistry

Microfluidic chips are a growing trend in the development of chemical and biochemical analyses and the detection of a wide range of analytes of relevance to many chemical processes.

Microfluidic surface-enhanced Raman spectroscopy—lab on a chip (SERS-LOC) is one of the most important systems in this field. In fact, LOC can enhance the efficiency, security and, reproducibility of SERS identification by employing a completely integrated platform. However, an important issue for the future of this technology is the elimination of challenges ahead, such as their lack of reusability and their need to be equipped with multifunctionality [9].

It seems that the Raman spectroscopy analytical technology will make significant progress in overcoming this problem in the near future, but just as some of the dysfunctional features of integrated microfluidic systems raise concerns about its prospects, its constituent parts continue to be improved.

Continuing progress in polymer-based microfluidic systems will enable improvements in single-cell analysis studies in the future. This development has been achieved by investing and striving for adequate training, establishing a comprehensive collaboration between cell biology scientists and chemical engineers to identify and design thermoplastic polymer materials as the basis of cost-effective and optimized production methods [10].

Many scientists in the field of chemistry research have addressed some important issues in this field and the need to look ahead. For example, Amir Ghasemi and his coworkers in an article suggested the need for new methods to incorporate carbon nanotubes (CNT) into LOC devices. New research could overcome the fragility problem of freshly grown CNT, and improve the hydrophobic properties of these materials [11].

14.4 Future industrial applications and commercialization

In recent years, the production of bio-diesel and bio-ethanol has faced problems such, as the need for screening of algae and yeast and their isolation and purification at a commercial scale, and some of these may be solved using microfluidics technology. Microfluidic systems have advantages, namely a higher level of throughput, improved efficiency despite low solvent consumption, and less consumption of energy and time. Areas for future research and prospects for use of this technology in the fuel industry still require more effort. The development of analytical interfaces in these systems is crucial for monitoring production conditions in practice. The development of microfluidic systems for analyzing the production of biodiesel could reduce the risk of microbial contamination in future studies [12].

Some attempts have been made to commercialize microfluidic technology up to now, and it is anticipated that more of them will achieve long-term utilization in the future. Although there are still many obstacles such as nonstandard user interfaces, more sophisticated control systems, will allow this equipment to become less costly and more user-friendly. The development and use of laminates is one way to advance the commercialization of microfluidic devices. Laminates are more efficient than their counterparts for the production on a large-scale, can have multimaterial compositions [13].

Another idea to encourage commercialization is to simplify the design of microfluidic structures. Although in some applications, for instance in tissue engineering systems, the designs have tended to become increasingly sophisticated, this is not necessarily the case for all applications. In the industrial sector, more simple designs would make the devices easier to use, which would ultimately increase the commercialization rate of the products [14].

14.5 Closing words

We hope that this book will serve as a guide for physicians, scientists, and engineers with an interest in the field to learn more about modern microfluidic systems. It will also provide an intellectual framework for the selection of more appropriate microfluidic devices for their particular research goal.

We believe that having a comprehensive book on various aspects of this technology and its future development, will enhance and accelerate much relevant research in the years to come.

References

[1] D. Liu, et al., Trends in miniaturized biosensors for point-of-care testing, TrAC Trends Anal Chem 122 (2020).

[2] B.C. Dhar, N.Y. Lee, Lab-on-a-chip technology for environmental monitoring of microorganisms, Biochip J 12 (3) (2018) 173–183.

[3] A. Kaushik, C.K. Dixit, Challenges and future, in: Microfluidics for biologists: fundamentals and applications, Springer, 2016, pp. 247–248.

[4] K. Payne, et al., Circulating tumour cell biomarkers in head and neck cancer: current progress and future prospects, Cancers 11 (8) (2019).

[5] S.B. Cheng, et al., Current techniques and future advance of microfluidic devices for circulating tumor cells, TrAC Trends Anal Chem 117 (2019) 116–127.

[6] Z. Zhou, et al., Development and prospects of microfluidic platforms for sperm inspection, Anal. Methods 11 (36) (2019) 4547–4560.

[7] S.T. Sanjay, et al., Recent advances of controlled drug delivery using microfluidic platforms, Adv Drug Deliv Rev 128 (2018) 3–28.

[8] L.J. van den Broek, et al., Progress and future prospectives in skin-on-chip development with emphasis on the use of different cell types and technical challenges, Stem Cell Rev Rep 13 (3) (2017) 418–429.

[9] J. Guo, et al., Preparation and application of microfluidic SERS substrate: challenges and future perspectives, J Mater Sci Technol 37 (2020) 96–103.

[10] H. Wu, et al., Microfluidic-based single-cell study: current status and future perspective, Molecules 23 (9) (2018).
[11] A. Ghasemi, et al., Carbon nanotubes in microfluidic lab-on-a-chip technology: current trends and future perspectives, Microfluid Nanofluid 21 (9) (2017).
[12] R. Banerjee, et al., Intervention of microfluidics in biofuel and bioenergy sectors: technological considerations and future prospects, Renew Sust Energ Rev 101 (2019) 548–558.
[13] B.K. Gale, et al., A review of current methods in microfluidic device fabrication and future commercialization prospects, Inventions 3 (3) (2018).
[14] J. Ahn, et al., Microfluidics in nanoparticle drug delivery; from synthesis to pre-clinical screening, Adv Drug Deliv Rev 128 (2018) 29–53.

Index

Note: Page numbers followed by *f* indicate figures and *t* indicate tables.

A

AAVs. *See* Adeno-associated viruses (AAVs)
Acoustophoresis, 121, 123*f*
Acute lymphoblastic leukemia (ALL), 107–108
Acute promyelocytic leukemia cells, 268
Acylation, 243
Additive manufacturing (AM), 7–8
Adeno-associated viruses (AAVs), 188
Affinity capture, 88
Affymetrix oligonucleotide microarrays, 84–85, 84*f*
Alkyl-ketene-dimer (AKD), 263
ALL. *See* Acute lymphoblastic leukemia (ALL)
AM. *See* Additive manufacturing (AM)
Anisotropic wet etching of silicon, 29–30
Antisense oligonucleotides (ASOs), 297, 300–304
Aptamer chemical structures, nucleic acids, 293–294
Atomic absorption spectroscopy, 279–280
Automated microinjection, 200
Autonomous drug delivery platforms, 178–179

B

BBB. *See* Blood-brain barrier (BBB)
BEP. *See* Bulk electroporation (BEP)
Bioengineered RNAs (BERAs), 295–296
Bioinformatics techniques, 109–110
Biomedical applications
  reusable microchannels, 66–69
  soft microchannels, 66
  transport phenomena, 62–64
Biosensors, 13–14, 121–124
Blood-brain barrier (BBB), 220–221
Blood vessel-on-a-chip, 103
Bone marrow stromal cells (BMSCs), 108
Bone marrow-tumor-on-a-chip, 107–108
Brain-on-a-chip, 220–221
Brain-tumor-on-a-chip, 108–110
Brain tumor stem cells (BTSC), 110
Breast cancer micrometastasis to bone, 226*f*
Bulk electroporation (BEP), 198

C

Cancer cells 2D and 3D culture and co-culture, 224
Cancer cell studies, 178
Cancer tissue
  cancer cells 2D and 3D culture and co-culture, 224
  multiorgans, in vitro models, 225–227
  tumor spheroids and tissue, 224–225
Capillary driven test strips, 5–6
Capillary tubes, 190–191
Capillary tube T-junctions, 191
Cardiomyocytes (CMs), 222
Carrier materials, 165–166
Cationic liposomes (CLs), 192
Cell biology, 12–13
Cell culture, 210
Cell microarrays, 88–89
Cell-penetrating peptides (CPPs), 295
Cell squeezing, 200
Centrifugal microfluidic devices, 5–6
CFD. *See* Computational fluid dynamics (CFD)
Chemical synthesis, 8–10
Chemical vapor deposition (CVD), 132
Chemiluminescence-based microfluidics, 125–127
Circulating tumor cells (CTCs), 12, 106
Cleanroom
  classification, 24
  concepts, 24–25
  equipment, 25
  laboratory, 24
CLs. *See* Cationic liposomes (CLs)
CMs. *See* Cardiomyocytes (CMs)
COC. *See* Cyclic olefin copolymer (COC)
Colorimetric-based microfluidics, 130–132
Computational fluid dynamics (CFD), 110
Computer-controlled microfluidic systems, 163
Continuous-flow electrotransfection system, 198
Continuous-flow emulsion-based droplet microfluidics, 5–6
Continuous-flow microfluidics, 5–6, 193
Continuous-flow polymerase chain reaction (PCR), 135–136
Continuous flow separation microfluidic approaches, 121, 122*f*
Continuous flow systems, 192–193, 198
Conventional bulk systems, 195
Conventional imaging techniques, 12–13
Conventional synthetic chemistry methods, 189
Covalent immobilization, 87
CPPs. *See* Cell-penetrating peptides (CPPs)
Cross-flow membrane emulsification (XME) process, 166
Cross-section geometry, microchannels, 38–50

CTCs. *See* Circulating tumor cells (CTCs)
CVD. *See* Chemical vapor deposition (CVD)
Cyclic olefin copolymer (COC), 155

D

ddPCR. *See* Droplet digital polymerase chain reaction (ddPCR)
Deoxyribonucleic acid (DNA), 159, 290
DEP. *See* Dielectrophoresis (DEP)
Deposition methods
  Si_3N_4 and SiO_2, 27
  thick metal layers, 28
  thin metal layers, 27–28
Di-acetylferrocene, 243
Didodecyldimethylammonium bromide (DDAB), 308
Dielectrophoresis (DEP), 6, 194–195
Digital light processing (DLP), 7–8, 33
Digital microfluidics (DMF), 6, 136
Digital micromirror display technology (DMD), 33
Direct drug delivery
  cellular and organ level
    on-site analysis, 175–176
    protein crystallization, 176–177
  localized drug delivery, 169–171
  skin anatomy and transdermal drug delivery, 171–175
DLP. *See* Digital light processing (DLP)
DMF. *See* Digital microfluidics (DMF)
DMPC. *See* Dynamic mask photocuring (DMPC)
DNA. *See* Deoxyribonucleic acid (DNA)
DNA chemical structure, nucleic acids, 292–293
DNA methylation, 293
DNA microarray
  antiinfective drugs, 81
  fabrication methods, 82–85
  gene expression, 80–82, 83*f*
  genomics, 81
  labeling approaches, 82
  nucleotide base sequences, 82
Driving forces, 5–6
Droplet-based carriers, 161–163
Droplet-based microfluidic devices, 193–196
Droplet-based microfluidic systems, 5–6, 163
Droplet digital polymerase chain reaction (ddPCR), 136
Droplet formation, 54*f*
Droplet microfluidic-based single-cell electroporation, 199
Droplet microfluidics, 7, 11, 136, 162–163
Drug delivery systems, 10–11
  benefits, microfluidics, 168–169
  drug carriers, 158
  immobilization of drugs, 167–168
  microfluidic devices, 157–158
  microfluidics in fabrication, 158–165
    droplet-based carriers, 161–163
    nonspherical carriers and particles, 163–165
    self-assembled drug carriers, 159–161
  microparticles and nanoparticles, 166
Drug encapsulation, 162, 167
Dry etching methods, 30
Dynamic mask photocuring (DMPC), 262

E

ECM. *See* Extracellular matrix (ECM)
EGF. *See* Epidermal growth factor (EGF)
Elastomers, 213
Electrochemical-based microfluidics, 132–134
Electro-chemiluminescent (ECL) detection technique, 95
Electrokinetic platforms, 5–6
Electropermeabilization, 198
Electroporation, 198–199
Electrowetting-based droplet microfluidics, 5–6
Electrowetting on dielectric (EWOD), 6
ELISA. *See* Enzyme-linked immunosorbent assay (ELISA)
Emulsion-based droplet microfluidic system, 195
Emulsion technology, 161–162
Encapsulation of doxorubicin (DOXO), 167
Encapsulation of drugs, 166
Enzyme-linked immunosorbent assay (ELISA), 276
Epidermal growth factor (EGF), 216
Etching techniques, 210–211
  anisotropic wet etching of silicon, 29–30
  dry etching methods, 30
  features, 29
  isotropic wet etching of silicon and glass, 29
  wet etching of thin films, 29
EWOD. *See* Electrowetting on dielectric (EWOD)
Extracellular matrix (ECM), 12, 100

F

Fabrication, microfluidic devices, 7–8
  drug delivery carriers, 158–165
  geometry, 155
  materials, 155–156
Fabrication of toroids, 163–165
Fabrication techniques
  chemical
    chemical vapor-phase deposition, 263
    inkjet printing, 263
    photolithography, 261–262
    plasma treatment, 262–263
    wet etching, 264

etching, 210–211
micromachining, 211
photolithography, 211–212
physical
flexographic printing, 259
inkjet etching, 258–259
ink stamping, 260
lacquer spraying, 260–261
laser treatment, 259
plotting, 258
screen printing, 261
shaping and cutting of paper, 260
wax printing, 258
polymer casting, 211–212
thermoforming, 211
three-dimensional (3D)
origami, 264
stacking technique, 264
FDM. *See* Fused deposition modeling (FDM)
FFP. *See* Flash flow pyrolysis (FFP)
Fibroblast growth factor-2 (FGF2), 216
Fibrous scaffolds, 214–215
Film hydration, 159
FLA. *See* Fragment length analysis (FLA)
Flash flow pyrolysis (FFP), 239
Flash vacuum pyrolysis (FVP), 239
Flow-3D software, 40
Flow-focusing geometry, 155
Flow lithography methods, 163–165
Flow lithography microfluidic platforms, 163–165
Flow regimes, 50–51
Flow types, 191–192
Fluid flows, 154
Fluorescence-based microfluidics, 125
Fluorescent microspheres (FMSs), 125
Fourier transform infrared (FT-IR), 9–10
Fragment length analysis (FLA), 110
Friction coefficient, effect, 60–62
Functional microfluidic device, 3
Fused deposition modeling (FDM), 7–8, 33–34
Fused filament fabrication (FFF), 33
Future perspective
biology and health, 319–320
chemistry, 321
industrial applications and commercialization, 321–322
FVP. *See* Flash vacuum pyrolysis (FVP)

G

GBM. *See* Glioblastoma multiforme (GBM)
Gelatin/nanoclay (GNC), 52–53
Gene and drug carriers, 160*f*
Genebank, 82–83
Gene delivery, 304–305, 309
continuous flow systems, 192–193
droplet-based microfluidic devices, 193–196
hydrodynamics-based transfection, 200–201
microinjection, 199–200
physical based microfluidic techniques, 202*t*
size, 188
Gene-modified cell therapy (GMCT), 200–201
Genes transfection, 196–199
Gene therapy, 187–189
Genetic agents, 187
Gene-Z system, 279
Glass, 26, 155
Glioblastoma multiforme (GBM), 108–109
GMCT. *See* Gene-modified cell therapy (GMCT)
Good manufacturing practice (GMP), 24
Gut-on-a-chip, 219–220

H

Heart-on-a-chip, 103–104, 222–223
Heavy Metal Water Test Kit, 279–280
Hematopoietic stem cells (HSCs), 216
Herringbone mixer, 191
hESCs. *See* Human embryonic stem cells (hESCs)
HFF. *See* Hydrodynamic flow focusing (HFF)
Homogeneous drug-loaded particles, 163
Hot embossing, 31
HSCs. *See* Hematopoietic stem cells (HSCs)
Human brain microvascular endothelial cells (hBMVECs), 220–221
Human embryonic stem cells (hESCs), 103–104, 217
Human foreskin fibroblast (HFF) cells, 200
Human serum albumin (HSA) microparticles, 167
Human umbilical vein endothelial cells (HUVEC), 218
HUVEC. *See* Human umbilical vein endothelial cells (HUVEC)
Hydrodynamic behavior of flow, 54–55
Hydrodynamic flow focusing (HFF), 159, 161, 191
Hydrodynamic focusing, 193*f*
Hydrodynamics-based transfection, 200–201
Hydrofluoric acid (HF), 29
Hydrogels, 213–215
Hydrophilic channels, 195
Hydrophilicity and hydrophobicity effects, 59–60
Hydroporator, 201

I

IDEAs. *See* Interdigitated microelectrode arrays (IDEAs)
IHC. *See* Immunohistochemistry (IHC)
IJP. *See* Inkjet printing (IJP)

Immiscible fluids, 6
Immobilization of drugs, 167–168
Immunohistochemistry (IHC), 109–110
Immunomagnetic separation (IMS), 120
Impedimetric method, 133
IMS. *See* Immunomagnetic separation (IMS)
Induced pluripotent stem cells (iPSCs), 215–216, 320
Injection molding, 31
Inkjet printing (IJP), 7–8
Inorganic chemistry, 189
Inorganic materials, 213
Interdigitated microelectrode arrays (IDEAs), 134
Internal microfluidic cell hydroporator (iMCH), 201
Intestine-on-a-chip, 102–103
iPSCs. *See* Induced pluripotent stem cells (iPSCs)
Isotropic wet etching of silicon and glass, 29

J

Junctions, 191*f*

K

Kidney-on-a-chip, 221–222

L

Lab-on-a-chip (LOC), 2–3, 93–95, 119–120, 153–154, 209–210, 239
Laminar flow in microfluidics, 3, 5–6
Laser printed microfluidic paper-based analytical devices (LP-μPAD), 132
Leukemia cells, 95
Lipid nanoparticles (LNPs), 159
Liposomes, 159, 161
Lithography techniques, 28–29, 154
Liver-on-a-chip, 104–106, 105*f*, 217–218
LNA. *See* Locked nucleic acids (LNA)
LNPs. *See* Lipid nanoparticles (LNPs)
LOC. *See* Lab-on-a-chip (LOC)
Localized drug delivery, 169–171
Locked nucleic acids (LNA), 295
Loop-mediated isothermal amplification (LAMP), 279
LP-μPAD. *See* Laser printed microfluidic paper-based analytical devices (LP-μPAD)
Lung-on-a-chip, 102

M

Machine learning technology, 110
Magnetic biosensors, 13
Magnetic nanoparticles, 13
Magnetic silica beads (MSBs), 120–121
Mass spectrometry (MS)-based microfluidics, 138–139
Materials, 155–156
  glass, 26
  metals, 26
  nonmetal thin films, 26
  polydimethylsiloxane, 25
  silicon, 25–26
  SU-8, 25
μCCA. *See* Microcell culture analog (μCCA)
Mechanisms in microfluidic systems, 305
MEMS. *See* Microelectromechanical systems (MEMS)
Mesenchymal stem cells (MSCs), 216–217
Metals, 26
Microarrays, 5
  applications, 77
  biosensing technology, 78
  capture molecules, 79
  classification, 80
  defined, 77
  diagnostic technology, 78
  dotted blot, 78–79
  immobilization, 79
  microfluidic arrays, 77
    advantages, 89–90
    automated (lab-on-a-chip systems), 93–95
    disadvantages, 90–91
    examples, 95
    fabrication, 91–93
  micro spots, 79, 80*f*
  platforms, 157
  single test chip, 78
  steps, 79
Microcell culture analog (μCCA), 225–227
Microchannel
  blood flow blocking mechanism, 53*f*
  cross-section geometry, 38–50
  flow regimes, 50–51
  junction characteristics, 40*f*
  microcapillaries, 5–6
  mixing profile simulation, 43*f*
  pathogen detection, nanotechnology, 64–66
  patterns of microfluidic devices, 39*f*
  phase study, 51–54
  physical specifications
    friction coefficient, effect, 60–62
    roughness effects, 62
  simulation of flow, 42*f*
  velocity development, 55–59
Microchannel emulsification-solvent evaporation method, 166
Microdroplets, 47–48, 195
Microelectromechanical systems (MEMS), 5, 153, 209
Microelectronics, 154

Microencapsulation of rifampicin, 166
Microfabrication principles, 101
Microfluidic-based diagnostic devices, 7
Microfluidic-based microfibrous structures, 214–215
Microfluidic-based microparticles, 215
Microfluidic-based POC devices, 7
Microfluidic biochips
 continuous flow, 94
 droplet-based, 94
 tasks, 93–94
Microfluidic cell culture, 12
Microfluidic-cis-coculture (MicroC3) system, 108
Microfluidic continuous flow, 5
Microfluidic electroporation, 307
Microfluidic flow, 3
Microfluidic paper-based analytical devices (μPADs), 4, 131–132
 advantages, 257
 applications
  biochemical detection, 265–267
  immunological detection, 267–269
  molecular detection, 269–270
 fabrication techniques, 257–264
 spectrophotometric detection, 270
Microfluidics
 advantages, 5–6
 applications, 3, 156
 design types, 6*f*
 development, 1–2
 in drug delivery systems, 157–158
 history, 2
 in organic chemistry (*see* Organic chemistry)
 organ-on-a-chip (*see* Organ-on-a-chip)
 for pathogen detection (*see* Pathogen detection)
 sample preparation, 120–121
Microfluidic single-cell nuclear translocation (μSCeNT), 108
Microinjection, 199–200
Micromachining technology, 173, 211
Micromixer device, 41–43
Micromolding, 215
Microneedles, 173–175
Micro/NPs production, microfluidic techniques, 190*t*
Microreactors, 190
MicroRNAs (miRNA), 299–300
Microscale and nanoscale drug carriers, 159
Microscale flows, 154
Microscale fluid mechanics, 38
Microtiter plate solid-phase assay, 79
MM. *See* Multiple myeloma (MM)
Molding-based microfluidic fabrication
 hot embossing, 31
 injection molding, 31
 soft lithography, 30–31
Monodisperse self-assembled liposomes, 161
MSBs. *See* Magnetic silica beads (MSBs)
μSCeNT. *See* Microfluidic single-cell nuclear translocation (μSCeNT)
MSCs. *See* Mesenchymal stem cells (MSCs)
Multientrance microchannel devices, 47–48
Multiple myeloma (MM), 108

N

NAFLD. *See* Nonalcoholic fatty liver disease (NAFLD)
Nanoparticle-based drug delivery, 10
Nanostructured materials, 9–10
Nanotechnology, 3, 47–50, 62–66
Neurovascular unit (NVU), 220–221
NISV. *See* Nonionic surfactant vesicles (NISV)
Nitrile synthesis, 237, 237*f*, 238*t*
Nonalcoholic fatty liver disease (NAFLD), 218
Noncontact dispensing systems, 5–6
Noncovalent adsorption, 88
Nonionic surfactant vesicles (NISV), 308
Nonspherical carriers and particles, 163–165
Nonviral gene delivery vectors, 307–308
Nonviral vectors, 188, 307–308
Nucleic acids, 187–188
 aptamer chemical structures, 293–294
 DNA-based approaches
  oligonucleotides and antisense oligonucleotides, 297
  plasmid, 296–297
 DNA chemical structure, 292–293
 hybridization, 269
 locked nucleic acids (LNA), 295
 pathogenesis and treatment of diseases, 295
 peptide nucleic acids, 294–295
 primary structure, 290
 quaternary structure, 291–292
 RNA-based approaches
  antisense oligonucleotides (ASOs), 300–304
  fluidic and microfluidic systems, 304–305
  microRNAs (miRNAs), 299–300
  short hairpin RNAs (shRNA), 299
  small interfering RNAs, 298–299
 RNA chemical structure, 293
 secondary structure, 290–291
 tertiary structure, 291
 transfer, 189

O

Oil-in-water (O/W) emulsions, 162
Oil-in-water-in-oil ($O_1/W/O_2$), 162

Oligodeoxynucleotide (ODN)-based therapeutics, 297
Oligonucleotides and antisense oligonucleotides, 297
On-site analysis, drug delivery, 175–176
Optical-based microfluidics, 124–125
Optofluidic channels, 277–278
Optofluidics, 125, 306–307
Organic chemistry
- β-amino alcohols, 239
- by-products, 242–243
- carbon monoxide (CO), 241
- control of conversion and selectivity, 246–247
- diethylaminosulfur trifluoride reagent, 239
- high-temperature synthesis, 245–246
- hydrogenations, 241
- layout diagram and epoxide setup, 239, 240*f*
- mass transfer, 236, 244
- microfluidic reactors, 235–236
- microparticles, 247, 248*f*
- molecules, 235
- nebulator, 236–237
- types, materials, 236

Organ-on-a-chip, 177
- biochemical and biological mechanistic studies, 111
- blood vessel-on-a-chip, 103
- bone marrow-tumor-on-a-chip, 107–108
- brain-on-a-chip, 220–221
- brain-tumor-on-a-chip, 108–110
- cell biology techniques, 99
- gut-on-a-chip, 219–220
- heart-on-a-chip, 103–104, 222–223
- intestine-on-a-chip, 102–103
- kidney-on-a-chip, 221–222
- liver-on-a-chip, 104–106, 105*f*, 217–218
- long-term reliability, 111
- lung-on-a-chip, 102
- microfabrication principles, 101
- microfluidic technology, 99
- tissue culture microenvironment, 99–100
- traditional systems drawbacks, 100–101
- tumor-on-a-chip, 106–107, 107*f*

Origami, 264
Ozonolysis, 241

P

PAbs. *See* Polyclonal antibodies (PAbs)
Packed-bed microfluidic reactor, 241–242
Paclitaxel (PAX), 11
Parvovirus B19 genotypes, 127, 128*f*
Passive microfluidic mixer, 159
Pathogen detection
- advantages and disadvantages, 118, 119*t*
- biosensor-based microfluidics, 121–124
- chemiluminescence-based microfluidics, 125–127
- colorimetric-based microfluidics, 130–132
- electrochemical-based microfluidics, 132–134
- fluorescence-based microfluidics, 125
- foodborne illnesses, 117–118
- infectious diseases, 117
- lab-on-a-chip (LOC), 119–120
- mass spectrometry (MS)-based microfluidics, 138–139
- materials, 139, 140–141*t*
- microchannel devices, 64–66
- nucleic acid-based-methods, 118
- optical-based microfluidics, 124–125
- plasmonic-based microfluidics, 127–130, 130*f*
- polymerase chain reaction (PCR)-based microfluidics, 134–138, 137*f*

Pathogenic microorganisms, 117
PCR. *See* Polymerase chain reaction (PCR)
PDGF. *See* Platelet-derived growth factor (PDGF)
PDMCs. *See* Placenta-derived multipotent stem cells (PDMCs)
PDMS. *See* Polydimethylsiloxane (PDMS)
PEEK. *See* Polyether ether ketone (PEEK)
PEGDA. *See* Polyethylene glycol diacrylate (PEGDA)
PEI. *See* Polyetherimide (PEI)
Peptide nucleic acids (PNAs), 294–295
PET. *See* Polyethylene terephthalate (PET)
Pharmaceutical industry, 156
Phospholipid nanoparticles, 166
Photolithography, 28–29, 132, 154, 211–212, 212*f*
Physical vapor deposition (PVD), 7–8
PIPR. *See* Polyimide plastic resin (PIPR)
Placenta-derived multipotent stem cells (PDMCs), 220
Plasmid DNA, 296–297
Plasmonic-based microfluidics, 127–130, 130*f*
Platelet-derived growth factor (PDGF), 216
PNAs. *See* Peptide nucleic acids (PNAs)
Point-of-care (POC) diagnostic devices, 7
Poly(methyl methacrylate) (PMMA), 190
Polycarbonate (PC), 155
Polyclonal antibodies (PAbs), 125
Polydimethylsiloxane (PDMS), 3–4, 25, 92, 101, 211, 258
Polyether ether ketone (PEEK), 155
Polyetherimide (PEI), 213
Polyethylene glycol diacrylate (PEGDA), 215
Polyethylene terephthalate (PET), 213
Polyimide plastic resin (PIPR), 155

Polylactic-*co*-glycolic acid-polyethylene glycol (PLGA-PEG) copolymer, 161
Polymer and paper-based microfluidic devices, 7
Polymerase chain reaction (PCR), 5, 134–138, 137*f*, 276, 294
Polymer casting, 211–212
Polymeric nanoparticles (PNPs), 11
Polymers, 213
Polymer-substrate microreactors, 190
Polymethylmethacrylate (PMMA), 155, 213
Poly(dimethylsiloxane) (PDMS) microfluidic chips, 154
Polystyrene (PS), 213
Poly-tetrafluoroethylene (PTFE) porous membrane, 109
Polyvinyl chloride (PVC), 213
Potentiometric assay/potentiometry, 134
Pressure-driven systems, 5–6
Production of drug and gene carriers, 165
Production of nonviral vectors (micro/NPs), 189–192
Protein crystallization, 176–177
Protein microarrays
  analytical, 85–86
  drug discovery, 81
  fabrication, 87–88
  functional, 86
  high throughput rapid analysis, 85
  proteomics, 85
  reverse phase, 87
PVD. *See* Physical vapor deposition (PVD)

Q

Quaternary structure of nucleic acids, 291–292

R

Rapid prototyping (RP), 7–8
Reactive oxygen species (ROS), 217
Recombinant tissue-type plasminogen activator (rt-PA), 167
Replica molding method, 101
Reusable microchannels in biomedical applications, 66–69
Reversed phase evaporation, 159
Reynolds (Re) number, 50–51, 191
Ribonucleic acid (RNA), 290
RNA chemical structure, nucleic acids, 293
ROS. *See* Reactive oxygen species (ROS)
Roughness effects in channels, 62
Routine clinical testing, 283–285

S

Salmonella typhimurium, 125, 126*f*, 133
Scaffold fabrication, microfluidics, 213–215
SDDS. *See* Smart drug delivery system (SDDS)
Segmented flow platforms, 5–6
Self-assembled drug carriers, 159–161
Semiconductor industry, 5
Serpentine type patterns, 47*f*
Sexually transmitted diseases (STDs), 278
Short hairpin RNAs (shRNA), 299
Silicon, 3–4, 25–26
SILP. *See* Supported ionic liquid phase (SILP)
Single-phase continuous-flow nested polymerase chain reaction (SP-CF-NPCR), 136, 137*f*
Single-phase microfluidic devices, 192
Skin anatomy and transdermal drug delivery, 171–175
SLA. *See* Stereolithography apparatus (SLA)
Small-angle X-ray scattering (SAXS) curves, 192
Small interfering RNAs (siRNA), 159, 298–299, 307
Smart drug delivery microfluidic devices, 179*f*
Smart drug delivery system (SDDS), 10
Smart integrated drug delivery microfluidic platforms, 178–179
Smartphone-based fluorescent microscopy system, 125
Smartphone-based microfluidic devices
  analysis of genes, 278–279
  biomedical diagnosis, 276
  food safety and environmental contamination
    bacterial contaminants, 281–282
    heavy metal pollution, 279–281
    pH, nitrate and nitrite, 282–283
  pathogens, 276–278
  routine clinical testing, 283–285
  software and hardware development, 275
Soft lithography, 30–31, 154–156
SP-CF-NPCR. *See* Single-phase continuous-flow nested polymerase chain reaction (SP-CF-NPCR)
Spiral microchannels, 49–50
Stacking technique, 264
STDs. *See* Sexually transmitted diseases (STDs)
Stem cell-based microfluidics systems, 215–217
Stereolithography apparatus (SLA), 7–8, 33
Stop-flow lithography, 163–165
Supported ionic liquid phase (SILP), 242
Suzuki-Miyaura cross-coupling reaction (SMC), 242
Synthesis
  polydimethylsiloxane (PDMS), 25
  silicon, 25–26
Synthetic chemistry, 9–10
Systematic evolution of ligands by exponential enrichment (SELEX), 293–294

T

Targeted delivery
T cell engineering, 200–201
3D cell culture, 210
3D-hydrodynamic flow for polyplex formation, 194*f*
3D microchannel electroporation (MEP)–magnetic tweezers (MT) system, 199
3D printing, 7–8, 31–32
Teflon, 4
Teflon AF-2400, 240
Teflon-hybrid chips, 4
Tetrahydrocarbazole, 246
Therapeutic moieties, 225–227
Therapeutic nucleic acids
  DNA-based approaches
    oligonucleotides and antisense oligonucleotides, 297
    plasmid, 296–297
  RNA- based approaches
    antisense oligonucleotides (ASOs), 300–304
    fluidic and microfluidic systems, 304–305
    microRNAs (miRNAs), 299–300
    short hairpin RNAs (shRNA), 299
    small interfering RNAs, 298–299
Thermoforming method, 211
Tissue engineering
  brain-on-a-chip, 220–221
  conventional methods, 210
  damaged tissues, 210
  fabrication techniques, 210–212
  gut-on-a-chip, 219–220
  heart-on-a-chip, 222–223
  kidney-on-a-chip, 221–222
  liver-on-a-chip, 217–218
  materials, microfluidic devices, 212–213
  scaffold fabrication
    microfluidic-based microfibrous structures, 214–215
    microfluidic-based microparticles, 215
  stem cell-based microfluidics systems, 215–217
T-junction geometry, 155
Transcatheter arterial chemoembolization (TACE) approach, 167
Transfer fluids, 5–6
Tree-shaped microchannels, 45–46
Tumor heterogeneity, 95
Tumor-on-a-chip, 106–107, 107*f*
Tumor spheroids, 224–225
Tumor tissue, 224–225
Tunica, 103
Two-dimensional (2D) monolayer cell cultures, 210
2D tissue culture, 210

V

Vector free methods, 188–189
Velocity development in microchannels, 55–59
Viral vectors, 188

W

Water-in-oil-in-water ($W_1/O/W_2$), 162
Wet etching of thin films, 29
WHO. *See* World Health Organization (WHO)
World Health Organization (WHO), 117–118

Y

Y-junctions, 191
Y-shaped microfluidic devices, 191

Kolibri 360 GmbH
Ferdinand-Jühlke-Straße 7
99095 Erfurt, Deutschland
produktsicherheit@kolibri360.de